PUBLIC HEALTH IN THE 21ST CENTURY

CORONAVIRUS DISEASE

FROM MOLECULAR TO CLINICAL PERSPECTIVES

PUBLIC HEALTH IN THE 21ST CENTURY

Additional books and e-books in this series can be found on Nova's website under the Series tab.

PUBLIC HEALTH IN THE 21ST CENTURY

CORONAVIRUS DISEASE

FROM MOLECULAR TO CLINICAL PERSPECTIVES

YILDIZ DINCER
EDITOR

nova
Medicine & Health

Library of Congress Cataloging-in-Publication Data

ISBN: 978-1-53619-296-4

Published by Nova Science Publishers, Inc. † New York

This book is dedicated to all COVID-19 victims and healthcare professionals serving in defiance of their lives

CONTENTS

PREFACE

The world is experiencing an unprecedented challenge due to coronavirus disease (COVID-19) pandemic. In December 2019, a novel severe acute respiratory syndrome coronavirus 2 (SARS-CoV-2), first emerged in a seafood wholesale market in Wuhan, China, caused an outbreak of COVID-19. Due to the rapid spread of COVID-19, on March 11, 2020, the WHO announced COVID-19 as a pandemic. As of January 13, 2021, a total of 92,138,941 laboratory-confirmed cases included 1,973,295 deaths reported globally. The majority of the infected individuals exhibit mild to moderate respiratory illness and recover without requiring special treatment. However, older people and those with underlying medical problems like cardiovascular disease, diabetes, chronic respiratory disease, and cancer may rapidly progress to acute respiratory distress syndrome, septic shock, coagulation disorders, multi-organ failure, and death. Although the course of COVID-19 is usually mild in children, in rare cases, children can be severely affected due to the development of the multisystem inflammatory syndrome. The worldwide spread of COVID-19 caused fear, anxiety, depression, panic attacks, and a general decrease in overall wellbeing in the population. Due to the high infectivity rate of COVID-19, the unexpected and rapid influx of large numbers of patients, especially patients who need intensive care, have caused great pressure on the health care systems. Healthcare professionals who occupy the front line during pandemics are at increased risk concerning their physical and mental health. Our knowledge of this novel virus is limited. A better understanding of the pathogenesis of COVID-19 will provide important insight into its management and reduce the mortality rate. In this book, based on the latest global scientific data as well as our experiences, we purposed to give the readers an overview of COVID-19 pathogenesis and transmission routes; anatomical basis and clinical aspects of the disease; current diagnostic and treatment strategies; intensive care management of COVID-19 patients; the clinical course of the disease in children and elderly patients; the genetic background of differences in the incidence of new SARS-CoV-2 infection; the impact of the COVID-19 pandemic on patients with chronic diseases such as diabetes, cancer, cardiovascular diseases, chronic respiratory diseases; ocular manifestation of the COVID-19; organization of ophthalmology and general surgery for the safe treatment during the pandemic period; overproduction of reactive oxygen species due to cytokine storm and their role in tissue damage leading acute respiratory distress syndrome and coagulopathies; role of antioxidant therapy to limit tissue damage; molecular approaches in COVID-19 treatment, and vaccine studies. I hope this book will be a valuable resource for researchers in the field of COVID-19 and will be helpful for medical doctors to deal with the pandemic.

Yildiz Dincer
Istanbul, January 2021

In: Coronavirus Disease
Editor: Yildiz Dincer
ISBN: 978-1-53619-296-4

Chapter 1

EPIDEMIOLOGY AND PATHOGENESIS OF COVID-19

Seda Salman Yılmaz*[1]*, PhD and Gökhan Aygün*[2,*]*, MD

[1]Istanbul University - Cerrahpasa, Cerrahpasa Medical Faculty, Department of Covid-19 Diagnosis Laboratory, Istanbul, Turkey

[2]Istanbul University - Cerrahpasa, Cerrahpasa Medical Faculty, Department of Medical Microbiology, Istanbul, Turkey

ABSTRACT

COVID-19 is a pandemic caused by the coronavirus, Severe Acute Respiratory Syndrome Coronavirus (SARS CoV-2), that affects the entire world, which can result in death, especially in the elderly and people with underlying disease (hypertension, diabetes mellitus, coroner artery disease). The number of patients and deaths continues to increase rapidly in the world. Today, the most important source of infection is sick people. Contagiousness in the asymptomatic and presymptomatic period is the most important problem in preventing the pandemic. The most important route of transmission is the droplets. Aerosols can be transmitted by aerosol- generating procedures in health-care. Fomites that spread to the immediate environment of sick people play a role in transmission through contact. There is insufficient data on other transmission routes. In the first period, COVID-19, which spread as a travel disease, spread to all societies in closed environments (home, meeting, public transportation, ceremonies, prisons, long-term care units...) where many people are together. Local outbreaks occur, especially in hospitals and health centers. There are many uncertainties in the pathophysiology of Covid-19. Studies at different stages of the disease and with different methodologies are published and this provides conflicting data. Lymphopenia, cytokine storm, ferritin elevation, and D-dimer elevation were found to be associated with poor prognosis. Acute respiratory distress syndrome (ARDS) and sepsis are the most important causes of

* Corresponding Author's Email: gokhanaygun67@yahoo.com.

mortality. In this section, a perspective for the future is presented by addressing the issues in the light of the available data.

Keywords: COVID-19, epidemiology, pathogenesis

INTRODUCTION

Coronaviruses; enveloped single-stranded, positive-sense RNA viruses. The coronavirus has a large genome of approximately 30 000 bases and an RNA polymerase activity with "proofreading" activity to correct mutations. This family is found in many mammals, especially cats, dogs, pigs, and bats, and includes important human pathogens. Viruses that adapt to new hosts with genetic recombination and variations in different hosts become important pathogens for humans when they gain the ability to be transmitted and spread from person to person. These viruses, which can settle in the respiratory and digestive systems in many mammals, were first identified as the agents with upper respiratory tract infection (HCoV-NL63, H.CoV229E, HCoV-OC43, HCoVHKU1). With the clinic of Severe Acute Respiratory Syndrome Coronavirus (SARS) in 2003 and Middle East Respiratory Syndrome (MERS) in 2012, it was observed that it could cause diseases and epidemics with high mortality in humans with pneumonia. SARS-CoV-2 is an agent with long spike structures (9-12 nanometers) in dimensions of 60-120 nanometers. Bats were found as the reservoir of this virus, and although pangolin as an intermediate host was identified as the most likely source, this issue has not been fully clarified. A new coronavirus was identified as the cause of a series of pneumonia cases at the end of 2019 in Wuhan, a city in China's Hubei province. This infection, which spread rapidly, resulted in an epidemic throughout China and then spread to other countries in the world, this epidemic was declared by WHO as a Public Health Emergency of International Importance (PHEIC). In February 2020, the World Health Organization took the name Covid-19 disease, which means coronavirus disease 19, and the virus that causes COVID-19 was named SARS-CoV-2. WHO declared COVID-19 as a pandemic on March 11, 2020. On September 25, 2020, a total of 32.110.656 detected cases and 980.031 COVID-19 deaths were recorded worldwide, and the numbers continue to increase [1].

EPIDEMIOLOGY

The global epidemiology of COVID-19 in the first phase of the pandemic was evaluated as a cross-sectional analysis using web-based surveillance [2]. In the web-based surveillance study, almost two-thirds of the COVID-19 cases first reported were those with travel links to China, Italy, or Iran. In the first period of the outbreak sixty-fixe studies were evaluated and most of these have been reported from China. It has been stated that most of these are due to family contacts. The major types of cluster infections were families, gatherings, religious organizations, transportation, community transmission, conferences, shopping malls, respectively [3]. Although there were many household contagion clusters among the early cases, the numbers in these clusters were low (2-22 cases) clusters in occupational or community settings tended to be larger (gathering 112, shopping mall 40, religion 53 cases was found to be affected) and physical distance was a possible risk to slow the progression of SARS-CoV-2 was supportive of its role [4]. A total of 161 studies (n = 17 648) provided data for the mode of transmission. The most common mode of transmission was travel-related (58.1%, 95% CI: 51.1-64.8), followed by close contacts (43.1%, 95% CI: 37.2-49.2), and finally community spread (27.4%, 95% CI: 18.4-38.7) [5]. At present, general findings show that test strategies, socioeconomic differences, and reporting systems of countries affect the spread in society.

In children, it is stated that the number of cases detected is less, the disease has a milder course, and asymptomatic cases are more common in this situation. In a systemic review and meta-analysis, it is stated that approximately 4% of patients with a diagnosis of COVID-19 are symptomatic, having underlying diseases play a role in this course [6].

Severe or critical illness has been reported among 2.5% to 5% of pediatric cases, and more recently, 4% of cases were reported as severe or critical, and pre-existing medical conditions have been suggested as a risk factor for severe disease and ICU admission in children and adolescents [7]. Several countries affected by the COVID-19 pandemic reported cases of children who were hospitalized in intensive care units due to a rare pediatric inflammatory multisystem syndrome (PIMS) or multisystem inflammatory syndrome in children (MIS-C) [8], characterized by a systemic disease involving persistent *fever*, *inflammation* and organ dysfunction following exposure to SARS-CoV-2 [9, 10].

COVID-19 course has not been shown to be worse in pregnant women. Pregnant women are often tested for SARS-CoV-2 infection at admission for hospital delivery. According to this may explain the high proportion of asymptomatic cases found among pregnant women in different countries. In addition, infants and newborns have been described as more vulnerable to severe COVID-19 than other pediatric groups [11, 12]. Although a low mortality rate (0.006%) has been reported for this group in most cases [13, 14]. Among the COVID-19 cases with serious illness and death and the rates of people with underlying health conditions are remarkable. Primary health conditions reported among COVID-19 patients and admitted to the intense care unit (ICU) include hypertension, diabetes, cardiovascular disease, chronic respiratory disease, immunocompromised status, cancer, and obesity. A high proportion of long-term care facilities and nursing homes in Europe and the world are also severely affected by

COVID-19. Consequently, high morbidity and mortality and high rates of absenteeism due to SARS-CoV-2 infections have been observed in residents [15-17]. In a systematic analysis study, 6007 articles, 212 studies from 11 countries/regions involving 281 461 individuals were analyzed (the mean age 46.7 years, and female-male ratio 49.2%-51.8%). Older age, male gender, diabetes, and hypertension were also associated with higher mortality with severe COVID-19, and the mortality rate was 5.6% and severe disease rate was 22.9% [5].

Health-care workers are at high risk of covid-19. Higher rates of cases are detected in contrast to other segments of society. This risk is thought to be caused by their exposure to higher concentrations of the virus. Since healthcare workers are younger and have fewer comorbidities, a milder disease picture is generally observed. Despite that, a large number of health-care workers died due to Covid-19. Mistakes in the use of personal protective equipment, problems with compliance with hand hygiene, intensive work, deficiencies related to hospital organization are factors that increase the risk of health-care workers [7]. Health-care worker's risk of Covid-19 transmission has been associated with the misuse of personal protective equipment during contact. In one study, 2% of the health-care workers who came into contact with Covid-19, and post-contact findings appeared within an average of 3.6 (0-17 days) days. In contamination, male gender, comorbidity, high-risk contact, and auxiliary personnel were identified as factors that increase the risk [18].

In a study, in our country, inappropriate use of personnel protective equipment, staying in the same personnel break room as an HCW without a medical mask, consuming food within, and failure to keep a safe social distance from an HCW were statistically significant risk factors for infection [19]. One of the studies concluded in our hospital, it was found that approximately half of the health-care workers with Covid-19 were infected with their colleagues in social areas (unpublished data).

The elderly in long-term care (LTC) and their caregiving staff are at elevated risk from COVID-19. Coronavirus disease (COVID19)-related deaths in LTCF residents represent 30-60% of all COVID-19 deaths in many European countries [20].

In all epidemiological studies, the reliability of the data is low due to the lack of genome data of the virus, the fact that many asymptomatic cases can be contagious, and the studies are generally conducted using cross-sectional data.

PATHOGENESIS

The high infectivity of the virus, the lack of effective antivirals and vaccines, and potentially large asymptomatic populations have made the management of COVID-19 extremely difficult. Continuous efforts to better understand the pathogenesis of this disease, in addition to rapid medical interventions, will undoubtedly shed light on the management of the growing pandemic.

SARS-CoV-2 first affects the respiratory tract cells and the first proliferation site is the nasal mucosa. Viral load reaches its highest level at the onset of symptoms, but its spread (viral shedding) begins about 2-3 days before symptoms. Clinical course viral load is determined by the complex processes of infective dose and immune system response. The virus binds to cells with the spike S-protein and its main receptor is the angiotensin-converting enzyme 2 (ACE-2) receptor [21].

In the disease course, COVID-19 of viral replication in the lower respiratory tract, and generates secondary viremia, followed by an extensive attack against target organs. SARS- CoV-2 extensive attack against target organs that express ACE2, such as heart, kidney, gastrointestinal tract [22]. When SARS-CoV-2 infects cells expressing the surface receptors angiotensin-converting enzyme 2 (ACE2). Transmembrane protease serine 2 (TMPRSS2) activates viral S protein (especially Furin-like cleavage region) and cleaves the ACE2 receptor to facilitate viral binding to the host cell membrane. This binding triggers endocytosis allowing SARS-CoV-2 to enter the cell type in the virion cell membrane. The virus enters the host cell via endocytosis releases its RNA, and uses cell machinery to replicate itself and assemble more virions. Bronchial epithelial cells, type I and type II alveolar pneumocytes, and capillary endothelial cells are infected, an inflammatory response ensues.

The active replication release of the virus causes the host cell damage and release damage-associated molecular patterns (ATP, nucleic acids, and caspase proteins). Antagonism of the interferon (IFN-α and IFN-β) response aids viral replication, resulting in increased release of pyroptosis products that can further induce aberrant inflammatory responses. These are recognized by neighboring epithelial cells, endothelial cells, and alveolar macrophages, triggering the generation of pro-inflammatory cytokines and chemokines (including IL-6, IP-10, macrophage inflammatory proteins, MCP1…). All these proteins attract monocytes, macrophages, and T cells to the site of infection, promoting further inflammation (with the addition of IFNγ). Continued inflammatory response results in alveolar interstitial mononuclear inflammatory infiltrate and edema develops and appears as ground-glass opacities on radiological imaging. In the late stage, thickened interstitium, hyaline membrane formation, the influx of monocytes and neutrophils, increased vascular permeability compatible with early-phase acute respiratory distress syndrome (ARDS) [19, 23].

When the immune response is excessive, it causes a cytokine storm with excessive production of proinflammatory cytokines in the lungs. This response can effectively lead to multiple organ damage in other organs. In addition, non-neutralizing antibodies produced by B cells may exacerbate antibody-dependent enhancement (ADE) organ damage. This process is mainly observed as clinical worsening observed 7-14 days following the onset of the disease. These findings show that the disease symptoms are particularly related to immune response, apart from viral damage. In severe and critically ill patients with COVID-19, two distinctive features of progressive increase in inflammation have been recognized. Possible pathways contributing to hyperactivation and hyperinflammation of monocyte-derived macrophages in COVID-19. Delayed type I interferon production, leading to increased cytopathic effects and greater perception of microbial threats, promote the increased release of monocyte chemoattractants by alveolar epithelial cells, leading to the continuous accumulation of monocytes into the lungs. Monocytes differentiate into proinflammatory macrophages through Janus kinase (JAK) activation. Activated natural killer (NK) cells and T cells further promote the recruitment and activation of macrophages through the production of granulocyte - macrophage-colony-stimulating factor (GM-CSF), tumor necrosis factor (TNF), and interferon-(IFNγ). The binding of Fc receptors (FcRs) by anti-spike protein IgG immune complexes may contribute to the increased inflammatory activation of monocyte-derived macrophages. Activated monocyte-derived macrophages contribute to the COVID-19 cytokine storm by secreting large amounts of pro-inflammatory cytokines [24].

Several factors may contribute to the hypercoagulability in COVID-19 patients. Certain cytokines including IL-6 could activate the coagulation system and suppress the fibrinolytic system. In the setting of COVID-19, activation of coagulation leads to microthrombus formation. COVID-19 patients elevated levels of D-dimer and fibrinogen associated with poor prognosis.

Lymphopenia is an important feature of patients with COVID-19. Lymphopenia is more common in patients with severe COVID-19, and this is an important sign of a poor prognosis [25, 26]. Declining lymphocyte groups are especially T lymphocytes and NK cells. Showed that T-lymphocyte count was inversely proportional to TNFa, IL-6, and IL-10 levels in particular and that an increase in inflammatory cytokine levels may promote depletion of T-cell populations along with disease progression [27]. Activation of CD14+CD16+ inflammatory monocytes was associated with an increase in IL-6, one of the key cytokines in the cytokine storm [28].

The clinical course of SARS-CoV-2 infection can be divided into three stages: the viremia stage, the acute stage (Immune response stage), and the progression or recovery stage. Patients with appropriate immune functions and without obvious risk factors (old age, comorbidities, genetic factors, etc.) can generate effective and sufficient immune responses to suppress the virus in the first or second stage without an excessive immune reaction. In contrast, patients with immune dysfunction may have a more severe clinical picture, intensive care admission, and a higher risk of death. There are no proven effective antivirals. Therefore, it mainly focuses on the close monitoring of disease stages and the application of ways of stopping or slowing the progression of the disease (IL-6 inhibition, corticosteroid, immune plasma). In contrast, in a healthy immune response, the initial inflammation draws virus-specific T cells to the site of infection and they can eliminate infected cells before the virus spreads. Neutralizing antibodies in these individuals can block viral infection and alveolar macrophages recognize neutralized viruses and apoptotic cells and clear them by phagocytosis. All of these processes result in recovery by causing the virus to be cleared and minimal lung damage [19, 28].

In a post-mortem study of 10 consecutive patients who died of COVID-19 in Germany (mean age 79, 70% male, mean time between hospitalization and mortality 7.5 days), significant ARDS findings were found in the lungs, especially in the middle and lower lobes. Organizing-stage diffuse alveolar damage with pronounced fibroblastic proliferation, partial fibrosis, pneumocyte hyperplasia leading to interstitial thickening and collapsed alveoli, and patchy lymphocyte infiltration was the predominant finding.

In a post-mortem study of 10 consecutive patients who died of COVID-19 in Germany (mean age 79, 70% male, mean time between hospitalization and mortality 7.5 days), significant ARDS findings were found in the lungs, especially in the middle and lower lobes. Neutrophil infiltration was also detected in five cases with suspected aspiration and secondary infection [29].

Grifoni et al. Found SARS-CoV-2-specific CD8 and CD4 cells between 70-100% in 20 COVID-19 patients. CD4 cell response was correlated with the magnitude of the IGg response to spike protein. Interestingly, in the study, CD4 T lymphocytes reacting with SARS-CoV-2 were detected in 40-60% of those who were not in contact with the virus. This finding suggests a cross-response. These findings may be related to some people and children having milder COVID-19 disease [30]. Virus-specific IgM and IgG are detectable in serum between 7 and 14 days after the onset of symptoms. Viral RNA is inversely correlated with neutralizing antibody titers. Higher titers have been observed in critically ill patients, but it is unknown whether antibody responses somehow contribute to pulmonary pathology. The SARS-CoV-1 humoral response is relatively short-lived, and memory B cells may disappear altogether, suggesting that immunity with SARS-CoV-2 may wane 1-2 years after primary infection [31].

Non-neutralizing virus-specific IgG facilitates the entry of virus particles into cells expressing the Fc receptor (FcR), particularly macrophages and monocytes, and can lead to inflammatory activation of these cells. This phenomenon is called antibody-dependent enhancement (ADE), it is a condition that needs attention for immunoglobulin treatments and vaccine studies [32].

Conclusion

The Covid-19 pandemic cannot be expected to end soon. It has been understood that personal protective measures (mask, social distance, and hand hygiene) are effective methods against pandemics. There are many uncertainties regarding pathogenesis. Studies on this subject provide important findings on treatment and vaccination. Learning to live with the virus and accessing new information about pathogenesis will be the primary goal of science.

References

[1] Tang D., Comish P. and Kang R. (2020). The hallmarks of COVID-19 disease. *PLoS Pathog*, 16(5).

[2] Dawood F. S., Ricks P., Njie G. J., Daugherty M., Davis W., Fuller J. A., Winstead A., McCarron M., Scott L. C., Chen D., Blain A. E., Moolenaar R., Li C., Popoola A., Jones C., Anantharam P., Olson N., Marston B. J. And Bennett S. (2020). Observations of the global epidemiology of COVID-19 from the prepandemic period using web-based surveillance: a cross-sectional analysis. *Lancet.* https://doi.org/ 10.1016/S1473-3099(20)30581-8.

[3] Liu T., Gong D., Xiao J., Hu J., He G., Rong Z. and Ma W. (2020). Cluster infections play important roles in the rapid evolution of COVID-19 transmission: A systematic review. *International Journal of Infectious Diseases*, 99: 374-380.

[4] Bi Q., Wu Y., Mei S., Ye C., Zou X., Zhang Z., Liu X., Wei L., Truelove S. A., Zhang T., Gao W., Cheng C., Tang X., Wu X., Wu Y., Sun B., Huang S., Sun Y., Zhang J., Ma T., Lessler J. and Feng T. (2020). Epidemiology and transmission of COVID-19 in 391 cases and 1286 of their close contacts in Shenzhen, China: a retrospective cohort study. *Lancet Infect Diseases*, 20:911-9.

[5] Li J., Huang D. Q., Zou B., Yang H., Hui W. Z., Rui F., Yee N. T. S., Liu C., Nerurkar S. N., Kai J. C. Y., Teng M. L. P., Li X., Zeng H., Borghi J. A., Henry L., Cheung R. and Nguyen M. H. (2020). Epidemiology of COVID-19: A systematic review and meta-analysis of clinical characteristics, risk factors, and outcomes. *J. Med. Virology*, https://doi.org/10.1002/jmv.26424.

[6] Götzinger F., Santiago-García B., Noguera-Julián A., Lanaspa M., Lancella L., Calò Carducci F. I., Gabrovska N., Velizarova S., Prunk P., Osterman V., Krivec U., Vecchio A. L., Shingadia D., Soriano-Arandes A., Melendo S., Lanari M., Pierantoni L., Wagner N, L'Huillier A. G., Heininger U., Ritz N., Bandi S., Krajcar N., Roglić S, Santos M., Christiaens C., Creuven M., Buonsenso D., Welch S. B., Bogyi M., Brinkmann F. and Tebruegge M. (2020). COVID-19 in children and adolescents in Europe: a multinational, multicentre cohort study. *Lancet Child Adolesc Health*, 4(9):653-661.

[7] https://www.ecdc.europa.eu/en/covid-19/latest-evidence/ epidemiology.

[8] World Health Organization (WHO). *Multisystem inflammatory syndrome in children and adolescents with COVID-19.* Geneva: WHO; 2020 [cited 21 July 2020]. https://www.who.int/publications/i/item/multisystem-inflammatory-syndrome-in-children-and-adolescents-with- covid-19.

[9] Riphagen S., Gomez X., Gonzalez-Martinez C., Wilkinson N. and Theocharis P. (2020). Hyperinflammatory shock in children during COVID-19 pandemic. *Lancet*, 395(10237):1607-8.

[10] Rowley A. H. (2020). Understanding SARS-CoV-2-related multisystem inflammatory syndrome in children. *Nature Reviews Immunology*, 2020:1-2.

[11] https://www.who.int/publications/i/item/multisystem-inflammatory-syndrome-in-children-and-adolescents-withcovid-19.

[12] Yu Y. and Chen P. (2020). Coronavirus Disease 2019 (COVID-19) in Neonates and Children from China: A Review. *Frontiers in Pediatrics*, 2020;8:287.

[13] Raba A. A., Abobaker A., Elgenaidi I. S. and Daoud A. (2020). Novel coronavirus infection (COVID-19) in children younger than one year: A systematic review of symptoms, management and outcomes. *Acta Paediatrica*, 109(10);1-8.

[14] Mantovani A., Rinaldi E., Zusi C, Beatrice G., Saccomani M. D. and Dalbeni A. (2020). Coronavirus disease 2019 (COVID-19) in children and/or adolescents: a meta-analysis. *Nature Pediatric Research*, doi: 10.1038/s41390-020-1015-2.

[15] Comas-Herrera A., Zalakain J., Litwin C., Hsu A. T. and Fernandez-Plotka J. L. (2020). Mortality associated with COVID-19 outbreaks in care homes: early international evidence. *International Long Term Care Policy Network*, https://ltccovid.org/2020/04/12/mortality-associated-with-covid19-outbreaks-in-care-homes-early-international-evidence/.

[16] McMichael T. M., Currie D. W., Clark S., Pogosjans S., Kay M., Schwartz N. G., Lewis J., Baer A., Kawakami V., Lukoff M. D., Ferro J., Brostrom-Smith C., Rea T. D., Sayre M. R., Riedo F. X., Russell D., Hiatt B., Montgomery P, Rao A. K., Chow E. J., Tobolowsky F., Hughes M. J, Bardossy A. C, Oakley L. P., Jacobs J. R., Stone N. D., Reddy S. C., Jernigan J. A., Honein M. A., Clark T. A, Duchin J. S., Public Health-Seattle and King County, EvergreenHealth, and CDC COVID-19 Investigation Team (2020). Epidemiology of Covid-19 in a Long-Term Care Facility in King County. *N. Engl. J. Med.*, 21;382(21):2005-2011.

[17] Gardner W., States D. and Bagley N. (2020). The Coronavirus and the Risks to the Elderly in Long-Term Care. *Journal of Aging & Social Policy*, 32(4-5):310-315.

[18] Maltezou H. C., Dedoukou X., Tseroni M., Tsonou E., Raftopoulos V., Papadima K., Elisavet Mouratidou E., Poufta S., Panagiotakopoulos G., Hatzigeorgiou D. and Sipsas N. (2020). SARS-CoV-2 infection in healthcare personnel with high-risk occupational exposure: evaluation of seven-day exclusion from work policy. *Clinical Infectious Diseases*, doi: 10.1093/cid/ciaa888.

[19] Celebi G., Piskin N., Beklevic A. C., Altunay Y., Keles A. S., Tuz M. A., Altinsoy B. and Haciseyitoglu D. (2020). Specific risk factors for SARS-CoV-2 transmission among health care workers in a university hospital. *American Journal of Infection Control*, 48(10): 1225-1230.

[20] ECDC Public Health Emergency Team, Danis K., Fonteneau L., Georges S., Daniau C., Bernard-Stoecklin S., Domegan L., O'Donnell J., Hauge S. H., Dequeker S., Vandael E. Van der Heyden J., Renard F., N. B. Sierra, Ricchizzi E., Schweickert B., Schmidt N., Sin M. A., Eckmanns T., Paiva J. A. and Schneider E. (2020). High impact of COVID-19 in long-term care facilities, suggestion for monitoring in the EU/EEA, May 2020. *Euro Surveill.* 25(22): 2000956.

[21] Tay M. Z., Poh C. M., Rénia L., MacAry P. A. and Ng L. F. P. (2020). The trinity of COVID-19: immunity, inflammation and intervention. *Nature Reviews Immunology*, 20(6):363-374.

[22] Cao W. and Li T. (2020). COVID-19: towards understanding of pathogenesis. *Nature*, 30:367-369.

[23] Wiersinga W. J., Rhodes A., Cheng A. C., Peacock S. J. and Prescoot H. C. (2020). Pathophysiology, Transmission, Diagnosis, and Treatment of Coronavirus Disease 2019 (COVID-19): A Review. *JAMA*, 324(8):782-793.

[24] Merad M. and Martin J. C. (2020). Pathological inflammation in patients with COVID-19: a key role for monocytes and macrophages. *Nature Reviews Immunology*. 355-362(2020).

[25] Lippi, G. and Plebani, M. (2020). Laboratory abnormalities in patients with COVID-2019 infection. *Clin. Chem Lab. Med.* 58:1131-1134.

[26] Zhang W., Li L., Liu J., Chen L., Zhou F., Jin T., Jiang L., L, X., Yang M. and Wang H. (2020). The characteristics and predictive role of lymphocyte subsets in COVID-19 patients. *International Journal of Infectious Diseases*, 99: 92-99.

[27] Moon C. (2020). Fighting COVID-19 exhausts T cells. *Nature Reviews Immunology*, 20:277 (2020).

[28] Zhou Y., Fu B., Zheng X., Wang D., Zhao C., Qi Y., Sun R., Tian Z., Xu X. And Wei H. (2020). *Aberrant pathogenic GM-CSF+T cells and inflammatory CD14+CD16+monocytes in severe pulmonary syndrome patients of a new coronavirus*. https://doi.org/10.1101/ 2020.02.12.945576.

[29] Schaller T., Hirschbüh K., Burkhardt K., Braun G., Trepel M., Märkl B. and Claus R. (2020). Postmortem Examination of Patients with COVID-19. *JAMA*, 323(24): 2518-2520.

[30] Grifoni A., Weiskopf D., Ramirez S. I, Mateus J., Dan J. M., Moderbacher C. R., Rawlings S. A., Sutherland A., Premkumar L., Jadi R. S., Marrama D., de Silva A. M., Frazier A., Carlin A. F., Greenbaum J. A., Peters B., Krammer F., Smith D. M., Crotty S. and Sette A. (2020). Targets of T Cell Responses to SARS-CoV-2 Coronavirus in Humans with COVID-19 Disease and Unexposed Individuals. *Cell*, 181(7):1489-1501.e15.

[31] Vabret N., Britton G. J., Gruber C., Hegde S., Kim J., Kuksin M., Levantovsky R., Malle L., Alvaro Moreira A., Park M. D., Pia L, Risson E., Saffern M., Salome′ B., Selvan M. E., Spindler M. P., Tan J., Heide V., Gregory J. K., Alexandropoulos K.,

Bhardwaj N., Brown B. D., Greenbaum B., Gumus Z. H., Homann D., Horowitz A., Kamphorst A. O., Lafaille M. A. C., Mehandru S., Merad M. and Samstein R. M. (2020). Immunology of COVID-19 Current State of the Science, *Immunity*, 52 (6): 910-941.

[32] Taylor A., Foo S. S., Bruzzone R., Dinh L. V., King N. J. C. and Mahalingam S. (2015). Fc receptors in antibody-dependent enhancement of viral infections. *Immunological Reviews*, 268(1):340-364.

In: Coronavirus Disease
Editor: Yildiz Dincer
ISBN: 978-1-53619-296-4

Chapter 2

TRANSMISSION OF SARS-COV-2 AND PREVENTION STRATEGIES

Bilgul Mete[1], MD, Ahmet Furkan Kurt[1], MD and Gökhan Aygün[2,*], MD

[1]Istanbul University-Cerrahpasa, Cerrahpasa Medical Faculty, Department of Infectious Diseases and Clinical Microbiology, Turkey

[2]Istanbul University-Cerrahpasa, Cerrahpasa Medical Faculty, Department of Medical Microbiology, Turkey

ABSTRACT

The main transmission routes of SARS-CoV-2 are through respiratory droplets and close contact with the index case but other possible routes are also reported. Although the virus may spread during aerosol-generating procedures, the probability of airborne transmission in other circumstances is controversial. Experimental studies demonstrated that SARS-CoV-2 remained viable in aerosols and on fomite surfaces up to 72 hours. However, no reports directly demonstrated transmission from the fomites. SARS-CoV-2 RNA was isolated in various biological specimens but currently, there is no report demonstrating direct transmission of SARS-CoV-2 apart from respiratory secretions except for two cases of vertical transmission.

The type, time, and duration of exposure, application of preventive measures, and the amount of the virus are among the most important predictors of the risk of transmission. Infectiousness begins approximately 3 days before symptom onset and peaks on the day of onset. The risk of transmission remains high in case of exposure to the index case within 5 days of symptom onset and is thought to continue until to10-20 days depending on the severity of the disease and presence of underlying immunosuppressive diseases.

Although the preventive measures may differ according to public and healthcare settings the main strategy is to accept everyone as potential COVID-19 patients. In public

* Corresponding Author's Email: gokhanaygun67@yahoo.com.

settings, everyone should be encouraged to wear a facemask, maintain social distance, apply hand hygiene, avoid touching mouth, nose, and eyes, keep clean high touch areas, and obey isolation rules in case of illness or contact with COVID-19 patient. Every healthcare center should redesign the structuring of its facility to maintain the physical distance and isolate COVID-19 patients. The administration should consider making arrangements regarding surgical and invasive procedures, outpatient and inpatient clinics in terms of COVID-19.

Patients and visitors should wear a facemask. *H*ealthcare workers who care for patients with suspected or confirmed COVID-19 should wear personal protective equipment.

Introduction

At the end of 2019, a new virus later named as SARS-CoV-2 was thought to be transmitted firstly in a seafood market where live animals were sold, in Wuhan. Later on, person to person transmission was reported to be the main route of spread [1]. The routes of transmission and prevention strategies will be mentioned in this chapter.

Routes of Transmission

Although the main transmission routes for SARS-CoV-2 are through droplets and close contact, many other ways also are reported [2-4]. Other possible routes consist of airborne, fomite, fecal-oral, bloodborne, vertical, and animal to human transmission [2].

Droplet and Contact Transmission

The primary means of transmission is via respiratory droplets (> 5 μm, not traveling more than 1-2 meters). Direct, indirect, or close contact with infected respiratory secretions or droplets may lead to transmission. Infected patients may spread the respiratory droplets including SARS-CoV-2 during coughing, sneezing, singing, or talking to people in a close range contact. The droplets may reach directly the mucous membranes (mouth, nose, or eyes) of a susceptible host [2, 4]. Indirect contact transmission may occur after contact with a contaminated object/surface and then spreading the virus to eyes, nose, or mouth by touching [3].

Airborne Transmission

Airborne transmission occurs when aerosols (droplet nuclei< 5 μm, traveling more than 2 meters) containing the microorganism suspended in air disseminate over a distance. Although SARS-CoV-2 may spread during aerosol-generating procedures; the probability of airborne transmission in other circumstances is controversial [2]. Various experimental studies evaluated this issue: some revealed that aerosols may develop during coughing or talking varying according to the modes of practices (such as loud speech, shouting), the others demonstrated that SARS-CoV-2 RNA may remain in aerosols generated via high-powered jet nebulizers for up to 3-16 hours and some investigators identified viral RNA in ventilation systems or air of COVID-19 patients' rooms. But the presence of a viable virus in air samples is reported only in a limited number of studies [2, 5-11]. Although outbreak reports in a closed, crowded, and poorly ventilated area (such as restaurants, buses) may suggest the probability of airborne transmission, the transmission in these cases may also be associated with droplet and fomite surfaces [2, 12, 13].

Until further research clarifies the possibility of airborne transmission in SARS-CoV-2 infection in the community, it would be reasonable to accept that the virus may be transmitted via droplet nuclei during aerosol-generating procedures.

Fomite Transmission

Respiratory droplets may contaminate the surfaces and the objects around the patients and touching mouth, eyes, or mouth after contact with these surfaces may lead to indirect transmission of the virus [2]. The virus may be disseminated all over the ward including bed handrails, doorknobs, trash cans, computer mouse, floor, shoe soles, and other surfaces. However, the detection of the nucleic acid over these surfaces does not indicate that the virus is viable [14]. The environment temperature and humidity and the type of surfaces are predictors of stability of the virus over the fomites [2]. Van Doremalen et al., in their experimental studies demonstrated that SARS-CoV-2 remained viable in aerosols, on copper, cardboard, plastic, and stainless steel up to 3, 4, 24, and 72 hours respectively while the virus titer reduced with time [7]. Although many studies evaluated the survival of the virus on environmental surfaces there are no reports directly demonstrating transmission from the fomites [2].

Other Modes of Transmission

SARS-CoV-2 RNA was isolated in other biological specimens such as urine, feces, semen, or ocular secretions, but the presence of viable viruses was reported only in some studies [11, 15-18]. Although there are various hypotheses, currently there is no report demonstrating direct transmission of SARS-CoV-2 via these routes [2]. Viral RNA was also detected in blood but the role of transmission via blood and blood products is controversial [15-19].

Nasopharyngeal specimens, umbilical cord blood, and placental specimens of neonates born to infected mothers were demonstrated to include viral RNA, however evidence of intrauterine transmission is sparse [20-22].

World Health Organization (WHO) in its scientific brief reported that viral RNA fragments have been found in breast milk samples of infected mothers. But since the viable virus could not be detected, WHO recommends that mothers with suspected or confirmed COVID-19 should be encouraged to breastfeed [23].

Dogs, cats, and farmed minks have been reported to be infected by humans but the probability of transmission of COVID-19 from infected animals to humans is unclear [24-26].

Period of Infectiousness

With the first report of transmission of SARS-CoV-2 after contact with an index case during the incubation period in Germany, the variability in the probability of transmission during COVID-19 has become a matter of interest [27]. He et al., in their experimental study demonstrated that infectiousness begins 5–6 days before symptom onset and peaks on the day of onset. Upon observation that 1% of transmissions would occur 5 days and 9% of transmissions 3 days before symptom onset, they concluded that 3 days before symptom onset is critical in terms of transmission [28]. In another study performed in Taiwan, 2500 close contacts of 100 patients were analyzed and a secondary clinical attack rate was found to be higher in case of exposure to the index case within 5 days of symptom onset [29].

Although viral RNA may be detected in biological specimens after months of SARS-CoV-2 infection, Wölfel et al., demonstrated that this may not mean that the virus is infectious if the RNA level was $< 10^6$ copies/mL [30, 31]. On the other hand viable viruses although not replication-competent, may be isolated after more than 10 days in some cases depending on the severity of the disease and underlying immunosuppression [30, 32, 33]. According to the Centers for Disease Control and Prevention (CDC), patients with mild to moderate disease and with more severe disease or immunosuppression most probably are not infectious for longer than 10 days and 20 days after symptom onset, respectively [33].

Prevention Strategies

The type, time, and duration of exposure, application of preventive measures, and the amount of the virus are among the most important predictors of the risk of transmission

[3, 28, 29]. The risk of transmission is high among household contacts where the secondary attack rate ranges between 15-38% [34, 35]. Besides household contacts and gathering activities, traveling with an index case without preventive measures or indoor activities are associated with a high risk of transmission. Since the probability of neglect of wearing a facemask or social distancing may be high while eating or drinking in indoor environments, the risk for transmission remains an important concern [36, 37]. Outdoor activities carry a low risk for transmission except for close contact with an index case [3].

The best way of prevention of transmission includes testing the suspected individuals, isolating the infected cases, determining all close contacts, and self/quarantine them [3].

The prevention strategies can be classified under 2 subgroups: public and healthcare settings.

Public Settings

On individual and public health basis, these measures should be applied by everyone in the public:

- *Washing hands with soap and water for at least 20 seconds or rubbing hands with hand antiseptic containing at least 65% alcohol, after being in a public area, before or after touching the face, after handling the mask, after sneezing or coughing, after touching surfaces, before eating or preparing food, after going to the restroom*
- *Avoiding touching eyes, nose, or mouth*
- *Avoiding close contact (maintaining a distance of 1-2 meters between people)*
- *Wearing a mask (facemask or cloth covering) covering the mouth and nose in public settings*
- *Using tissues to cover mouth and nose during coughing and sneezing and throwing them into the trash can or bent elbow when coughing or sneezing*
- *Cleaning and disinfecting touched surfaces daily [38].*
- *Individuals having close contact (< 2 meters for ≥ 15 minutes) with people having COVID-19 symptoms (laboratory-confirmed or clinically compatible) 2 days before symptom onset and until discontinuation of isolation are accepted to have a high risk for exposure. They should quarantine themselves for 14 days after the last exposure, maintain social distance between people, self-monitor for symptoms of COVID-19 [39].*

Each country can make different arrangements to re-organize environmental conditions in schools, workplaces, prisons, dormitories, nursing homes, shopping centers, fitness centers, restaurants, and other indoor areas, and ameliorates travel conditions, taking into account the number of confirmed cases, current resources, and sociocultural characteristics.

Healthcare Settings

Every healthcare center should implement its prevention strategies to the utmost to protect its workers and patients. These measures should include some major principles:

General Principles

- Telemedicine policies should be implemented if possible, to eliminate the unnecessary admission of patients to the centers and transmission of SARS-CoV-2. Besides telemedicine, general information about the facilities' strategies during the pandemic period should be mentioned on the website. If the patients have to apply to the healthcare center, they should be questioned about the signs and symptoms of COVID-19. Patients without compatible symptoms should be advised to cover their mouth and nose with a facemask or cloth covering upon admission.
- Every healthcare center should redesign the structuring of the facility to maintain the physical distance, constitute separate entrances for patients admitted with signs and symptoms of COVID-19 and separate outpatient clinics, wards, or buildings for COVID-19 patients, and display (posters and visuals) information at the entrance to direct the patients to these designated areas.
- Posters and visuals should be placed at the entrance and in common places to mention the use of facemasks and proper hand hygiene.
- Rearrangements should be made to maintain social distance in strategic places such as waiting areas, elevators, and cafeterias to prevent crowding. Regular cleaning and disinfection of these areas should be provided.
- All staff in the institution should be educated in terms of prevention measures.
- The administration should consider postponing elective procedures, outpatient admissions, and surgeries if relevant and update the decisions when convenient.
- Patients and visitors should wear facemask or cloth face-covering upon arrival to the hospital. If facemasks or cloth coverings are not worn facemasks should be provided at the entry.
- Every patient admitted to the healthcare facility for any reason should be screened for COVID-19 signs and symptoms (the body temperature should be actively measured) and questioned for exposure to COVID-19 patients within the

last 14 days upon entry. In case of suspicion, the patients should be transferred to a special area dedicated to COVID-19 patients.

- Restrictions to visitors should be applied. They should also be screened for COVID-19 symptoms and questioned for exposure to COVID-19 patients within the last 14 days. Those with symptoms and with a history of exposure should not be permitted to enter the healthcare centers and directed to the COVID-19 outpatient clinic.
- Environmental and engineering controls should provide adequate ventilation, structural design, environmental cleaning. Air conditioners should not be run in areas where more than one person is present.
- Commonly used and frequently touched surfaces (push buttons, door handles,etc.) should be cleaned and disinfected regularly. Equipment such as stretchers and wheelchairs used by patients should be disinfected after each patient use.
- Disinfection of devices such as phones, computers, etc. should be provided by the handler (70% of alcohol).
- Communication and transfer with paper, cardboard files, etc. should be minimized in the whole facility and online communication should be encouraged.
- All scientific and educational meetings should be held online at the utmost.

Outpatient Clinics

- Arrangements should be made to provide 1.5-2 meters of distance between healthcare workers (HCW) and patients in outpatient clinics.
- Alcohol-based hand antiseptics and substances required for the disinfection of the surfaces should be provided.
- The patients should wear facemasks and the HCWs should wear medical masks and goggles/face shields.
- Disinfection of common equipment after each use (70% alcohol) should be provided.

Inpatient Clinics

- All wards should be rearranged to place patients in a single room, if not possible, the patients should be separated by 2 meters from each other to prevent the transmission.
- COVID-19 patients should be followed up in a well ventilated private room with the bathroom placed within and the door closed. If isolation of the patient is not possible, confirmed COVID-19 patients may be cohorted.
- Inpatients should be provided facemasks. Patients may remove their masks when in their rooms but should put on when leaving their room, or when HCWs, other

staff, or visitors enter their room. Alcohol-based hand antiseptics should be available in every patient room and common areas.

- Equipment used for patients should be patient-specific and shared equipment should be disinfected (70% alcohol) after use.
- Patient rooms should be cleaned every day and in case of contamination.

Healthcare Workers

- Besides standard precautions, contact and droplet prevention measures should be taken during the care of suspected or confirmed COVID-19 patients.
- All HCWs who care for patients with suspected or confirmed COVID-19 should wear personal protective equipment (PPE). Standard PPE includes the use of a respirator or medical mask, goggles or face shield, a gown, and gloves.
- In conventional settings HCWs caring for patients with suspected or known COVID-19, should use a medical mask (CDC recommends the use of a medical mask or N95 or equivalent or higher level respirator; in case of respirator shortages, medical mask or reprocessed respirator can be used).
- Gloves and gowns are recommended in procedures carrying the risk of exposure to body fluids. They should always be changed after each patient contact. In case of heavy exposure to body fluids waterproof gowns may be preferred.
- HCWs should wear medical masks the day in the healthcare center including breakrooms or meeting areas since they may be exposed to asymptomatic or presymptomatic people.
- HCWs should avoid touching their face to eliminate the risk of self-contamination.
- Aerosol-generating procedures may lead to airborne transmission. These procedures include the following:

  - Endotracheal intubation and extubation
  - Manual ventilation before intubation
  - Noninvasive ventilation
  - Filter changes on the ventilator
  - Bronchoscopy (including mini bronchoalveolar lavage)
  - Cardiopulmonary resuscitation
  - Sputum induction
  - Open suctioning of airways
  - Tracheotomy
  - High-flow oxygen
  - Nasal endoscopy
  - Upper endoscopy (including transesophageal echocardiogram)
  - Use of nebulizer

  - Colonoscopy
  - Autopsies

- Aerosol-generating procedures should be carried out in a negative pressure room if possible or in a single room with the door kept closed and the room should be ventilated after the procedure.
- HCWs should wear an N95 (or equivalent or higher level) respirator, goggles or face shield, gloves, and gowns during these procedures. If N95 respirators are not available reprocessed respirators should be reused or a face shield or medical mask should be put on the respirator as a cover for extended use.
- Respirators with exhalation valves are not recommended.
- Hand hygiene should be performed before and after patient contact, after exposure to infectious material, before wearing and after removing all PPE.
- *Alcohol-based hand antiseptics containing 65-95% of alcohol should be used for hand hygiene or the hands should be washed with soap and water* [40-45].
- *Although* nasopharyngeal specimen collection is not considered as aerosol-generating procedure CDC recommends the use of respirator, face shield or goggles, gloves, and gowns [40].
- Exposure of contaminated material to HCW's eyes nose or mouth during aerosol-generating procedures is defined as high-risk exposure if the HCW has no any PPE.
- The HCW should be excluded from work for 14 days after last exposure in case of a prolonged and close contact ($<$ 2 meters for $\geq$ 15 minutes) with a confirmed COVID-19 patient before 2 days of symptom onset until the end of the isolation period:
- if the HCW does not wear a medical mask or respirator or
- if the HCW does not have eye or face protection when the patient does not wear a mask or
- if the HCW does not wear all PPE during aerosol-generating procedures (any duration of the contact is accepted as prolonged and close contact)
- In the case of the staffing shortage, HCW with a history of exposure can be allowed to work as long as he/she obeys preventive measures strictly. The HCW should monitor him/herself for signs and symptoms for the next 14 days after exposure.

Surgical Procedures

- Elective surgeries should be postponed. If the surgical procedures can not be postponed patients should be screened for COVID-19 signs and symptoms and in the presence of symptoms they should be tested for COVID-19 by molecular methods. If the suspicion level for COVID-19 is high and the nasopharyngeal swab test result by polymerase chain reaction (PCR) is negative, a second test may be performed. Some centers may consider testing all patients before surgery independent of symptoms. However, delays in results and the probability of negative results during the incubation period should be taken into consideration.

- COVID-19 patients should wear a medical mask and transport staff should apply droplets and contact prevention measures during transfer to the operating room.
- All HCWs in the operation team should wear N95, FFP2, or equivalent or higher level respirators, waterproof sterile gown, sterile gloves, goggles/face shield during the operation of a suspected or confirmed COVID-19 patients.
- Even if COVID-19 is excluded at the end of the evaluation, general contact and droplet precautions should be taken in operating rooms during the pandemic period.

Environmental Cleaning and Disinfection

- Surfaces should be cleaned with water and detergent firstly. Then application of 0.1% (1000ppm) sodium hypochlorite or 70-90% ethanol is effective. In the case of contamination with blood or body fluids, a concentration of 0.5% (5000ppm) sodium hypochlorite should be used.
- For sensitive surfaces and screens, 70% of alcohol can also be used for surface disinfection.
- Cleaning staff should use PPE [40-45].

CONCLUSION

COVID-19 pandemic continues all over the world. Although investigations in the fields of vaccination and treatment continue, the pandemic is not expected to end in a short time. Except for aerosol-generating procedures, the main route of transmission is thought to be through droplets and close contact. Considering all these factors, the use of masks, social distance, and hand hygiene should be provided based on the public setting. In the healthcare settings, except for aerosol-generating procedures, HCWs should take standard, contact, and droplet precautions.

REFERENCES

[1] World Health Organization. *Novel coronavirus situation report -2.* January 22, 2020. https://www.who.int/docs/default-source/coronaviruse/situation-reports/20200122-sitrep-2-2019-ncov.pdf.

[2] https://www.who.int/news-room/commentaries/detail/transmission-of-sars-cov-2-implications-for-infection-prevention-precautions.

[3] Mclntosh, K. (2020). *Coronavirus disease 2019 (COVID-19): Epidemiology, virology and prevention*. UpToDate. Version 111.0.

[4] Wiersinga, W. J., Rhodes, A., Cheng, A. C., Peacock, S. J., Prescott, H. C. (2020). Pathophysiology, Transmission, Diagnosis and Treatment of Coronavirus Disease 2019 (COVID-19) A Review. *JAMA*. 324: 782-93.

[5] Somsen, G. A., van Rijn, C., Kooij, S., Bem, RA., Bonn, D. (2020). Small droplet aerosols in poorly ventilated spaces and SARS-CoV-2 transmission. *Lancet Respir. Med*. 8:658-59.

[6] Asadi, S., Wexler, A. S., Cappa, C D., Barreda, S., Bouvier, N. M., Ristenpart, W. D. (2019). Aerosol emission and superemission during human speech increase with voice loudness. *Sci. Rep*. 9:2348.

[7] Van Doremalen, N., Bushmaker, T., Morris, D. H., Holbrook, M. G., Gamble, A., Williamson, B. N., Tamin, A., Harcourt, J. L., Thornburg N. J., Gerber S. I., Lloyd-Smith J. O., de Wit E., Munster V. J. (2020). Aerosol and surface stability of SARS-CoV-2 as compared with SARS-CoV-1. *N. Engl. J. Med*. 382:1564-67.

[8] Fears, A. C., Klimstra, W. B., Duprex, P., Weaver, S. C., Plante, J. A., Aguilar, P. V., Fernandez, D., Nalca, A., Totura, A., Dyer, D., Kearney, B., Lakemeyer, M., Bohannon, J. K., Johnson, R., Garry, R. F. Reed, D. S. Roy, C. J. (2020). Persistence of Severe Acute Respiratory Syndrome Coronavirus 2 in Aerosol Suspensions. *Emerg. Infect. Dis*. 26: 2168-71.

[9] Zhou, J., Otter, J. A., Price, J. R., Cimpeanu, C., Garcia, D. M., Kinross, J., Boshier, P. R., Mason, S., Bolt, F., Holmes, A. H., Barclay, W. S. (2020). Investigating SARS-CoV-2 surface and air contamination in an acute healthcare setting during the peak of the COVID-19 pandemic in London. *Clin. Infect. Dis*. ciaa905.

[10] Lednicky, J. A., Lauzardo, M., Hugh Fan, Z., Jutla, A., Tilly, T. B., Gangwar, M., Usmani, M., Shankar, S. N., Mohamed, K., Eiguren-Fernandez, A., Stephenson, C. J., Alam, M. M., Elbadry, M. A., Loeb, J. C., Subramaniam, K., Waltzek, T. B., Cherabuddi, K., Glenn Morris, J. Jr., Wu, C. Y. (2020). Viable SARS-CoV-2 in the air of a hospital room with COVID-19 patients. *Int. J. Infect. Dis*. 9712:30739-6.

[11] Anfinrud, P., Stadnytskyi, V., Bax, C. E., Bax, A. (2020). Visualizing Speech-Generated Oral Fluid Droplets with Laser Light Scattering. *N. Engl. J. Med*. 382:2061-63.

[12] Lu, J., Gu, J., Li, K., Xu, C., Su, W., Lai, Z., Zhou, D., Yu, C., Xu, B., Yang, Z. (2020). COVID-19 Outbreak Associated with Air Conditioning in Restaurant, Guangzhou, China, 2020. *Emerg. Infect. Dis*. 26:1628-31.

[13] Shen, Y., Li, C., Dong, H., Wang, Z., Martinez, L., Sun, Z., Handel, A., Chen, Z., Chen, E., Ebell, M. H., Wang, F., Yi, B., Wang, H., Wang, X., Wang, A., Chen, B., Qi, Y., Liang, L., Li, Y., Ling, F., Chen, J., Xu, G. (2020). Community Outbreak

Investigation of SARS-CoV-2 Transmission Among Bus Riders in Eastern China. *JAMA. Intern. Med.* e205225.

[14] Guo, Z-D., Wang, Z-Y., Zhang, S-F., Li, X., Li, L., Li, C., Cui, Y., Fu, R-B., Dong, Y-Z., Chi, X-Y., Zhang, M-Y., Liu, K., Cao, C., Liu, B., Zhang, K., Gao, Y-W., Lu, B., Chen, W. (2020). Aerosol and Surface Distribution of Severe Acute Respiratory Syndrome Coronavirus 2 in Hospital Wards, Wuhan, China, 2020. *Emerg. Infect. Dis.* 26:1583-91.

[15] Wang, W., Xu, Y., Gao, R., Lu, R., Han, K., Wu, G., Tan, W. (2020). Detection of SARS-CoV-2 in Different Types of Clinical Specimens. *JAMA.* 323:1843-44.

[16] Zheng, S., Fan, J., Yu, F., Feng, B., Lou, B., Zou, Q., Xie, G., Lin, S., Wang, R., Yang, X., Chen, W., Wang, Q., Zhang, D., Liu, Y., Gong, R., Ma, Z., Lu, S., Xiao, Y., Gu, Y., Zhang, J., Yao, H., Xu, K., Lu, X., Wei, G., Zhou, J., Fang, Q., Cai, H., Qiu, Y., Sheng, J., Chen, Y., Liang, T. (2020). Viral load dynamics and disease severity in patients infected with SARS-CoV-2 in Zhejiang province, China, January-March 2020: retrospective cohort study. *BMJ.* 369:m1443.

[17] Colavita, F., Lapa, D., Carletti, F., Lalle, E., Bordi, L., Marsella, P., Nicastri, E., Bevilacqua, N., Giancola, ML., Corpolongo, A., Ippolito, G., Capobianchi, M. R., Castilletti, C. (2020). SARS-CoV-2 Isolation From Ocular Secretions of a Patient With COVID-19 in Italy With Prolonged Viral RNA Detection *Ann. Intern. Med.* 173(3):242.

[18] Xiao, F., Sun, J., Xu, Y., Li, F., Huang, X., Li, H., Zhao, J., Huang, J., Zhao J. (2020). Infectious SARS-CoV-2 in Feces of Patient with Severe COVID-19. *Emerg. Infect. Dis.* 26:1920-22.

[19] Chen, W., Lan, Y., Yuan, X., Deng, X., Li, Y., Cai, X., Li, L., He, R., Tan, Y., Deng, X., Gao, M., Tang, G., Zhao, L., Wang, J., Fan, Q., Wen, C., Tong, Y., Tang, Y., Hu, F., Li, F., Tang, X. (2020). Detectable 2019-nCoV viral RNA in blood is a strong indicator for the further clinical severity. *Emerg. Microbes. Infect.* 9:469-73.

[20] Kotlyar, A. M, Grechukhina, O., Chen, A., Popkhadze, S., Grimshaw, A., Tal, O., Taylor, H. S., Tal, R. (2020). Vertical transmission of coronavirus disease 2019: a systematic review and meta-analysis. *Am. J. Obstet. Gynecol.* 9378(20)30823-1.

[21] Kirtsman, M., Diambomba, Y., Poutanen, S. M., Malinowski, A. K., Vlachodimitropoulou, E., Parks, W. T., Erdman, L., Morris, S. K., Shah, P. S. (2020). Probable congenital SARS-CoV-2 infection in a neonate born to a woman with active SARS-CoV-2 infection *CMAJ.* 2020;192:E647-50.

[22] Vivanti, A. J., Vauloup-Fellous, C., Prevot, S., Zupan, V., Suffee, C., Do Cao, J., Benachi, A., De Luca, D. (2020). Transplacental transmission of SARS-CoV-2 infection. *Nat. Commun.* 11:3572.

[23] Breastfeeding and COVID-19. Geneva: *World Health Organization; 2020* (available at https://www.who.int/news-room/commentaries/ detail/breastfeeding-and-covid-19).

[24] [24] Sit, T. H., Brackman, C. J., Ip, S. M., Tam, K.W., Law, P.Y., To, E. M. W., Yu, V. Y. T., Sims, L. D., Tsang, D. N. C., Chu, D. K. W., Perera, R. A. P. M., Poon, L. L. M., Peiris, M. (2020). Infection of dogs with SARS-CoV-2. *Nature.*

[25] Newman, A. (2020). First Reported Cases of SARS-CoV-2 Infection in Companion Animals—New York, March–April 2020. MMWR *Morbid. Mortal. Wkly. Rep.* 69:710–713.

[26] Oreshkova, N., Molenaar, R-J., Vreman, S., Harders, F., Munnink, B. B. O., van der Honing, R. W. H., Gerhards, N., Tolsma, P., Bouwstra, R., Sikkema, R. S., Tacken, M. Gj., Mt de Rooij, M., Weesendorp, E., Engelsma, M. Y., Bruschke, C. J., Smit, L. A., Koopmans, M., van der Poel, W. H., Stegeman, A. (2020). SARS-CoV2 infection in farmed mink, Netherlands, April 2020. *Euro. Surveill.* 25:2001005.

[27] Rothe, C., Schunk, M., Sothmann, P., Bretzel, G., Froeschl, G., Wallrauch, C., Zimmer, T., Thiel, V., Janke, C., Guggemos, W., Seilmaier, M., Drosten, C., Vollmar, P., Zwirglmaier, K., Zange, S., Wölfel, R., Hoelscher, M. (2020).Transmission of 2019-nCoV Infection from an Asymptomatic Contact in Germany. *N. Engl. J. Med.* 2020; 382:970-71.

[28] He, X., Lau, E. H. Y., Wu, P., Deng, X., Wang, J., Hao, X., Lau, Y. C., Wong, J., Y., Guan, Y., Tan, X., Mo, X., Chen, Y., Liao, B., Chen, W., Hu, F., Zhang, Q., Zhong, M., Wu, Y., Zhao, L., Zhang, F., Cowling, B. J., Li, F., Leung, G. M. (2020)Temporal dynamics in viral shedding and transmissibility of COVID-19. *Nat. Med.* 26:672-75.

[29] Cheng, H-Y., Jian, S-W., Liu, D-P., Ng, T-C., Huang, W-T., Lin, H-H., Taiwan COVID-19 Outbreak Investigation Team. (2020). Contact Tracing Assessment of COVID-19 Transmission Dynamics in Taiwan and Risk at Different Exposure Periods Before and After Symptom Onset. *JAMA. Intern. Med.* 180: 1156-63.

[30] Xiao, A. T., Tong, Y. X., Zhang, S. (2020). Profile of RT-PCR for SARS-CoV-2: a preliminary study from 56 COVID-19 patients. *Clin. Infect. Dis.* ciaa460.

[31] Wölfel, R., Corman, V. M., Guggemos, W., Seilmaier, M., Zange, S., Müller, M. A., Niemeyer, D., Jones, T., C., Vollmar, P., Rothe, C., Hoelscher, M., Bleicker, T., Brünink, S., Schneider, J., Ehmann, R., Zwirglmaier, K., Drosten, C., Wendtner C. (2020). Virological assessment of hospitalized patients with COVID-2019. *Nature.* 2020; 581:465-69.

[32] Jeong, H. W., Kim, S. M., Kim, H. S., Kim, Y. I., Kim, J. H., Cho, J. Y., Kim, S. H., Kang, H., Kim, S. G., Park, S. J., Kim, E. H., Choi, Y. K. (2020). Viable SARS-CoV-2 in various specimens from COVID-19 patients. *Clin. Microbiol. Infect.* 743:30427-4.

[33] Centers for Disease Control and Prevention. *Symptom-Based Strategy to Discontinue Isolation for Persons with COVID-19: Decision Memo.*

https://www.cdc.gov/coronavirus/2019-ncov/community/strategy-discontinue-isolation.html.

[34] Park, S. Y., Kim, Y. M., Yi, S., Lee, S., Na, B. J., Kim, C. B., Kim, J. I., Kim, H. S., Kim, Y. B., Park, Y., Huh, I. S., Kim, H. K., Yoon, H. J., Jang, H., Kim, K., Chang, Y., Kim, I., Lee, H., Gwack, J., Kim, S.S., Kim, M., Kweon, S., Choe, Y.J., Park, O., Park, Y.J., Jeong, E. K. (2020). Coronavirus Disease Outbreak in Call Center, South Korea. *Emerg. Infect. Dis.* 26:1666-70.

[35] Rosenberg, E. S., Dufort, E. M., Blog, D. S., Hall, E. W., Hoefer, D., Backenson, B. P., Muse, A. T., Kirkwood, J. N., George, K. S., Holtgrave, D. R., Hutton, B. J., Zucker, H. A., New York State Coronavirus 2019 Response Team. (2020). COVID-19 Testing, Epidemic Features, Hospital Outcomes, and Household Prevalence, New York State-March 2020. *Clin. Infect. Dis.* ciaa549.

[36] Fisher, K. A., Tenforde, M. W., Feldstein, L. R.,Lindsell, C. J., Shapiro, N. I., Files, D. C., Gibbs, K. W., Erickson, H. L., Prekker, M. E., Steingrub, J. S., Exline, M., C., Henning, D. J., Wilson, J., G., Brown, S. M., Peltan, I. D., Rice, T. W., Hager, D. N., Ginde, A. A., Talbot, H. K., Casey, J. D., Grijalva, C., G., Flannery, B., Patel, M. M., Self, W. H., IVY Network Invevestigators; CDC COVID-19 Response Team. (2020). *Community and Close Contact Exposures Associated with COVID-19 Among Symptomatic Adults ≥ 18 Years in 11 Outpatient Health Care Facilities* — United States, July 2020. MMWR. Morb. Mortal. Wkly. Rep.

[37] Khanh, N.C., Thai, P.Q., Quach, H.L., Thi, N. H., Dinh, P. C., Duong, T. N., Mai, L. T. Q., Nghia, N. D., Tu, T. A., Quang, N., Quang, T. D., Nguyen, T. T., Vogt, F., Anh, D. D. (2020). Transmission of Severe Acute Respiratory Syndrome Coronavirus 2 During Long Flight. *Emerg. Infect. Dis.* 26.

[38] https://www.cdc.gov/coronavirus/2019-ncov/prevent-getting-sick/prevention.html.

[39] https://www.cdc.gov/coronavirus/2019-ncov/php/public-health-recommendations.html.

[40] https://www.cdc.gov/coronavirus/2019-ncov/hcp/infection-control-recommendations.html.

[41] World Health Organization. *Infection prevention and control during health care when novel coronavirus (nCoV) infection is suspected.* January 25, 2020. https://www.who.int/publications-detail/infection-prevention-and-control-during-health-care-when-novel-coronavirus-(ncov)-infection-is-suspected-20200125.

[42] Palmore, T. N. (2020). *Coronavirus disease 2019 (COVID-19): Infection control in health care and home settings.* UpToDate. Version 111.0.

[43] Lynch, J. B., Davitkov, P., Anderson, D. J., Bhimraj, A., Cheng,V. C., Guzman-Cottrill, J., Dhindsa, J., Duggal, A., Jain, M. K., Lee, G. M., Liang, S. Y., McGeer, A., Lavergne, V., Murad, M. H., Mustafa, R. A., Morgan, R. L., Falck-Ytter, Y., Sultan, S. (2020). Infectious Diseases Society of America Guidelines on Infection

Prevention for Health Care Personnel Caring for Patients with Suspected or Known COVID-19. *Clin. Infect. Dis.* ciaa1063.

[44] https://www.ecdc.europa.eu/en/publications-data/infection-prevention-and-control-and-preparedness-covid-19-healthcare-settings

[45] https://www.cdc.gov/coronavirus/2019-ncov/hcp/guidance-risk-assesment-hcp.htm.

In: Coronavirus Disease
Editor: Yildiz Dincer

ISBN: 978-1-53619-296-4

Chapter 3

CLINICAL ASPECT OF COVID-19

Aslıhan Demirel[1], MD and Fehmi Tabak[2,*], MD
[1]Florence Nightingale Hospital, Department of Infectious Diseases and Clinical Microbiology, Turkey
[2]Istanbul University-Cerrahpasa, Cerrahpasa Medical Faculty, Department of Infectious Diseases and Clinical Microbiology, Turkey

ABSTRACT

COVID-19, named by the World Health Organization in February 2020, is an infectious and fatal disease that first started in China in December 2019 by the determination of pneumonia cases secondary to severe acute respiratory syndrome coronavirus 2 (SARS-CoV-2) and has been rapidly spreading all over the world since then. Although COVID-19 was first thought to be a disease manifested only by respiratory symptoms at the beginning of the outbreak, we learned in time that it is a disease that can develop symptoms in a wide spectrum from asymptomatic infection to cardiovascular complications. Experience in the diagnosis, clinical characteristics and treatment of COVID-19 has been accumulating in the time since it is a new disease. The severity of the disease might be variable according to the viral load received and the immune response of the individual. The frequency of asymptomatic disease is substantially high. The most commonly seen complaints in symptomatic disease are fever, cough, fatigue, and myalgia, while nausea, vomiting, and loss of taste and smell can also be seen. The longer the duration of the symptoms, the higher is the risk of developing a more severe disease necessitating hospital admission and intensive care, and invasive ventilation. Solid knowledge of clinical symptoms and diagnostic tests is important since early diagnosis may prevent the spread and intensification of the disease.

Keywords: COVID-19, SARS-CoV-2, coronavirus, clinical findings, laboratory findings

---

* Corresponding Author's Email: fehmitabak@yahoo.com.

Introduction

COVID-19 infection has caused a fatal outbreak which started in the Wuhan City of China and spread all over the world from there. COVID-19 developed secondary to SARS-CoV-2 has been officially declared to be a pandemic by the World Health Organization on March 11, 2020 [1]. The clinical picture is variable from a completely asymptomatic one to a rapidly destructive course. The clinical picture of COVID-19 including the incubation period, asymptomatic patients, symptoms, risk factors for severe disease, and complications will be reviewed in this chapter.

Incubation Period

The incubation period of COVID-19 disease is 2-14 days in 98% of the patients with a mean duration of 4-5 days [2-5]. The symptoms were reported to begin in 11.5 days (8.2-15.6) in 97.5% of the patients in a modeling study including 181 patients with a definitive diagnosis of Covid-19, while the mean duration of incubation was determined as 5.1 days [5]. Typically, the period from the initiation of symptoms and the development of the severe disease is a week [2]. The mean duration of incubation was predicted to be 5 days (4.4-5.6 days) in an analysis performed at a center out of Wuhan including 158 definitive cases [6].

It was reported in a striking study that the duration between the exposure and initiation of contagiousness (latent period) might be shorter [7]. Another study revealed that the viral load was high 2-3 days before the symptoms with a peak value of 0.7 days before the start of symptoms [8]. Therefore, it is important to screen the contacts of patients diagnosed to have COVID-19 and to consider the period before the start of symptoms.

Asymptomatic Infections

Asymptomatic infections and infections that are not symptomatic at the time of the diagnosis (pre-symptomatic) have been documented thoroughly in several studies [9-21]. Knowledge of the frequency of asymptomatic infections is crucial to understand the spread of the virus and the dynamics of the disease. Asymptomatic infections were reported to constitute 40-45% of SARS-CoV-2 infections in a study based on the data obtained from three major cohort studies [21]. However, no longitudinal follow-up was performed in that above mentioned and other similar studies to observe the development of symptoms. The prevalence of asymptomatic infections and the diagnosis of presymptomatic infections has yet to be understood since asymptomatic individuals are not routinely tested. The definition of asymptomatic is variable in several studies due to the specific symptoms evaluated. For example; 328 out of 634 (51.7%) cases were found to be asymptomatic in the Diamond Princess cruise in which all passengers and crew were quarantined in the Yokohama City of Japan. Considering the incubation period varying between 5.5 and 9.5 days, the authors calculated the actual rate of asymptomatic cases as 17.9% [14]. The rate of asymptomatic cases was 26% in an observational cohort study conducted on 199 infected patients in an inpatient treatment center in South Korea [22]. The percentage of patients tested positive for SARS-CoV-2 but without any symptoms was reported to be 44% in a screening study performed in Ireland; however, some of them might be pre-symptomatic [20]. Higher rates of asymptomatic cases have been reported in some studies. For example, 29 out of 210 pregnant women (14%) admitted to two New York hospitals for childbirth at the time of the peak of the pandemic were tested to be positive for SARS-CoV-2 using polymerase chain reaction (RT-PCR). Other than those, four women who were tested positive for SARS-CoV-2 had a fever and other symptoms. Therefore, 29 out of 33 women with a positive test for SARS-CoV-2 (88%) were asymptomatic at the time of presentation to the hospital [19]. The rate of asymptomatic patients was around 20-40% in all those studies, while this wide range might be due to the different properties of the populations analyzed.

Asymptomatic patients might present clinically objective findings [10, 23]. An example of this is a study including 24 patients with asymptomatic infection; 50% of the patients had typical CT involvement of COVID-19 and another 20% of them had atypical radiological abnormalities [10]. In another study including 55 patients with asymptomatic infection, pneumonia was detected by CT in 67% of the patients at presentation; only two patients developed hypoxia, and all patients recovered (23). Cases that were asymptomatic at the time of the diagnosis as the cases mentioned above can be classified as pre-symptomatic infections. The initiation of symptoms was seen as a mean of 4 days (3-7 days) after the first positive RT-PCR test in a study performed [24].

Clinical Presentation

Differentiating the first symptoms of COVID-19 from other viral upper respiratory infections is almost impossible. However, with the accumulating experience, it has now been acknowledged that COVID-19 infection is not a disease of the respiratory tract alone, but it is a disease involving many organs and is manifested with different symptoms according to the organ involved and the degree of the immune response [25].

The most frequent symptoms seen in COVID-19 infection are as follows [3, 26-31]:

- Fever
- Cough
- Dyspnea or difficulty in breathing
- Fatigue, weakness
- Muscle pain (myalgia) or the ache of body parts
- Headache
- Loss of smell (anosmia) and taste (ageusia)
- Sore throat
- Nasal congestion
- Nausea or vomiting
- Diarrhea

Symptoms vary according to the severity of the disease. For example, fever, cough, and dyspnea were reported to be more common in hospitalized patients with COVID-19 compared to patients with less severe disease and thus not admitted to the hospital. Atypical symptoms might be seen in the elderly and patients with comorbidities, and the manifestation of fever and respiratory symptoms might be delayed [32, 33]. Fever was reported to be present in 44% of 1099 patients at admission to the hospital and 89% had fever rising after admission in a study performed in China [3]. No differentiation between mild and severe cases and prediction of the clinical course can be made according to the presence or absence of fever and cough [34, 35]. Dyspnea was demonstrated in larger studies to be a powerful predictor of severe disease. Respiratory distress might be developed generally during the second week of the disease and might progress to hypoxemia [3]. A clinical picture of viral pneumonia predominates and may include fever, cough, and hypoxia. Imaging of the lungs reveals bilateral ground-glass imaging and infiltrations [36].

Fatigue, headache, and myalgia are the most commonly reported symptoms with an incidence of 15-40% among outpatients with COVID-19 [37, 38]. These symptoms, although frequently disturbing, are not indicators of a severe clinical picture. Headache is bilateral with an intermediate severity and experienced in the temporo-parietal, frontal or periorbital areas [39]. A part of the patients may present with gastrointestinal symptoms such as nausea, vomiting, or diarrhea before the development of fever and lower respiratory tract signs and symptoms [31]. Diarrhea and nausea and vomiting were observed in 24% and 19%, respectively among the first 393 patients admitted to two hospitals in New York [40]. Enteric symptoms are generally seen together with fever and respiratory tract complaints. Among the 18,605 patients presenting to the hospital in the United Kingdom, 29% had enteric symptoms, generally together with respiratory symptoms, while only 4% of all patients reported enteric symptoms alone [38].

Symptoms of the upper respiratory tract such as nasal congestion, nasal discharge, sneezing, and sore throat are quite rare in COVID-19 infection.

On the other hand, loss of taste (ageusia) and smell (anosmia) has been reported widely before the start of the symptoms in young women and young and middle-aged individuals who needed no hospitalization [41, 42]. The largest study on this subject revealed the loss of smell in 1754 (87%) and loss of taste in 1136 (56%) out of 2013 patients [43].

Although most symptoms of COVID-19 are common in other respiratory tract infections or viral diseases, anosmia seems to be a more specific sign of COVID-19 [42]. In conclusion, the presence of anosmia and ageusia demonstrate no severe disease; however, they might be important indicators of SARS-CoV-2 infection.

Clinical Course of the Disease

The severity of COVID-19 infection might be variable from mild to critical. The course is frequently mild [9, 26, 27, 28, 41, 44]. Currently, there is no definitively accepted clinical classification for COVID-19. The following classification including four categories has been used by some authors [45].

- Mild cases: symptomatic cases with no observed pneumonia with imaging.
- Ordinary cases: Fever and signs of pneumonia with imaging.
- Severe cases: Dyspnea, hypoxia ($SpO2 \leq 93\%$), abnormal blood gas analysis $PaO2 < 60mmHg$, $PaCO2 > 50mmHg$).
- Critical cases: Respiratory failure necessitating mechanical ventilation, shock, other organ failure requiring admission to ICU.

A similar classification was used in the study of Chinese Disease Control Center including 44.500 confirmed infections; however, item 1 and 2 were combined, such as;

- Mild to intermediate disease (pneumonia is mild or absent), reported in 81%
- Severe disease (dyspnea, hypoxia or findings such as more than 50% lung involvement in imaging studies in 24 to 48 hours) in 14%
- Critical disease (clinical pictures such as respiratory failure, shock, or multiorgan dysfunction), reported in 5%.

No death was seen in non-critical patients in that study. The General case fatality rate was reported to be 2.3% [46]. Asymptomatic/mild-intermediate disease, respiratory failure and death were seen in 80.5%, 19.5% and 5.5%, respectively in a meta-analysis including 38 studies [47]. The rate of critical disease and death are higher in hospitalized patients [34, 35, 48, 49]. Some 665 patients (24%) died or were referred to nursing care in a study including 2741 patients hospitalized due to COVID-19 in New York [35]. The clinical course of the disease and death rates are variable according to the region. The rate of admission to the intensive care unit was 12% among all cases with COVID-19 and 16% among all patients hospitalized in Italy with an estimated case fatality rate of 7,2% in mid-March [50, 51]. In contrast, the estimated case fatality rate in mid-March in South Korea was 0,9% [52]. This might be due to the demographic variability of the infections such as the median age of the infected patients (64 years in Italy and 40 years in Korea).

Clinical Progression

The clinicians must be careful on clinical progression since it generally occurs a week after the initiation of the disease. Mean duration between the initiation of symptoms to development of dyspnea among patients who develop severe disease has been reported to be 5-8 days, between the start of the disease to the development of acute respiratory distress syndrome (ARDS) as 8-12 days and from the initiation of symptoms or the disease to the admission to intensive care unit (ICU) as 10-12 days in the studies performed [27, 28, 32, 41]. The rate of admission to ICU among hospitalized patients has been reported to be 26-32% [28, 41]. The mortality rate in patients admitted to the ICU, depending on the study and the properties of the population is 39-72% [27, 30, 32, 41]. The mean duration of hospital stay in surviving patients has been 10-13 days in the studies performed [3, 28, 30].

Risk Factors for Severe Illness

Advanced age; is a powerful risk factor for severe disease, and the development of complications and mortality [3, 28, 30, 46, 53, 54, 55]. Mortality rate among more than 44.000 confirmed COVID-19 cases in China was reported as 14.8%, 8%, 3.6%, 1.3%, 0.4% and 0.2% in patients aged 80 years and above, 70-79 years, 60-69 years, 50-59 years, 40-49 years and <40 years, respectively [56, 57]. Advanced age has been defined as a serious risk factor for severe disease and death rates in recent literature from all over the world. One example of these studies is a large one evaluating the outbreak in 20.133 patients in the United Kingdom and the mean age of 5.165 patients who died in the hospital (26%) due to COVID-19 was reported as 80 years in that study [58]. A dramatic increase was observed among the group of patients with advanced age among 5700 patients in New York and the mortality rate reached up to 61% (122/199) in males and 48% (115/242) in females with the age of more than 80 years [34].

The mortality rate was markedly higher among the elderly patients (>63 years) compared to young patients (36% and 15%) in 1.591 patients admitted in the ICU in Italy. The mortality rate in 362 patients with an age above 70 years was reported to be 41% [59].

Other risk factors: Initial studies from China revealed that diseases such as hypertension, cardiovascular disease, and diabetes were associated with severe disease and mortality [3]. Later, other studies from various regions have demonstrated that the risk of development of severe disease and mortality was higher in patients with comorbidities [32, 46, 35, 60, 61, 62, 63].

- Cardiovascular disease
- Diabetes mellitus
- Hypertension
- Chronic lung disease
- Cancer (in particular hematologic malignancies, lung cancer, and metastatic disease)
- Chronic kidney disease
- Obesity
- Smoking

Individuals with hypertension, cardiovascular disease, and chronic lung disease were reported to carry a higher risk of having a severe course in a meta-analysis evaluating 46.248 confirmed cases of COVID-19 in eight studies [64]. The mortality rate was 12-fold among patients with reported comorbidities compared to the ones with no comorbidities in a study from the United States of America including 300.000 confirmed COVID-19 cases [65].

In conclusion; advanced age and presence of comorbidity, alone or combined, are marked risk factors for severe disease and mortality.

Complications

Patients with a mild course are generally not hospitalized. The treatment of most patients can be managed at home. The decision for hospitalization depends on the clinical picture, necessity of supportive care, potential risk factors for severe disease, and the ability of the patient for self -isolation. Patients with risk factors should be closely followed-up especially during the second week since there is a risk of advancement to severe disease. Patients with COVID-19 with initially mild symptoms may deteriorate during the first week [66]. Dyspnea was reported to develop mean five days after the start of the symptoms and admission to hospital was required a mean of seven days after the initiation of symptoms in a study including 138 patients admitted to the hospital with pneumonia secondary to SARS-CoV-2 in Wuhan [28].

The most significant complications of COVID-19 can be defined as:

Respiratory Failure

Acute respiratory distress syndrome (ARDS) is the most important complication in patients with COVID-19 and might be observed a short period after the initiation of dyspnea. ARDS develops on day 8-14 in 10-20% of the patients [67, 68]. Non-cardiogenic pulmonary edema develops in those patients and mechanical ventilation might be required. Hypertension, diabetes mellitus, and cardiovascular and cerebrovascular diseases have been reported to be a risk factor for ARDS [68]. Retrospective studies on patients with critical illness established that initiation of dyspnea was average 6.5 days after the start of the disease; however, the development of ARDS was seen even in a shorter period after the start of dyspnea (mean 2 days) [28, 32, 41, 55]. Some 12-24% of the hospitalized patients required mechanical ventilation according to the studies performed in the USA [34, 35].

Cardiac and Cardiovascular Complications

Arrhythmia, acute cardiac damage, and shock are reported complications [28, 55, 69]. The rate of these complications was reported to be 17%, 7%, and 9%, respectively in a study [28]. On the other hand, acute cardiac damage and heart failure was seen in 77% (72/94) and 49% (41/83), respectively in a retrospective study evaluating 113 patients who died due to COVID-19 infection [69]. The development of cardiomyopathy was reported in one-third of the patients in a series including 21 severe cases admitted to the ICU in the USA [55].

Thromboembolic Complications

Coagulation disorders that complicate the clinical management of the disease are seen in some patients with COVID-19. These patients carry a high risk for arterial and venous thrombosis of small and large vessels due to hypercoagulation [70, 71]. SARS-CoV-2 directly invades endothelial cells and causes cell damage. Endothelial damage, microvascular inflammation, endothelial exocytosis, and/or endothelitis play a central role in the pathogenesis of acute respiratory distress syndrome and organ failure according to some experts [72, 73]. Induction of endothelial cells due to infection causes excess production of thrombin and fibrinolysis is prevented. Also, patients are prone to venous and arterial thromboembolic events due to hypoxia, increased inflammation, and immobilization. Commonly observed laboratory findings among hospitalized patients with COVID-19-associated coagulopathy are mild thrombocytopenia, increased level of D-dimer, fibrin degradation products, and prothrombin time. High levels of D-dimer have been highly associated with a higher death rate [70, 74, 75, 76]. Pulmonary embolism, deep venous thrombosis, myocardial infarct, ischemic events, or systemic arterial embolism can be frequently seen in these patients. Cases with severe COVID-10 have been generally shown in the studies performed to be complicated with coagulopathies and DIC has been demonstrated in most cases of mortality.

Inflammatory Complications

A "cytokine storm" including an increase in the levels of inflammatory cytokines such as IL-1, IL-6, IL-8, and levels of TNF-α and IFN-γ is present in the pathogenesis of COVID-19 disease [77, 78]. Persistent high fever and high levels of inflammatory markers (i.e., D-dimer and ferritin) and increased proinflammatory cytokines have proven a marked inflammatory response on a laboratory basis and these laboratory values have been associated with critical and fatal diseases [27, 79, 80]. Levels of many cytokines such as C-reactive protein (CRP), ferritin, and IL-6 were reported to increase in severe disease in a meta-analysis [32]. Decreased interleukin-6 (IL-6) levels were revealed to be closely associated with treatment efficacy, while increased levels of IL-6 demonstrated exacerbation of the disease in a retrospective observational analysis including 69 cases with severe COVID-19 [81]. The authors concluded that the dynamic changes in the IL-6 levels could be used as a marker during the follow-up of the disease in patients with severe COVID-19. Finally, cytokine storm should be considered in patients with persistent fever despite treatment, increased D-dimer, ferritin, and CRP levels, decreased lymphocyte and platelet counts, increased fibrinogen levels, and deteriorated liver function tests. Early diagnosis of this clinical picture is substantial since it is a condition that needs emergency treatment. Patients demonstrating signs of severe COVID-19 infection should be daily monitored for markers of a cytokine storm. Other inflammatory complications and auto-antibody mediated signs have been defined other than the cytokine storm [82, 83]. Myasthenia gravis is one of them [82]. Guillain-Barré syndrome can be developed 5-10 days after the initial symptoms [84]. In addition, a multi-system inflammatory syndrome with similar clinical properties with Kawasaki disease and toxic shock syndrome has been defined in children with COVID-19. This syndrome, rarely reported in adults also has been characterized with markedly increased inflammatory markers and multi-organ dysfunction (especially cardiac dysfunction) and minimal pulmonary involvement [85].

Secondary Infections

Secondary infections don't seem to be a common complication of COVID-19, although the data is limited [86, 87]. The rate of the reported bacterial or fungal infections was 8% in a publication evaluating nine studies, mostly from China and they mainly included respiratory tract infections and bacteremia [86]. Possible invasive aspergillosis has been reported among the patients with ARDS secondary to COVID-19 and no immune suppression; however, the incidence of this complication is unknown [88, 89, 90, 91].

Recovery and Long-Term Sequela

According to the World Health Organization (WHO), the period of recovery seems to be almost two weeks for mild disease and three to six weeks for the severe disease [92]. Nevertheless, the period of recovery varies based on age and previously present additional diseases in addition to the severity of the disease.

A survey on 350 patients with COVID-19 in the United States of America revealed that only 39% of the patients admitted to a hospital had a full recovery 14-21 days after the diagnosis [93]. Similarly, only 13% of 143 patients admitted to the hospital (7 of them were intubated) due to COVID-19 in Italy were without symptoms after a mean of 60 days starting from the initiation of the disease [94]. The most common persistent symptoms were fatigue (53%), dyspnea (43%), joint pain (27%), and chest pain (22%); however, none of the patients had a fever or acute findings of the disease. On the other hand, persistent severe disease together with persistent fever for weeks and pneumonia associated with underlying immunosuppression has been reported in another study [95].

Symptoms may persist for a long time also in patients with COVID-19 and milder symptoms [98, 96]. In a survey with 292 participants diagnosed to have COVID-19 and were treated on an outpatient basis, 65% of the patients reported being as healthy as before they had the disease 14-21 days after the diagnosis [96]. Individuals with full recovery recovered in a mean of 7 days after the diagnosis. The symptoms that patients most possibly continued to have 14-21 days after the diagnosis were cough (43%) and fatigue (35%).

As of the established data, a potential of respiratory insufficiency and the cardiac sequel has been suggested, although the evaluation of long-term sequela of COVID-19 has not been adequately evaluated yet [97-102].

Laboratory Findings

The most common laboratory findings seen in patients hospitalized with the diagnosis of COVID-19 are lymphopenia, high levels of serum aminotransferase, lactate dehydrogenase, and inflammatory markers (i.e., ferritin, C-reactive protein, and erythrocyte sedimentation rate), and abnormalities in coagulation tests. [28, 3, 40, 27, 30].

Lymphopenia is the most common laboratory finding of COVID-19 and is present in 83% of hospitalized patients [3, 27]. High D-dimer levels and lymphopenia are associated with mortality [30, 46].

Although procalcitonin level is normal at presentation; its level is possibly increased in patients admitted to the ICU [27, 26, 28]. Cardiac troponin I levels were found to be substantially high only in patients with severe COVID-19 in addition to low level of lymphocytes, high levels of LDH, and D-dimer in a meta-analysis evaluating 341 patients [103].

Conclusion

COVID-19 disease is a contagious and fatal infection that has spread all over the world in a short time. We have observed up to now that the infection is mostly asymptomatic; symptomatic and severe infection develops less frequently. The incubation period is 2-14 days with an average of 4-5 days. The most commonly seen complaints are fever, cough, myalgia, fatigue, diarrhea, and loss of taste and smell. Pneumonia is the most common sign of serious infection and severe infection is developed in approximately 15% of the patients with hypoxia, dyspnea, or diffuse pulmonary involvement. ARDS is the main complication in patients with severe disease and it might be observed a short while after the start of dyspnea. Many other complications including thromboembolic events, acute cardiac damage, and inflammatory complications have been reported. The risk of developing severe disease and mortality is high in elderly individuals and individuals with comorbidities. Laboratory parameters and imaging studies will be of guidance in the course of the disease. A good understanding of the clinical and laboratory findings of the COVID-19 disease will play a major role in the early diagnosis of the disease and the control of the outbreak.

References

[1] *World Health Organization*. Director-General's remarks at the media briefing on 2019-nCoV on 11 February 2020. http://www. who.int/dg/speeches/detail/who-director-general-s-remarks-at-the-media-briefing-on-2019-ncov-on-11-february-2020.

[2] Ortiz-Prado, E., Simbaña-Rivera, K., Gómez- Barreno, L., Rubio-Neira M., P. Guaman, L., C Kyriakidis, N., Muslin, C., Gómez Jaramillo, A. M., Barba-Ostria, C., Cevallos-Robalino, D., Sanches-SanMiguel, H., Unigarro, L., Zalakeviciute, R., Gadian, N., López-Cortés, A. 2020. Clinical, molecular, and epidemiological characterization of the SARS-CoV-2 virus and theCoronavirus Disease 2019 (COVID-19), a comprehensive literature review. *Diagn Microbiol Infect Dis.* 98(1): 115094.

[3] Guan, WJ., Ni, ZY., Hu, Y., Liang, WH., Ou, CQ., He, JX., Liu, L., Shan, H., Lei, CL., Hui, DSC., Du, B., Li, LJ., Zheng, G., Yuen, KY., Chen, RC., Thang, CL., Wang, T., Chen, PY., Xiang, J., Li, SY., Wang, JL., Liang, ZJ., Peng, YX., Wei, L., Liu, Y., Hu, YH., Peng, P., Wang, JM., Liu, JY., Chen, Z., Li, G., Zheng, ZJ., Qie, SQ., Luo, J., Ye, CJ., Zhu, SY., Zhong, NS., for the China Medical Treatment Expert Group for Covid-19 (2020). Clinical Characteristics of Coronavirus Disease 2019 in China. *N Engl J Med*. 382:1708-20.

[4] Li, Q., Guan, X., Wu, P., Wang, X., Zhou, L., Tong, Y., Ren, R., Leung, KSM., Lau, EHY., Wong, JY., Xing, X., Xiang, N., Wu, Y., Li, C., Chen, Q., Li, D., Liu, T., Zhao, J., Liu, M., Tu, W., Chen, C., Jin, L., Yang, R., Wang, Q., Zhou, S., Wang, R., Liu, H., Luo, Y., Liu, Y., Shao, G., Li, H., Tao, Z., Yang, Y., Deng, Z., Liu, B., Ma, Z., Zhang, Y., Shi, G., Lam, TTY., Wu, JT., Gao, GF., Cowling, BJ., Yang, B., Leung, GM., Feng, Z. (2020). Early Transmission Dynamics in Wuhan, China, of Novel Coronavirus-Infected Pneumonia. *N Engl J Med.* 382:1199-207.

[5] Lauer, SA., Grantz, KH., Bi, Q., Jones, FK., Zheng, Q., Meredith, HR., Azman, HS., Reich, NG., Lessler, J. (2020). The Incubation Period of Coronavirus Disease 2019 (COVID-19) From Publicly Reported Confirmed Cases: Estimation and Application. *Ann Intern Med*. 172(9):577-582.

[6] Linton, NM., Kobayashi, T., Yang, Y., Hayashi, K., Akhmetzhanov, AR., Jung, SM., Yuan, B., Kinoshita R., Nishiura, H. (2020). Incubation Period and Other Epidemiological Characteristics of 2019 Novel Coronavirus Infections with Right Truncation: A Statistical Analysis of Publicly Available Case Data. *J Clin Med.* 17;9(2).

[7] Li, P., Fu, JB., Li, KF., Liu, JN., Wang, HL., Liu, LJ., Chen, Y., Zhang, YL., Liu, SL., Tang, A., Tong, ZD., Yan, JB. (2020). Transmission of COVID-19 in the terminal stage of incubation period: a familial cluster. *Int J Infect Dis.* 96:452-453.

[8] He, X., Lau, EHY., Wu, P., Deng, X., Wang, J., Hao, X., Lau, YC., Wong, JY., Guan, Y., Tan, X., Mo, X., Chen, Y., Liao, B., Chen, W., Hu, F., Zhang, Q., Zhong, M., Wu, Y., Zhao, L., Zhang, F., Cowling, BJ., Li, F., Leung, GM. (2020) Temporal dynamics in viral shedding and transmissibility of COVID-19. *Nat Med.* 26:672-675.

[9] Chan, JF., Yuan, S., Kok, KH., Wang, KK., Chu, H., Yang J., Xing, F., Liu, J., Yip, CC., Poon, RW., Tsoi, HW., Lo, SK., Chan, KH., Poon, WK., Chan, WM., Ip, JD., Cai, JP., Cheng, VC., Chen H., Hui, CK., Yuen, KY. (2020). A familial cluster of pneumonia associated with the 2019 novel coronavirus indicating person-to-person transmission: a study of a family cluster. *Lancet.* 395:514-23.

[10] Wang, Y., Liu, Y., Liu, L., Wang, X., Luo, N., Ling, L. (2020). Clinical outcome of 55 asymptomatic cases at the time of hospital admission infected with SARS-Coronavirus-2 in Shenzhen, China. *J Infect Dis*. 221.1770-1774.

[11] Pan, X., Chen, D., Xia, Y., Wu, X., Li, T., Ou, X., Zhou, L., Liu, J. (2020). Asymptomatic cases in a family cluster with SARS-CoV-2 infection. *Lancet Infect Dis.* 20:410-1.

[12] Bai, Y., Yao, L., Wei, T., Tian, F., Jin, DY., Chen, L., Wang, M. (2020). Presumed Asymptomatic Carrier Transmission of COVID-19. *JAMA*. 323:1406-1407.

[13] Kam, KQ., Yung, CF., Cui, L., Lin, RTP., Mak, TZ., Maiwald M., Li, J., Chong, CY., Nadua, K., Tan, NWH., Thoon, KC. (2020). A Well Infant with Coronavirus Disease 2019 (COVID-19) with High Viral Load. *Clin Infect Dis*. 71:847-849.

[14] Mizumoto, K., Kagaya, K., Zarebski, A., Chowell, G. (2020). Estimating the asymptomatic proportion of coronavirus disease 2019 (COVID-19) cases on board the Diamond Princess cruise ship, Yokohama, Japan, 2020. *Euro Surveill.* 25:2000180.

[15] Wei, WE., Li, Z., Chiew, CJ., Yong, SE., Toh, MP., Lee, VJ. (2020). Presymptomatic Transmission of SARS-CoV-2 – Singapore, January 23-March 16, 2020. *MMWR Morb Mortal Wkly Rep*. 69:411-5.

[16] Tong, ZD., Tang, A., Li, KF., Li, P., Wang, HL., Yi, JP., Zhang, YL., Yan, JB. (2020). Potential Presymptomatic Transmission of SARS-CoV-2, Zhejiang Province, China, 2020. *Emerg Infect Dis*. 26:1052-4.

[17] World Health Organization. *Coronavirus disease 2019* (COVID-19) Situation Report – 28. February 18, 2020. https://www.who.int/docs/default-source/coronaviruse/situation-reports/20200217-sitrep-28-covid-19.pdf?sfvrsn=a19cf2ad_2.

[18] Kimball, A., Hatfield, KM., Arons, M., James, A., Taylor J., Spicer, K., Bardossy, AC., Oakley, LP., Tanwar, S., Chisty, Z., Bell, JM., Methner, M., Harney, J., Jacobs, JR., Carlson, CM., McLaughlin, HP., Stone, N., Clark, S., Smith, CB., Page, LC., Kay, M., Lewis, J., Russel, D., Hiatt, B., Gant, J., Duchin, JS., Clark, TA., Honein, MA., Reddy, SC., Jernigan, JA., Public Helath-Seattle & King

County; CDC COVID-19 Investigation Team. Asymptomatic and Presymptomatic SARS-CoV-2 Infections in Residents of a Long-Term Care Skilled Nursing Facility- King County, Washington, March 2020. (2020). *MMWR Morb Mortal Wkly Rep*. 69:377.

[19] Sutton, D., Fuchs, K., D'Alton, M., Goffman, D. Universal Screening for SARS-CoV-2 in Women Admitted for Delivery. (2020). *N Engl J Med.* 382:2163.

[20] Gudbjartsson, DF., Helgason, A., Jonsson, H., Magnusson, OT., Melsted, P., Norddahl, GL., Saemundsdottir, J., Sigurdsson, A., Sulem, P., M. D., Agustsdottir, AB., Eiriksdottir, B., Fridriksdottir, R., Gardarsdottir, EE., Georgsson, G., Gretarsdottir, OS., Gudmundsson, KR., Gunnarsdottir, TR., Gylfason, A., Holm, H., Jensson, BO., Jonasdottir, A., Jonsson, F., Josefsdottir, KS., Kristjansson, T., Magnusdottir, DN., Roux, L., Sigmundsdottir, G., Sveinbjornsson, G.,. Sveinsdottir, KE., Sveinsdottir, M., Thorarensen, EA., Thorbjornsson, B., Löve, A., Masson, G., Jonsdottir, I., Möller, AD., Gudnason, T., Kristinsson, KG., Thorsteinsdottir, U., Stefansson, K. (2020). Spread of SARS-CoV-2 in the Icelandic Population. *N Engl J Med*. 382:2302.

[21] Oran, DP., Topol, EJ. (2020). Prevelance of Asymptomatic SARS-CoV-2 Infection: A Narrative Review. *Ann Intern Med.* 173:362.

[22] Noh, JY., Yoon, JG., Seong, H., Choi, WS., Sohn, JW., Cheong, HJ., Kim, WJ., Song, JY. (2020) Asymptomatic infection and atypical manifestations of COVID-19: Comparison of viral shedding duration. *J Infect.* 81:816-846.

[23] Hu, Z., Song, C., Xu, C., Jin, G., Chen, Y., Xu, X., Ma, H., Chen, W., Lin, Y., Zheng, Y., Wang, J., Hu, Z., Yi, Y., Shen, H. (2020) Clinical chracteristics of 24 asymptomatic infections with COVID-19 screened among close contacts in Nanjing, China. *Sci China Life Sci China Life Sci*. 63:706.

[24] Sakurai, A., Sasaki, T., Kato, Hayashi, M., Tsuziki, SI., Ishihara, T., Iwata, M., Morise, S., S., Doi, Y. (2020) Natural History of Asymptomatic SARS-CoV-2 Infection. *N England J Med.* 383:885.

[25] Mancia, G., Rea, F., Ludergnani, M., Apolone, G., Corrao, G. (2020). Renin–angiotensin–aldosteronesystem blockers and the risk of Covid-19. *New England Journal of medicine.* 382:2431-2440.

[26] Chen, N., Zhou, M., Dong, X., Qu, J., Gong, F., Han, Y., Qiu, Y., Wang, J., Liu, Y., Wei, Y., Xia, J., Yu, T., Zhang, X., Zhang, L. (2020). Epidemiological and clinical characteristics of 99 cases of 2019 novel coronavirus pneumonia in Wuhan, China: a descriptive study. *Lancet*. 395:507-13.

[27] Huang, C., Wang, Y., Li, X., Ren, L., Zhao, J., Hu, Y., Zhang, L., Fan, G., Xu, J., Gu, X., Cheng, Z., Yu, T., Xia, J., Wei, Y., Wu, W., Xie, X., Yin, W., Li H., Liu, M., Xiao, Y., Gao, H., Guo, L., Xie, J., Wang, G., Jiang, R., Gao, Z., Jin, Q., Wang, J., Cao, B. (2020) Clinical features of patients infected with 2019 novel coronavirus in Wuhan, China. *Lancet*. 395:497-506.

[28] Wang, D., Hu, B., Hu, C., Zhu, F., Liu, X., Zhang, J., Wang, B., Xiang, H., Cheng, Z., Xiong, Y., Zhao, Y., Li, Y., Wang, X., Peng, Z. (2020). Clinical Characteristics of 138 Hospitalized Patients with 2019 Novel Coronavirus-Infected Pneumonia in Wuhan, China. *JAMA*. 323:1061-1069.

[29] Xu, XW., Wu, XX., Jiang, XG., Xu, K., Ying, LJ., Ma, CL., Li, SB., Wang, HY., Zhang, S., Gao, H., Sheng, JF., Cai, HL., Qui, YK., Li, LJ. (2020). Clinical findings in a group of patients infected with the 2019 novel coronavirus (SARS-Cov-2) outside of Wuhan, China: retrospective case series. *BMJ*. 368:m606.

[30] Wu, C., Chen, X., Cai, Y., Xia, J., Zhou, X., Xu, S., Huang, H., Zhang L., Zhou, X., Du, C., Zhang, Y., Song, J., Wang, S., Chao, Y., Yang, Z., Xu, J., Zhou, X., Chen, D., Xiong, W., Xu, L., Zhou, F., Jiang, J., Bai, C., Zheng, J., Song, Y. (2020). Risk Factors Associated With Acute Respiratory Distress Syndrome and Death in Patients With Coronavirus Disease 2019 Pneumonia in Wuhan, China. *JAMA Intern Med*. 180:934-943.

[31] Pan, L., Mu, M., Yang, P., Sun, Y., Wang, R., Yan, J., Li, P., Hu, B., Wang, J., Hu, C., Jin, Y., Niu, X., Ping, R., Du, Y., Li, T., Xu, G., Hu, Q., Tu, L. (2020) Clinical Characteristics of COVID-19 Patients With Digestive Symptoms in Hubei, China: A Descriptive, Cross-Sectional, Multicenter Study. *Am J Gastroenterol*. 115:766-773.

[32] Zhou, F., Yu, T., Du, R., Fan, G., Liu, Y., Liu, Z., Xiang J., Wang, Y., Song, B., Gu, X., Guan, L., Wei, Y., Li, H., Wu, X., Xu, J., Tu, S., Zhang, Y., Chen, H., Cao, B. (2020). Clinical course and risk factors for mortality of adult inpatients with COVID-19 in Wuhan, China: a retrospective cohort study. *Lancet*. 395:1054-1062.

[33] Dong, Y., Mo, X., Hu, Y., Qi, X., Jiang, F., Jiang, Z., Tong, S. (2020). Epidemiology of COVID-19 among Children in China. *Pediatrics*. 145(6):e20200702.

[34] Richardson, S., Hirsch, J. S., Narasimhan, M., Crawford, J. M., McGinn, T., Davidson, K. W., Barnaby, D. P., Becker, L. B., Chelico, J. D., Cohen, S. L., Cookingham, J., Coppa, K., Diefenbach, M. A., Dominello, A. J., Duer-Hefele, J., Falzon, L., Gitlin, J., Hajizadeh, N., & Harvin, T. G. (2020). Presenting characteristics, comorbidities, and outcomes among 5700 patients hospitalized with COVID-19 in the New York City area. *JAMA*. 323(20): 2052.

[35] Petrilli, C. M., Jones, S. A., Yang, J., Rajagopalan, H., O'Donnell, L., Chernyak, Y., Tobin, K. A., Cerfolio, R. J., Francois, F., & Horwitz, L. I. (2020). Factors associated with hospital admission and critical illness among 5279 people with coronavirus disease 2019 in New York City: Prospective cohort study. *BMJ*. 369:m1966.

[36] Yang, W., Cao, Q., Qin, L., Wang, X., Cheng, Z., Pan, A., Dai, J., Sun, Q., Zhao, F., Qu, J., & Yan, F. (2020). Clinical characteristics and imaging manifestations of

the 2019 novel coronavirus disease (COVID-19):a multi-center study in Wenzhou city, Zhejiang, China. *Journal of Infection*. 80(4):388-393.

[37] Argenziano, M. G., Bruce, S. L., Slater, C. L., Tiao, J. R., Baldwin, M. R., Barr, R. G., Chang, B. P., Chau, K. H., Choi, J. J., Gavin, N., Goyal, P., Mills, A. M., Patel, A. A., Romney, M. S., Safford, M. M., Schluger, N. W., Sengupta, S., Sobieszczyk, M. E., Zucker, J. E., Asodourian, PA., Bell, FM., Boyd, R., Cohen, MF., Colquohun, MI., Colville, LA., Jonge, JH., Dershowitz, LB., Dey, SA., Eiseman, KA., Girvin, ZP., Goni, DT., Harb, AA., Herzik, N., Householder, S., Karaaslan, LE., Lee, H., Lieberman, E., Ling, A., Lu, R., Shou, AY., Sisti, AC., Snow, ZE., Sperring, CP., Xiong, Y., Zhou, HW., Natarajan, K., Hripcsak, G., Chen, R. (2020). Characterization and clinical course of 1000 patients with coronavirus disease 2019 in New York: Retrospective case series. *BMJ*. 369: m1996.

[38] Docherty, A. B., Harrison, E. M., Green, C. A., Hardwick, H. E., Pius, R., Norman, L., Holden, K. A., Read, J. M., Dondelinger, F., Carson, G., Merson, L., Lee, J., Plotkin, D., Sigfrid, L., Halpin, S., Jackson, C., Gamble, C., Horby, P. W., Nguyen-Van-Tam, J. S., Dunning, J., Openshaw, PJM., Baillie, JK., Semple, M. G. (2020). Features of 20 133 UK patients in hospital with COVID-19 using the ISARIC WHO clinical characterisation protocol: Prospective observational cohort study. *BMJ*. 369:m1985.

[39] Bolay, H., Gül, A., Baykan, B. (2020). COVID-19 is a real headache! *Headache: The Journal of Head and Face Pain*. 60 (7):1415-1421.

[40] Goyal, P., Choi, J. J., Pinheiro, L. C., Schenck, E. J., Chen, R., Jabri, A., Satlin, M. J., Campion, T. R., Nahid, M., Ringel, J. B., Hoffman, K. L., Alshak, M. N., Li, H. A., Wehmeyer, G. T., Rajan, M., Reshetnyak, E., Hupert, N., Horn, E. M., Martinez, F. J., Gulick, RM., Safford, M. M. (2020). Clinical characteristics of COVID-19 in New York City. *New England Journal of Medicine*. 382 (24):2372-2374.

[41] Yang, X., Yu, Y., Xu, J., Shu, H., Xia, J., Liu, H., Wu, Y., Zhang, L., Yu, Z., Fang, M., Yu, T., Wang, Y., Pan, S., Zou, X., Yuan, S., & Shang, Y. (2020). Clinical course and outcomes of critically ill patients with SARS-Cov-2 pneumonia in Wuhan, China: A single-centered, retrospective, observational study. *The Lancet Respiratory Medicine*. 8(5):475-481.

[42] Giacomelli, A., Pezzati, L., Conti, F., Bernacchia, D., Siano, M., Oreni, L., Rusconi, S., Gervasoni, C., Ridolfo, A. L., Rizzardini, G., Antinori, S., & Galli, M. (2020). Self-reported olfactory and taste disorders in patients with severe acute respiratory coronavirus 2 infection: A cross-sectional study. *Clinical Infectious Diseases*. 71(15): 889-890.

[43] Lechien, J. R., Chiesa-Estomba, C. M., Hans, S., Barillari, M. R., Jouffe, L., & Saussez, S. (2020). Loss of smell and taste in 2013 European patients with mild to moderate COVID-19. *Annals of Internal Medicine*. 173(8): 672-675.

[44] Liu, K., Fang, Y., Deng, Y., Liu, W., Wang, M., Ma, J., Xiao, W., Wang, Y., Zhong, M., Li, C., Li, G., & Liu, H. (2020). Clinical characteristics of novel coronavirus cases in tertiary hospitals in Hubei province. *Chinese Medical Journal*. 133(9):1025-1031.

[45] Wang, Y., Lu, X., Li, Y., Chen, H., Chen, T., Su, N., Huang, F., Zhou, J., Zhang, B., Yan, F., & Wang, J. (2020). Clinical course and outcomes of 344 intensive care patients with COVID-19. *American Journal of Respiratory and Critical Care Medicine*. 201(11):1430-1434.

[46] Wu, Z., & McGoogan, J. M. (2020). Characteristics of and important lessons from the coronavirus disease 2019 (COVID-19) outbreak in China. *JAMA*. 323(13): 1239.

[47] Zhu, J., Ji, P., Pang, J., Zhong, Z., Li, H., He, C., Zhang, J., & Zhao, C. (2020). Clinical characteristics of 3062 COVID-19 patients: A meta-analysis. *Journal of Medical Virology*. 92(10):1902-1914.

[48] Myers, L. C., Parodi, S. M., Escobar, G. J., & Liu, V. X. (2020). Characteristics of hospitalized adults with COVID-19 in an integrated health care system in California. *JAMA*. 323(21):2195.

[49] Cummings, M. J., Baldwin, M. R., Abrams, D., Jacobson, S. D., Meyer, B. J., Balough, E. M., Aaron, J. G., Claassen, J., Rabbani, L. E., Hastie, J., Hochman, B. R., Salazar-Schicchi, J., Yip, N. H., Brodie, D., & O'Donnell, M. R. (2020). Epidemiology, clinical course, and outcomes of critically ill adults with COVID-19 in New York City: A prospective cohort study. *The Lancet*. 395(10239): 1763-1770.

[50] Grasselli, G., Pesenti, A., & Cecconi, M. (2020). Critical care utilization for the COVID-19 outbreak in Lombardy, Italy. *JAMA*. 323(16):1545.

[51] Onder, G., Rezza, G., & Brusaferro, S. (2020). Case-fatality rate and characteristics of patients dying in relation to COVID-19 in Italy. *JAMA*. 323:1775-1776.

[52] KCDC. *Updates on COVID-19 in Korea*. March 14, 2020. https:// www.cdc.go.kr/board/board.es?mid=a30402000000&bid=0030 (Accessed on March 14, 2020).

[53] Li, R., Pei, S., Chen, B., Song, Y., Zhang, T., Yang, W., Shaman, J. (2020). Substantial undocumented infection facilitates the rapid dissemination of novel coronavirus (SARS-Cov-2). *Science*. 368(6490):489-493.

[54] Bialek, S., Boundy, E., Bowen, V., Chow, N., Cohn, A., Dowling, N., Ellington, S., Gierke, R., Hall, A., MacNeil, J., Patel, P., Peacock, G., Pilishvili, T., Razzaghi, H., Reed, N., Ritchey, M., Sauber-Schatz, E. (2020). Severe outcomes among

patients with coronavirus disease 2019 (COVID-19) — United States, February 12–March 16, 2020. *MMWR. Morbidity and Mortality Weekly Report*. 69(12):343-346.

[55] Arentz, M., Yim, E., Klaff, L., Lokhandwala, S., Riedo, F. X., Chong, M., & Lee, M. (2020). Characteristics and outcomes of 21 critically ill patients with COVID-19 in Washington State. *JAMA*. 323(16), 1612.

[56] To, K. K., Tsang, O. T., Leung, W., Tam, A. R., Wu, T., Lung, D. C., Yip, C. C., Cai, J., Chan, J. M., Chik, T. S., Lau, D. P., Choi, C. Y., Chen, L., Chan, W., Chan, K., Ip, J. D., Ng, A. C., Poon, R. W., Luo, C., … Yuen, K. (2020). Temporal profiles of viral load in posterior oropharyngeal saliva samples and serum antibody responses during infection by SARS-Cov-2: An observational cohort study. *The Lancet Infectious Diseases*. 20(5):565-574.

[57] Livingston, E., & Bucher, K. (2020). Coronavirus disease 2019 (COVID-19) in Italy. *JAMA*. 323(14):1335.

[58] Docherty, A. B., Harrison, E. M., Green, C. A., Hardwick, H. E., Pius, R., Norman, L., Holden, K. A., Read, J. M., Dondelinger, F., Carson, G., Merson, L., Lee, J., Plotkin, D., Sigfrid, L., Halpin, S., Jackson, C., Gamble, C., Horby, P. W., Nguyen-Van-Tam, J. S., … Semple, M. G. (2020). Features of 20 133 UK patients in hospital with COVID-19 using the ISARIC WHO clinical characterisation protocol: Prospective observational cohort study. *BMJ*. 369:m1985.

[59] Grasselli, G., Zangrillo, A., Zanella, A., Antonelli, M., Cabrini, L., Castelli, A., Cereda, D., Coluccello, A., Foti, G., Fumagalli, R., Iotti, G., Latronico, N., Lorini, L., Merler, S., Natalini, G., Piatti, A., Ranieri, M. V., Scandroglio, A. M., Storti, E. (2020). Baseline characteristics and outcomes of 1591 patients infected with SARS-Cov-2 admitted to ICUs of the Lombardy region, Italy. *JAMA*. 323(16): 1574.

[60] Liang, W., Guan, W., Chen, R., Wang, W., Li, J., Xu, K., Li, C., Ai, Q., Lu, W., Liang, H., Li, S., & He, J. (2020). Cancer patients in SARS-Cov-2 infection: A nationwide analysis in China. *The Lancet Oncology*. 21(3): 335-337.

[61] Chow, N., Fleming-Dutra, K., Gierke, R., Hall, A., Hughes, M., Pilishvili, T., Ritchey, M., Roguski, K., Skoff, T., & Ussery, E. (2020). Preliminary estimates of the prevalence of selected underlying health conditions among patients with coronavirus disease 2019 — United States, February 12–March 28, 2020. *MMWR. Morbidity and Mortality Weekly Report*. 69(13): 382-386.

[62] Lighter, J., Phillips, M., Hochman, S., Sterling, S., Johnson, D., Francois, F., & Stachel, A. (2020). Obesity in patients younger than 60 years is a risk factor for COVID-19 hospital admission. *Clinical Infectious Diseases*. 71(15):896-897.

[63] Williamson, E. J., Walker, A. J., Bhaskaran, K., Bacon, S., Bates, C., Morton, C. E., Curtis, H. J., Mehrkar, A., Evans, D., Inglesby, P., Cockburn, J., McDonald, H. I., MacKenna, B., Tomlinson, L., Douglas, I. J., Rentsch, C. T., Mathur, R., Wong,

A. Y., Grieve, R., … Goldacre, B. (2020). Factors associated with COVID-19-related death using OpenSAFELY. *Nature*. 584(7821): 430-436.

[64] Yang, J., Zheng, Y., Gou, X., Pu, K., Chen, Z., Guo, Q., Ji, R., Wang, H., Wang, Y., & Zhou, Y. (2020). Prevalence of comorbidities and its effects in patients infected with SARS-Cov-2: A systematic review and meta-analysis. *International Journal of Infectious Diseases*. 94: 91-95.

[65] Stokes, E. K., Zambrano, L. D., Anderson, K. N., Marder, E. P., Raz, K. M., El Burai Felix, S., Tie, Y., & Fullerton, K. E. (2020). Coronavirus disease 2019 case surveillance — United States, January 22–May 30, 2020. *MMWR. Morbidity and Mortality Weekly Report*. 69(24):759-765.

[66] Cohen, P. A., Hall, L. E., John, J. N., & Rapoport, A. B. (2020). The early natural history of SARS-Cov-2 infection. *Mayo Clinic Proceedings*. 95(6): 1124-1126.

[67] Tian, S., Hu, N., Lou, J., Chen, K., Kang, X., Xiang, Z., Chen, H., Wang, D., Liu, N., Liu, D., Chen, G., Zhang, Y., Li, D., Li, J., Lian, H., Niu, S., Zhang, L., & Zhang, J. (2020). Characteristics of COVID-19 infection in Beijing. *Journal of Infection*. 80(4): 401-406.

[68] Liu, Y., Yan, L., Wan, L., Xiang, T., Le, A., Liu, J., Peiris, M., Poon, L. L., & Zhang, W. (2020). Viral dynamics in mild and severe cases of COVID-19. *The Lancet Infectious Diseases*. 20(6): 656-657.

[69] Chen, T., Wu, D., Chen, H., Yan, W., Yang, D., Chen, G., Ma, K., Xu, D., Yu, H., Wang, H., Wang, T., Guo, W., Chen, J., Ding, C., Zhang, X., Huang, J., Han, M., Li, S., Luo, X., … Ning, Q. (2020). Clinical characteristics of 113 deceased patients with coronavirus disease 2019: Retrospective study. *BMJ*, m1091.

[70] Tang, N., Li, D., Wang, X., & Sun, Z. (2020). undefined. *Journal of Thrombosis and Haemostasis*. 18(4): 844-847.

[71] American Venous Forum. *Considerations in prophylaxis and treatment of VTE in COVID-19 Patients*. (202). Accessed April 2020 at https://www.veinforum.org/covid-19/external icon.

[72] Teuwen, L., Geldhof, V., Pasut, A., & Carmeliet, P. (2020). COVID-19: The vasculature unleashed. *Nature Reviews Immunology*. 20(7): 389-391.

[73] Lowenstein, C. J., & Solomon, S. D. (2020). Severe COVID-19 is a Microvascular disease. *Circulation*. 142(17): 1609-1611.

[74] Klok, F., Kruip, M., Van der Meer, N., Arbous, M., Gommers, D., Kant, K., Kaptein, F., Van Paassen, J., Stals, M., Huisman, M., & Endeman, H. (2020). Incidence of thrombotic complications in critically ill ICU patients with COVID-19. *Thrombosis Research*. 191:145-147.

[75] Helms, J., Tacquard, C., Severac, F., Leonard-Lorant, I., Ohana, M., Delabranche, X., Merdji, H., Clere-Jehl, R., Schenck, M., Fagot Gandet, F., Fafi-Kremer, S., Castelain, V., Schneider, F., Grunebaum, L., Anglés-Cano, E., Sattler, L., Mertes, P., & Meziani, F. (2020). High risk of thrombosis in patients with severe SARS-

Cov-2 infection: A multicenter prospective cohort study. *Intensive Care Medicine*. 46(6): 1089-1098.

[76] Grillet, F., Behr, J., Calame, P., Aubry, S., & Delabrousse, E. (2020). Acute pulmonary embolism associated with COVID-19 pneumonia detected with pulmonary CT angiography. *Radiology*. 296(3): E186-E188.

[77] Wong, C. K., Lam, C. W., Wu, A. K., Ip, W. K., Lee, N. L., Chan, I. H., Lit, L. C., Hui, D. S., Chan, M. H., Chung, S. S., & Sung, J. J. (2004). Plasma inflammatory cytokines and chemokines in severe acute respiratory syndrome. *Clinical & Experimental Immunology*. 136(1), 95-103.

[78] Conti, P., Ronconi, G., Caraffa, A., Gallenga, C., Ross, R., Frydas, A., Kritas S. (2020). Induction of proinflammatory cytokines (IL-1 and IL-6) and lung inflammation by Coronavirus-19 (COVI-19 or SARS-CoV-2): anti-inflammatory strategies. *J of Bio Reg and Homeo Agents*. 34(2):327-331.

[79] Mehta, P., McAuley, D. F., Brown, M., Sanchez, E., Tattersall, R. S., & Manson, J. J. (2020). COVID-19: Consider cytokine storm syndromes and immunosuppression. *The Lancet*. 395(10229): 1033-1034.

[80] Wang, C., Kang, K., Gao, Y., Ye, M., Lan, X., Li, X., Zhao, M., & Yu, K. (2020). Cytokine levels in the body fluids of a patient with COVID-19 and acute respiratory distress syndrome: A case report. *Annals of Internal Medicine*. 173(6): 499-501.

[81] Liu, T., Zhang, J., Yang, Y., Ma, H., Li, Z., Zhang, J., Cheng, J., Zhang, X., Zhao, Y., Xia, Z., Zhang, L., Wu, G., & Yi, J. (2020). *The potential role of IL-6 in monitoring severe case of coronavirus disease* 2019. https://doi.org/10.1101/2020.03.01.20029769.

[82] Restivo, D. A., Centonze, D., Alesina, A., & Marchese-Ragona, R. (2020). Myasthenia gravis associated with SARS-Cov-2 infection. *Annals of Internal Medicine*. https://doi.org/10.7326/l20-0845.

[83] Berzuini, A., Bianco, C., Paccapelo, C., Bertolini, F., Gregato, G., Cattaneo, A., Erba, E., Bandera, A., Gori, A., Lamorte, G., Manunta, M., Porretti, L., Revelli, N., Truglio, F., Grasselli, G., Zanella, A., Villa, S., Valenti, L., & Prati, D. (2020). Red cell–bound antibodies and transfusion requirements in hospitalized patients with COVID-19. *Blood*. 136(6): 766-768.

[84] Toscano, G., Palmerini, F., Ravaglia, S., Ruiz, L., Invernizzi, P., Cuzzoni, M. G., Franciotta, D., Baldanti, F., Daturi, R., Postorino, P., Cavallini, A., & Micieli, G. (2020). Guillain–Barre syndrome associated with SARS-Cov-2. *New England Journal of Medicine*. 382(26): 2574-2576.

[85] Morris, S. B., Schwartz, N. G., Patel, P., Abbo, L., Beauchamps, L., Balan, S., Lee, E. H., Paneth-Pollak, R., Geevarughese, A., Lash, M. K., Dorsinville, M. S., Ballen, V., Eiras, D. P., Newton-Cheh, C., Smith, E., Robinson, S., Stogsdill, P., Lim, S., Fox, S. E., … Godfred-Cato, S. (2020). Case series of Multisystem

inflammatory syndrome in adults associated with SARS-Cov-2 infection — United Kingdom and United States, March–August 2020. *MMWR. Morbidity and Mortality Weekly Report*. 69(40): 1450-1456.

[86] Rawson, T. M., Moore, L. S., Zhu, N., Ranganathan, N., Skolimowska, K., Gilchrist, M., Satta, G., Cooke G., Holmes, A. (2020). Bacterial and fungal coinfection in individuals with coronavirus: A rapid review to support COVID-19 antimicrobial prescribing. *Clinical Infectious Diseases*. https://doi.org/10.1093/cid/ciaa530.

[87] Sepulveda, J., Westblade, L. F., Whittier, S., Satlin, M. J., Greendyke, W. G., Aaron, J. G., Zucker, J., Dietz, D., Sobieszczyk, M., Choi, J. J., Liu, D., Russell, S., Connelly, C., & Green, D. A. (2020). Bacteremia and blood culture utilization during COVID-19 surge in New York City. *Journal of Clinical Microbiology*. 58(8).

[88] Koehler, P., Cornely, O. A., Böttiger, B. W., Dusse, F., Eichenauer, D. A., Fuchs, F., Hallek, M., Jung, N., Klein, F., Persigehl, T., Rybniker, J., Kochanek, M., Böll, B., & Shimabukuro-Vornhagen, A. (2020). COVID-19 associated pulmonary aspergillosis. *Mycoses*. 63(6): 528-534.

[89] Blaize, M., Mayaux, J., Nabet, C., Lampros, A., Marcelin, A., Thellier, M., Piarroux, R., Demoule, A., & Fekkar, A. (2020). Fatal invasive aspergillosis and coronavirus disease in an immunocompetent patient. *Emerging Infectious Diseases*. 26(7), 1636-1637.

[90] Van Arkel, A. L., Rijpstra, T. A., Belderbos, H. N., Van Wijngaarden, P., Verweij, P. E., & Bentvelsen, R. G. (2020). COVID-19–associated pulmonary aspergillosis. *American Journal of Respiratory and Critical Care Medicine*. 202(1): 132-135.

[91] Bartoletti, M., Pascale, R., Cricca, M., Rinaldi, M., Maccaro, A., Bussini, L., Fornaro, G., Tonetti, T., Pizzilli, G., Francalanci, E., Gıntoli, L., Rubin, A., Moroni, A., Ambretti, S., Trapani, F., Vatamonu, O., Ranieri, VM., Castelli, A., Baiocchi, M., Lewis, R., Gianella, M., Viale, P., and PREDICO study group. (2020). Epidemiology of invasive pulmonary aspergillosis among COVID-19 intubated patients: a prospective study. *Clin Infect Dis*. doi: 10.1093/cid/ciaa1065.

[92] World Health Organization Director-General's opening remarks at *the media briefing on COVID-19* - 24 February 2020. Available at: https://www.who.int/dg/speeches/detail/who-director-general-s-opening-remarks-at-the-media-briefing-on-covid-19---24-february-2020 (Accessed on February 26, 2020).

[93] Tenforde, M. W., Billig Rose, E., Lindsell, C. J., Shapiro, N. I., Files, D. C., Gibbs, K. W., Prekker, M. E., Steingrub, J. S., Smithline, H. A., Gong, M. N., Aboodi, M. S., Exline, M. C., Henning, D. J., Wilson, J. G., Khan, A., Qadir, N., Stubblefield, W. B., Patel, M. M., & Self, W. H. (2020). Characteristics of adult outpatients and inpatients with COVID-19 — 11 academic medical centers, United States, march–May 2020. *MMWR. Morbidity and Mortality Weekly Report*. 69(26): 841-846.

[94] Carfì, A., Bernabei, R., & Landi, F. (2020). Persistent symptoms in patients after acute COVID-19. *JAMA*. 324(6): 603.

[95] Helleberg, M., Niemann, C. U., Moestrup, K. S., Kirk, O., Lebech, A., Lane, C., & Lundgren, J. (2020). Persistent COVID-19 in an Immunocompromised patient temporarily responsive to two courses of Remdesivir therapy. *The Journal of Infectious Diseases*. 222(7): 1103-1107.

[96] Tenforde, M. W., Kim, S. S., Lindsell, C. J., Billig Rose, E., Shapiro, N. I., Files, D. C., Gibbs, K. W., Erickson, H. L., Steingrub, J. S., Smithline, H. A., Gong, M. N., Aboodi, M. S., Exline, M. C., Henning, D. J., Wilson, J. G., Khan, A., Qadir, N., Brown, S. M., & Peltan, I. D. (2020). Symptom duration and risk factors for delayed return to usual health among outpatients with COVID-19 in a Multistate health care systems network — United States, March–June 2020. *MMWR. Morbidity and Mortality Weekly Report*. 69(30): 993-998.

[97] Huang, Y., Tan, C., Wu, J., Chen, M., Wang, Z., Luo, L., Zhou, X., Liu, X., Huang, X., Yuan, S., Chen, C., Gao, F., Huang, J., Shan, H., & Liu, J. (2020). Impact of coronavirus disease 2019 on pulmonary function in early convalescence phase. *Respiratory Research*. 21:1-9.

[98] You, J., Zhang, L., Ni-Jia-Ti, MY., Zhang, J., Hu, F., Chen, L., Dong, Y., Yang, K., Zhang, B., Zhang, S. (2020). Anormal pulmonary function and residual CT abnormalities in rehabilitating COVID-19 patients after discharge. *J Infect*. 81:E150.

[99] Mo, X., Jian, W., Su, Z., Chen, M., Peng, H., Peng, P., Lei, C., Chen, R., Zhong, N., & Li, S. (2020). Abnormal pulmonary function in COVID-19 patients at time of hospital discharge. *European Respiratory Journal*. 55(6): 2001217.

[100] Hui, D. S., Wong, K. T., Ko, F. W., Tam, L. S., Chan, D. P., Woo, J., & Sung, J. J. (2005). The 1-Year impact of severe acute respiratory syndrome on pulmonary function, exercise capacity, and quality of life in a cohort of survivors. *Chest*. 128(4): 2247-2261.

[101] Puntmann, V. O., Carerj, M. L., Wieters, I., Fahim, M., Arendt, C., Hoffmann, J., Shchendrygina, A., Escher, F., Vasa-Nicotera, M., Zeiher, A. M., Vehreschild, M., & Nagel, E. (2020). Outcomes of cardiovascular magnetic resonance imaging in patients recently recovered from coronavirus disease 2019 (COVID-19). *JAMA Cardiology*. doi: 10.1001/jamacardio.2020.3557.

[102] Rajpal, S., Tong, M. S., Borchers, J., Zareba, K. M., Obarski, T. P., Simonetti, O. P., & Daniels, C. J. (2020). Cardiovascular magnetic resonance findings in competitive athletes recovering from COVID-19 infection. *JAMA Cardiology*. doi: 10.1001/jamacardio.2020.4916.

[103] Lippi, G., Lavie, C. J., & Sanchis-Gomar, F. (2020). Cardiac troponin I in patients with coronavirus disease 2019 (COVID-19): Evidence from a meta-analysis. *Progress in Cardiovascular Diseases*. 63(3): 390-391.

In: Coronavirus Disease
Editor: Yildiz Dincer

ISBN: 978-1-53619-296-4

Chapter 4

DIAGNOSIS OF COVID-19

Mert A. Kuskucu[1], PhD and Fehmi Tabak[2,*], MD
[1]Department of Clinical Microbiology, Cerrahpasa School of Medicine, Istanbul University-Cerrahpasa, Istanbul, Turkey
[2]Department of Infectious Diseases and Clinical Microbiology, Cerrahpasa School of Medicine, Istanbul University-Cerrahpasa, Istanbul, Turkey

ABSTRACT

The pandemic that emerged at the beginning of this year spread rapidly all over the world. The most effective way to combat such a large-scale epidemic is to quickly diagnose infected individuals and take necessary isolation measures. Although rapid antigen tests used in the first stage in the diagnosis of COVID-19, they have quickly left their places to molecular-based real-time PCR tests due to sensitivity problems. Antibody response based diagnosis can be problematic because those found can become detectable as early as 2 weeks after the onset of infection, which is not a suitable acquisition for the diagnosis of acute infection. In this article, applications and methods used for the diagnosis of COVID-19, will be discussed.

Keywords: SARS-CoV-2, COVID-19, real-time PCR, diagnosis

INTRODUCTION

At the end of 2019, a new type of pneumonia caused by a novel coronavirus emerged in the city of Wuhan, China. Then this virus has spread rapidly worldwide. The World

* Corresponding Author's Email: femitabak@yahoo.com.

Health Organization (WHO) named the disease Coronavirus Disease 2019 (COVID-19) and the virus called severe acute respiratory syndrome coronavirus 2 (SARS-CoV-2). SARS-CoV-2 infections can cause common symptoms of viral pneumonia, like cough, fever, dyspnea, and myalgia. These symptoms are not specific for COVID-19. Therefore, patient history (contact with a suspicious or confirmed case, travel, etc.) constitutes the starting point for the diagnosis of COVID-19. The diagnostic algorithm of COVID-19 initially includes epidemiological history, clinical signs, CT scan, blood count, and biochemistry test results. Following these routine tests, showing the viral genome by nucleic acid amplification techniques (NAT) (like real-time PCR) may prove the diagnosis. Besides NAT, detection of IgM/IgG responses by serological tests and viral antigens by point-of-care tests (POCT) may be helpful.

Computed Tomography and Other Biochemical Properties

Computed tomography (CT) results may give information about the severity of SARS-CoV-2 infection and be used for rapid pre-diagnosis and prognosis prediction. Abnormal CT scans with bilateral patchy shadows or ground-glass opacity, bilateral pulmonary parenchymal involvement, and consolidative pulmonary opacities in the lungs found around 86% of the patients at the time of their hospital admission. Besides these findings no radiographic or CT abnormality was found in 3% of patients with severe disease and 18% of patients with mild disease also had no radiological sign. Nevertheless, there is a limitation in these early reports in regards to severity classification because the criteria were not well defined. However, these findings cannot be differentiated from other viral pneumonia, and in some different clinical situations, they have similar images. It should not be forgotten that it can be obtained [1-4].

The most common finding in hemogram is lymphopenia. It may occur in 70-83% of patients. Detoloration and persistence of lymphopenia combination with high levels of inflammatory cytokines, correlated with disease severity and mortality. Coagulopathy and disseminated intravascular coagulation related to other biomarkers like D-dimer and fibrinogen, procalcitonin, and troponin, also strongly correlated with clinical severity and mortality [4-6].

Sample Collection

The virus begins to spread in the upper respiratory tract 1-3 days before onset of the symptoms. Virus especially has high titers in the first week of the disease. The virus load in the upper respiratory tract decreases in the second week and it is found in greater amounts in the lower respiratory tract samples. For the diagnosis of COVID-19, upper respiratory samples are the most common samples, but sputum (who can produce sputum) or lower respiratory tract samples such as bronco alveolar lavage fluid (BAL), endotracheal aspirate can also be taken in patients. In the second week of the disease, lower respiratory tract samples can be preferred. Nasopharyngeal and oropharyngeal swab samples (alone or, preferably, in a combination of them) nasopharyngeal irrigation and nasal aspiration fluids are samples of upper airways. A healthcare professional can take these samples or the patient can give these samples to himself. Similar results reported both nasopharyngeal swabs and nasal swabs that the person obtains himself. Apart from this, more reproducible results can be obtained, especially with saliva samples originating from the pharynx posterior wall. Because of a high risk of aerosol generation, infection control measures should be taken when collecting lower respiratory tract samples such as induced sputum, BAL, or endotracheal aspirates. In the first 14 days after the onset of the disease, the most reliable example to detect SARS-CoV-2 is nasopharyngeal swab after sputum and then throat swab. In addition, the virus begins to be excreted with feces, especially from the second week and continues to be excreted with feces for a long time. Since viral excretion in upper respiratory tract samples may be low or irregular, especially in advanced stages of the disease, stool samples samples can be useful for diagnosis. However, since the viral load varies according to the samples and the severity/period of the disease, the negative test result obtained with samples taken from the upper respiratory tract does not exclude the disease, and in case of clinical suspicion, the test should be repeated a second time or by taking a different sample that may have higher sensitivity [6-8]. Single nasopharyngeal swab samples are becoming more preferred because they have better tolerated by the patient and safer for the sampler.

Timing and technique of sample collection have grand effect on the sensitivity of molecular tests. Yang et al. found the highest positivity rates in the first 7 days and samples taken from seriously ill patients. They obtained the highest positivity rates in BAL samples (78.6-100%) in severe patients [9]. In another study conducted in China, the positivity rates were 93% for BAL, 72% for sputum, 63% for nasal swabs, 32% for pharynx swabs, and around 29% for feces [10]. In contrast, besides more frequent usage of oropharyngeal swabs, compared to nasopharyngeal swab samples, SARS-CoV2 RNA was detected in only 32% of oropharyngeal swabs, which is significantly lower than the detection rate (63%) of nasopharyngeal swab samples [6, 9, 10]. Sampling technique (depend on the experience of health care worker), timing, quantity, so many other factors such as where the sample is taken, the transport and storage of the sample, the performance of the molecular test used, and the severity of the disease can seriously affect the test results.

Molecular and Serological Methods

The widely used technology for SARS-CoV-2 is reverse transcription followed by real-time polymerase chain reaction (RT-PCR) technology. RT-PCR is currently used in many microbiology laboratories in a very wide range from detection and quantification of the single pathogen to syndromic approaches and panels for the diagnosis of different infectious agents [1, 7]. Following the emergence and rapid spread of SARS-CoV-2 in China, many organizations have published their diagnostic protocols and then different commercial companies have released RT-PCR test kits for diagnosis, and some of these have been pre-approved or approved by different organizations such as the FDA and WHO.

The first step in RT-PCR is the synthesis of complementary DNA (cDNA) from the RNA genome. Then, the cDNA is amplified and detected using unique primer and probe systems. The development process of these tests generally involves two main steps, i. selection of suitable gene regions means the selection of conserved regions in known sequences and performing primer/probe design ii. Optimization and validation of the developed test. In a study by Corman et al., viral genomes associated with SARS include the RdRP gene (RNA-linked RNA polymerase gene), open reading frame ORF1ab region, E gene (envelope protein gene), and N gene (nucleocapsid protein gene) are reported as conserved regions, and these regions are still frequently used target regions for RT-PCR [5, 6, 8, 11]. Studies on these gene regions have also reported that both RdRP and E genes have high analytical sensitivity (3.6 and 3.9 copies per reaction) and the N gene has weaker analytical sensitivity (8.3 copies per reaction). At the same time, the reaction buffers used in the tests, sample collection, and nucleic acid extraction methods, the devices used for performing RT-PCR and detection can affect the test's performance [7, 8, 12]. In the United States, CDC recommends two nucleocapsid protein targets [N1 and N2], while WHO recommends an initial screening with the E gene followed by a confirmatory test using the RdRp gene for more sensitive and specific results. Since the viral genes have equal copy numbers, the test should be well optimized as the test performance is usually determined not by the target itself but by the reagent design. At least two molecular targets should be included in the analysis to prevent false positive or negative results from potential genetic alterations of SARS-CoV-2, as well as potential cross-reactions with other endemic coronaviruses [6]. However, the WHO should include single target test formats with high specificity, especially during the epidemic period.

It is developed and evaluated in molecular methods worldwide other than RT-PCR. These include loop-mediated isothermal amplification, multiplex isothermal amplification methods, followed by microarray detection and CRISPR/Cas systems [30]. Cas13-based SHERLOCK (specific high-sensitivity enzymatic reporter unlocking) platform, that tested for detection of ZIKA and Deng viruses in patient samples. This method could detect at concentrations as low as 1 copy per microliter. Currently, Zhang et al. have adopted this technology to detect SARS-CoV-2, and the test has received FDA pre-approval [13].

According to WHO, the urgent priority for COVID-19 diagnostic research is the development of nucleic acid and protein tests and providing the opportunity to test at the bedside of patients (point of care tests, POC). The longer-term priority is to integrate these tests into multiple panels, as the leading multi-parametric respiratory pathogens panel manufacturers are adding SARS-CoV-2 to their panels. To improve surveillance efforts, serological tests using proteins are needed in addition to nucleic acid tests. These tests, unlike nucleic acid tests, have post-recovery detection advantages. This allows clinicians to monitor both sick and recovered patients, providing a better estimate of total SARSCoV-2 infections. POC tests are cost-effective devices used to diagnose patients outside of central facilities. These can be employed in areas such as community centers to reduce the burden on clinical laboratories [8].

Although RT-qPCR is specific for the diagnosis of COVID-19, false negativities cannot be ignored. The sensitivity of RT-PCR was found around 89% in a meta-analysis [14]. Since the sensitivity changes depending on the samples, their sensitivity in practice is even lower. Because of mild or asymptomatic cases with infection, the number of COVID-19 infections reported around the world so far does not reflect the actual infected people. For example, asymptomatic cases were reported to be 17.9% in the Diamond Princess ship study. All of these findins point to be considered in preventing the spread of the disease, as asymptomatic individuals constitute a serious source of transmission [8]. In this regard, the deficiencies of nucleic acid detection and CT scans for the diagnosis of COVID-19 and the fact that they are more applicable in central institutions. Considering that, there is a need for test formats that can work with samples that can be taken quickly and easily in the field. Immunologically based tests that can detect antigens or antibodies in cases where no results obtained with PCR tests may work in practice.

For the rapid detection of SARS-CoV-2 antigens or antibodies, some serological tests have been developed, and some of them have been approved by many institutions. Many different commercial companies develop serological tests for detection of SARS-CoV-2 infection in lateral flow tests, automated chemiluminescence immunoassay systems (CLIA), ELISA, and other formats. Although antibodies reach the detectable level from the seventh day of the disease during COVID-19, generally IgM responses can be detectable in the second week and IgG responses start from the 3rd week safely. Antibody responses can also be affected by several factors such as disease severity and host immune status. Although IgM responses remain positive for a shorter time, IgG positivity may persist for a long time. The level and duration of protection of antibody responses that develop after SARS-2 virus infections are not yet known. Its protection is estimated not to be very long (longer than 6 months). It is attractive that rapid antigen tests will theoretically allow low-cost and rapid detection of SARS-CoV2, but as with influenza (Flu) viruses, their sensitivity will be lower than molecular tests. The sensitivity of an antigen test approved by the FDA is 80%. Especially with the development of monoclonal antibodies, more and more sensitive antigen tests are being developed [6, 15]. Considering the variability of viral loads and sample diversity in COVID-19 patients, the problem of sensitivity of antigen tests will be better understood. Antibody tests that examine the host's response to the agent, on the other hand, maybe more useful in showing the previous infection. They can also be used as additional tests in confirming COVID-19 infection; However, in a situation where the prevalence is low, the false positivity rates of these tests will be very high despite their high specificity (for example, if the seroprevalence in the population is 1%, the probability of antibody positivity obtained with a specificity of 99% will remain around 50%. Therefore, it is recommended that they be used carefully, considering the limitations mentioned in auxiliary tests and seroepidemiological studies. The use of antibody tests for purposes such as investigating the presence of protective antibodies in individuals should be avoided. Previously, this type of serological testing has played an important role in the epidemiology of SARS and other coronavirus outbreaks. Rapid lateral flow tests that can detect both IgM and IgG antibodies will undoubtedly play an important role in COVID-19. However, there are specificity problems in IgM responses and the development of specific IgG response takes time. In this regard, serology tests do not seem likely to play a role in active case management, apart from tasks such as diagnosing/confirming late COVID-19 cases or determining individual immunity [1, 6, 8]. Serological tests can be used as an IVD test to complement existing RT-PCR tests, this can also lead to a much better diagnosis of COVID-19 and provide additional information about the immune status of suspected cases. However, the clinical accuracy of rapid tests must be rigorously evaluated before they can be authorized for mass screening of COVID19. Recent reports from many European countries suggest that most rapid tests for COVID-19 sourced from China did not show good analytical performance and did not work in more than 70% of COVID-19 cases. Besides, due to the late development of IgM and IgG responses, there is a need to include other biomarkers of the early stage of SARS-CoV-2 infection to develop practical COVID-19 rapid tests [5].

Although its use in the diagnosis of SARS-CoV-2 is limited due to its high cost, next-generation DNA sequence analysis is used especially for understanding and monitoring viral evolution and for genoepidemiological studies. At the same time, the US Food and Drug Administration granted Emergency Use Authorization (EUA) for Illumina's next-generation sequencing (NGS) test for COVID-19, in June. This is the first such authorization for an NGS diagnostic. The testing yield was reported as 3,000 tests of nasopharyngeal or oropharyngeal samples with a 24-hour turnaround. The detection performance was reported at least 1,000 copies of the viral genome per milliliter and displays 98% sensitivity and 97% specificity by the company literature [5, 6, 8, 16, 17].

REFERENCES

[1] Li X., Geng M, Peng Y, Meng L, and Lu, S. "Molecular immune pathogenesis and diagnosis of COVID-19," *Journal of Pharmaceutical Analysis*, vol. 10, no. 2. Xi'an Jiaotong University, pp. 102-108, Apr. 01, 2020, doi: 10.1016/j.jpha.2020.03.001.

[2] Niemeyer D, et al. "Middle East Respiratory Syndrome Coronavirus Accessory Protein 4a Is a Type I Interferon Antagonist," *J. Virol.*, vol. 87, no. 22, pp. 12489-12495, Nov. 2013, doi: 10.1128/jvi.01845-13.

[3] Pan Y, et al. "Initial CT findings and temporal changes in patients with the novel coronavirus pneumonia (2019-nCoV): a study of 63 patients in Wuhan, China," *Eur. Radiol.*, vol. 30, no. 6, 2020, doi: 10.1007/s00330-020-06731-x.

[4] Fang B and Meng QH. "The laboratory's role in combating COVID-19," *Crit. Rev. Clin. Lab. Sci.*, vol. 57, no. 6, pp. 400-414, Aug. 2020, doi: 10.1080/10408363.2020.1776675.

[5] Vashist SK. "*In Vitro* Diagnostic Assays for COVID-19: Recent Advances and Emerging Trends," *Diagnostics*, vol. 10, no. 4, p. 202, Apr. 2020, doi: 10.3390/diagnostics10040202.

[6] Tang YW, Schmitz JE, Persing DH, and Stratton CW. "The Laboratory Diagnosis of COVID-19 Infection: Current Issues and Challenges," *J. Clin. Microbiol.*, vol. 58, no. 6, Apr. 2020, doi: 10.1128/JCM.00512-20.

[7] Corman VM, et al. "Detection of 2019 novel coronavirus (2019-nCoV) by real-time RT-PCR," *Eurosurveillance*, vol. 25, no. 3, Jan. 2020, doi: 10.2807/1560-7917.ES.2020.25.3.2000045.

[8] Udugama B, et al., "Diagnosing COVID-19: The Disease and Tools for Detection," *ACS nano*, vol. 14, no. 4. NLM (Medline), pp. 3822–3835, Apr. 28, 2020, doi: 10.1021/acsnano.0c02624.

[9] Yang Y, et al. "Evaluating the accuracy of different respiratory specimens in the laboratory diagnosis and monitoring the viral shedding of 2019-nCoV infections," *medRxiv*. Cold Spring Harbor Laboratory Press, p. 2020.02.11.20021493, Feb. 17, 2020, doi: 10.1101/2020.02.11.20021493.

[10] Wang W, et al. "Detection of SARS-CoV-2 in Different Types of Clinical Specimens," *JAMA - Journal of the American Medical Association*, vol. 323, no. 18. American Medical Association, pp. 1843-1844, May 12, 2020, doi: 10.1001/jama.2020.3786.

[11] Wu F, et al. "A new coronavirus associated with human respiratory disease in China," *Nature*, vol. 579, no. 7798, pp. 265-269, Mar. 2020, doi: 10.1038/s41586-020-2008-3.

[12] "*Diagnostic detection of Wuhan coronavirus 2019 by real-time RT-PCR - Charité, Berlin Germany* (pdf)." https://www.who.int/nepal/activities/supporting-

elimination-of-kala-azar-as-a-public-health-problem/docs/default-source/coronaviruse/protocol-v2-1 (accessed May 28, 2020).

[13] Jin Y, et al. "Virology, epidemiology, pathogenesis, and control of covid-19," *Viruses*, vol. 12, no. 4. MDPI AG, 2020, doi: 10.3390/ v12040372.

[14] Kim H, Hong H, and Yoon SH. "Diagnostic Performance of CT and Reverse Transcriptase-Polymerase Chain Reaction for Coronavirus Disease 2019: A Meta-Analysis," *Radiology*, p. 201343, Apr. 2020, doi: 10.1148/radiol.2020201343.

[15] Diao B, et al. "Diagnosis of Acute Respiratory Syndrome Coronavirus 2 Infection by Detection of Nucleocapsid Protein," *medRxiv*, p. 2020.03.07.20032524, Mar. 2020, doi: 10.1101/2020.03. 07.20032524.

[16] Jiang C, et al. "Comparative review of respiratory diseases caused by coronaviruses and influenza A viruses during epidemic season," *Microbes Infect.*, May 2020, doi: 10.1016/j.micinf.2020.05.005.

[17] "First NGS-based COVID-19 diagnostic," *Nature biotechnology*, vol. 38, no. 7. NLM (Medline), p. 777, Jul. 01, 2020, doi: 10.1038/ s41587-020-0608-y.

In: Coronavirus Disease
Editor: Yildiz Dincer
ISBN: 978-1-53619-296-4

Chapter 5

TREATMENT OPTIONS FOR COVID-19 PATIENTS

Hakan Yavuzer[1,*], MD and Pınar Arman[1], MD
[1]Istanbul University - Cerrahpasa, Cerrahpasa Medical Faculty,
Department of Internal Medicine, Division of Geriatrics, Istanbul, Turkey

ABSTRACT

COVID-19 disease was first defined in December 2019, and its causative agent was determined as SARS-COV-2 in January 2020.

There is no specific treatment for this infection that affects more than one organ system, especially the pulmonary system. Many medical treatments have been tried until today, and studies on their efficacy and safety have been published.

Anti-malarial drugs; anti-retrovirals, ribavirin, remdesivir, favipiravir, and other antiviral agents; corticosteroids; anti-cytokines and immunomodulatory agents; immunoglobulins are listed among the drugs evaluated. The mechanism of action, pharmacokinetic and pharmacodynamic properties, and side effects of each drug group are different. Medical treatment should be individualized considering these differences.

Keywords: Covid-19 treatment, chloroquine, ribavirin, remdesivir, favipiravir, corticosteroids

INTRODUCTION

Coronavirus-19 disease (COVID-19) was first reported in the Wuhan province of China in December 2019. Then, it was declared as a pandemic threatening the whole

* Corresponding Author's E-mail: drhakanyavuzer@gmail.com.

world by WHO on March 11, 2020. The causative agent, SARS-COV-2, belongs to the beta-coronaviridae family and has a single-stranded RNA structure. SARS-COV-2 encodes the S protein that binds human angiotensin-converting enzyme 2 (ACE2), thus membrane fusion occurs and the virus is allowed to enter the cell [1, 2]. Once inside the cell, SARS-COV-2, like other coronaviruses, controls the cell's synthesis mechanisms for the synthesis of viral proteins and viral replication [3].

Once the virus enters the human body, it usually induces a range of host responses such as autophagy, apoptosis, stress response, and innate immunity [4].

Some of these immune responses can be protective for patients, while others can be harmful. The protective immune response allows the patients to go through the disease with asymptomatic or mild symptoms. It has been found that approximately 80% of people infected with SARS-COV-2 developed a protective immune response. Providing interferon synthesis by stimulating the natural immune system including natural killer cells and T cells plays an important role in the formation of a protective immune response [5, 6].

In elderly, immunosuppressed patients or individuals with diabetes, hypertension, obesity, chronic obstructive pulmonary disease (COPD), pulmonary fibrosis, asthma and interstitial diseases, COVID-19 progresses with more severe respiratory symptoms and acute respiratory distress syndrome (ARDS), and may even result in death. SARS-CoV and MERS-CoV, which are members of the coronavirus family, have mechanisms that reduce or delay interferon production; this leads to increased inflammatory response and exacerbation of lung damage [7, 8]. Cytokine storm, known as overproduction of inflammatory cytokines, is associated with increased disease severity and poor prognosis [4, 9].

An increase in cytokine production, indicative of cytokine storm, has been detected in the bronchoalveolar lavage fluid and peripheral mononuclear blood cells of COVID-19 patients [10]. Besides the lungs, SARS-Cov-2 also affects other organs, especially the heart and brain. There is no specific drug or vaccine for SARS-Cov-2 yet. Therefore, the treatment of severe cases is challenging. Until specific drugs or vaccines are found, it is recommended to use other drug groups that have been shown to be effective in studies.

Current Drugs in the Treatment of COVID-19

Since there is no specific drug for treatment; early diagnosis, isolation of patients and rapid provision of supportive treatments are life-saving. Treatment of COVID-19 patients is based on the reassessment of existing medications and, primarily, improvement of symptoms. Since ARDS and secondary bacterial infections frequently develop in patients; antibacterial, anti-inflammatory, and immunomodulatory drugs take their place in the treatment in addition to antiviral agents.

ANTIMALARIAL AGENTS

Chloroquine and hydroxychloroquine have been developed for the treatment of malaria and have proven effective in the treatment of chronic inflammatory diseases such as rheumatoid arthritis (RA) and systemic lupus erythematosus (SLE). By inhibiting the glycosylation of host receptors, proteolysis and endosomal acidification prevent viruses from entering the cell. In addition, they decrease cytokine production and regulate immunomodulation by inhibiting autophagy and lysosomal activity. In a multi-center, randomized study, it was shown that the anti-inflammatory effect of hydroxychloroquine may be beneficial in COVID-19 patients [11].

However, hydroxychloroquine added to standard therapy does not increase the virus response; it decreases inflammation and the severity of lymphopenia and accelerates the regression of symptoms. It is thought that the patient group benefitting the most from hydroxychloroquine is the patients with high CRP and lymphopenia.

A meta-analysis of 42 studies showed that hydroxychloroquine was not associated with overall mortality [11]. In the same meta-analysis, it was shown that the fever response developed more rapidly in patients using hydroxychloroquine.

For the treatment of COVID-19, the chloroquine dose is 500mg orally, once or twice a day [12]. However, there are very few data proving the safety and efficacy of these doses. The recommended dose of hydroxychloroquine is 2 x 200mg per day after a 2 x 400mg loading dose [13].

Antimalarial drugs are generally well tolerated. QT prolongation, hypoglycemia, neuropsychiatric effects, and retinopathy are rare (10%) but serious side effects of hydroxychloroquine. QT prolongation; especially in patients with advanced age, female patients, individuals with a history of heart disease, hypokalemia or kidney and liver failure, patients using diuretics, such as furosemide and thiazide, and other drugs that prolong the QT interval is more frequently observed. ECG should be taken before treatment to evaluate and follow-up on the QT prolongation. No significant side effects of chlorokinin used at the indicated doses and duration for the treatment of COVID-19 have been reported. These drugs are safe during pregnancy.

In a review evaluating 12 studies, it was found that chloroquine and hydroxychloroquine used during pregnancy do not cause ocular toxicity in the newborn [14].

Antiviral Agents

Favipiravir

Favipiravir is used in the treatment of avian influenza or influenza that is resistant to neuraminidase inhibitors. It is a guanine analog, its antiviral activity is reduced by competition in the presence of purine nucleosides. Favipiravir is taken up into the infected cell by endocytosis and transforms into the active form by phosphoribosylation and phosphorylation. It targets the catalytic part of the RNA-dependent RNA polymerase, thus, it shows antiviral activity by disrupting the nucleotide sequence during viral RNA replication. It has been used in the treatment of RNA virus infections such as influenza, Ebola, and norovirus [15]. There are in- vitro and human studies which is used experimentally in the treatment of SARS-CoV-2. In a randomized controlled study comparing favipiravir and umifenovir, it was reported that the recovery rate was higher (71.4%) and the recovery time of fever and cough symptoms was shorter in the favipiravir group [16]. In another study, significant radiological improvement, faster reduction in viral load, and fewer side effects were observed in patients who received favipiravir compared to the control group [17].

The dose of favipiravir varies according to the viral agent detected. For example, in influenza treatment, lower doses are sufficient compared to ebola and SARS-Cov-2 treatment. The high dose range is also considered for the treatment of COVID-19 [18]. After a loading dose of 2400-3000 mg given every 12 hours on the first day, a maintenance dose of 2 x 1200-1800 mg/day is recommended. Its side effects are mild and can be treated. An increase in liver enzymes, hyperuricemia, psychiatric symptoms, and gastrointestinal side effects are seen.

Lopinavir/Ritonavir

Lopinavir is a protease inhibitor with a high affinity for HIV-1 protease. It is used in combination with ritonavir to increase the oral bioavailability and effectiveness of lopinavir. Since SARS-CoV-2 is an RNA virus like HIV, lopinavir/ritonavir has been used in the treatment of this infection. It has also been recommended in the treatment of COVID-19 due to the existence of studies that have found that it reduces the mortality in patients infected with SARS-CoV-1 [19]. Preliminary studies are showing increased viral clearance in COVID-19 patients treated with lopinavir/ritonavir [20]. However, a meta-analysis showed that this combination did not reduce the time of hospitalization and mortality compared to the control group [21]. The dose of lopinavir/ritonavir in the treatment of COVID-19 is 400mg/100mg twice a day. The duration of treatment is 14 days. Since there are prominent drug-drug reactions and side effects, the drugs used by the patients should be reviewed before the treatment and their side effects should be closely monitored. The most common side effects are nausea, vomiting, and hepatotoxicity. Approximately 50% of patients using lopinavir/ritonavir experience side effects; the rate of quitting the drug due to these side effects is 14% [22].

Ribavirin

Ribavirin is a guanine analog that inhibits RNA-dependent RNA polymerase. Although its effectiveness against other coronaviruses is known, its in-vitro activity against SARS-CoV2 is limited and requires higher doses. It is not recommended in first-line therapy. The efficacy of ribavirin has mostly been evaluated in combination therapy. In a multicentre, prospective, open-label, randomized controlled trial, it was shown that lopinavir and ribavirin combination therapy resulted in better compliance, faster viral clearance, and shorter hospital stay compared to lopinavir/ritonavir and ribavirin combination or ribavirin monotherapy [23]. In a systematic review that included 30 studies evaluating the effectiveness of ribavirin in COVID-19, inadequate results were obtained in 26 studies; severe hematological and hepatic side effects were reported in 4 studies [24]. The recommended dose of ribavirin is 1000-1500mg per day [25]. It is administered intravenously, the maximum duration of treatment is 10 days [25]. Ribavirin commonly has haematologic and hepatic side effects. Its hematological side effects are dose-dependent. It has been reported that hemolytic anemia developed in 60% of the patients and increased transaminases in 75% of the patients who received high-dose ribavirin for the treatment of SARS [24]. Also, ribavirin is teratogenic and should not be used during pregnancy [26].

Remdesivir

Remdesivir is the first antiviral drug developed for Ebola virus treatment [27]. It is an adenosine analog and a prodrug that disrupts viral RNA synthesis. In addition to the Ebola virus, it is effective against different virus families including Filoviridae, Paramyxoviridae, Pneumoviridae, and Orthocoronovirina. In animal studies evaluating its efficacy on SARS-COV-2, remdesivir has been observed to reduce viral load, rate of disease progression, and improve pulmonary function [28]. A randomized, double-blind, placebo-controlled trial demonstrated that the duration of clinical recovery was similar in the remdesivir and control groups [29]. A limitation of this study was that lopinavir/ritonavir, corticosteroid, and/or interferon could be used in both remdesivir and control groups. There are also studies proving the opposite. In another randomized controlled study comparing 538 patients treated with remdesivir and 521 patients treated with placebo, the mean recovery time in the remdesivir group was four days shorter than the control group [30]. Remdesivir is the first antiviral agent approved recently by the FDA for the treatment of COVID-19.

For the currently studied therapeutic dose of remdesivir; after a single loading dose of 200 mg on the first day, the maintenance dose is 100mg once a day. It is administered as an IV infusion. There are no clear data on the duration of treatment, and no significant difference was found between the two treatment durations in the Phase III study evaluating the 5 and 10-day treatment durations (NCT04292899). The most common side effects are constipation, hypokalemia, anemia, thrombocytopenia, and increased bilirubin levels. It is not recommended for use in patients with liver and kidney failure.

Antibacterial Agents

Azithromycin

In vitro efficacy of azithromycin, an antibiotic from the macrolide group, against the Ebola virus has been demonstrated [31]. It is also effective in preventing severe pulmonary infections in patients with viral infections. In a study evaluating the combined regimen with hydroxychloroquine in 20 COVID-19 patients, azithromycin was shown to increase the efficacy of hydroxychloroquine [32]. However, the risk of QT prolongation should be considered in combination with hydroxychloroquine.

Teicoplanin and Other Glycopeptides

Another antibacterial agent that stands out in the treatment of coronavirus infections is teicoplanin. It has been shown in vitro that teicoplanin prevents the entry of other coronaviruses such as Ebola, MERS, and SARS into the cell [33]. However, there is no study showing its effectiveness on SARS-CoV-2.

Immunmodulator and Immunsupressif Agents

Interleukin-6 Inhibitors

Tocilizumab is a human IL-6 receptor antagonist; it is used in the treatment of RA and cytokine release syndrome (CRS). It is observed that IL-2 receptor, IL-6, IL-8, IL-10, and TNF-alpha levels are increased in COVID-19 patients with cytokine storm. Increased cytokine release is associated with increased disease symptoms. Since IL-6 may play an important role in stimulating the excessive inflammatory response in the lungs with COVID-19 involvement, tocilizumab is thought to be effective in the treatment of this infectious disease. In a multi-center study, it was observed that 75% of the patients with severe COVID-19 disease experienced an improvement in fever and a decrease in oxygen demand [34]. In the same study, regression was found in CT findings and improvement was seen in CRP increase and lymphopenia [34]. The mortality rate was also significantly lower in the tocilizumab group compared to the control group. However, the most important disadvantage of this study is that it was not randomized and double-blind.

The dose of tocilizumab with demonstrated efficacy in the treatment of COVID-19 is a single 400mg IV infusion [35]. If fever persists within 12 hours after the first dose, a second dose may be administered. Its known side effects include increased risk of bacterial infection, gastrointestinal perforations, infusion-related reactions such as hypertension, headache, skin reactions, anaphylaxis, thrombocytopenia, increased liver enzymes, and hyperlipidemia [36]. The same side effects are seen in the treatment of COVID-19 [37]. Sarilumab is another human monoclonal IL-6 receptor blocker. The multi-center, double-blind, phase II/III study (NCT04315298) evaluating the effectiveness of this molecule, which has been developed for the treatment of RA, in COVID-19 treatment has not yet been concluded. Nevertheless, it showed that it may be more effective to reduce CRP than placebo. However, no data is showing the benefit of sarilumab in severe disease. It is not recommended for the treatment of COVID-19 for now due to insufficient efficacy and safety studies.

IL-1 Receptor Antagonists

Anakinra is a recombinant human IL-1 receptor antagonist and is used in the treatment of RA. Studies are showing that it is effective in macrophage activation syndrome (MAS) in which severe cytokine storm is observed [38]. Therefore, it is thought that anakinra may prevent symptoms of COVID-19 related cytokine release syndrome. Use of anakinra improved survival in patients with sepsis in a phase III, randomized controlled trial [39]. Currently, no randomised controlled studies are evaluating the efficacy and safety of its use in the treatment of COVID-19. In case series and cohort studies published so far, anakinra has been shown to improve clinical and laboratory markers, reduce the need for mechanical ventilation and mortality rates [40, 41].

Janus Kinase Inhibitors

It is suggested that Janus kinase (JAK) inhibitors may be effective in the treatment of CRS in severe COVID-19 disease by inhibiting the JAK-signal converting activator (JAK-STAT) pathway. Ruxolitinib is a potent and selective oral JAK1 and JAK2 protein kinase inhibitor. It is indicated for intermediate and high-risk myelofibrosis, polycythemia vera, steroid-resistant graft versus host disease. There is not yet sufficient data regarding the use of ruxolitinib and other JAK inhibitors in the treatment of COVID-19. In ongoing phase III studies (RUXOCOVID, RUXCOVID-DEVENT), the efficacy of ruxolitinib in the treatment of COVID-19 associated CRS and ARDS patients in need of mechanical ventilation is evaluated.

Anti-tumor Necrosis Factor-α

Tumor necrosis factor-α (TNFα) plays a role in all acute inflammations induced by acute stress and inflammation. TNFα is a molecule produced mainly in macrophages, monocytes, B cells, and other tissues. With the activation of TNFα, IL-1 and IL-6 begin to be produced. Plasma and tissue TNF levels were found to be high in COVID-19 patients [42]. Anti-TNFα agents such as adalimumab and infliximab are indicated for the treatment of inflammatory and autoimmune diseases such as RA, inflammatory bowel disease, and ankylosing spondylitis. Experimental studies are showing the effectiveness of anti-TNFα in the treatment of viral pneumonia [43].

The ability of a single dose of anti-TNFα to significantly lower blood TNFα levels suggests that it may be useful in the treatment of COVID-19 [44]. However, it should be considered that anti-TNFα therapy causes an increased risk of bacterial and fungal infections [44].

Intravenous Immunoglobulin

Intravenous immunoglobulin (IVIG) includes Ig G subtypes obtained by pooling from human plasma. It was used to provide immunity in the treatment of SARS, but thromboembolic complications were reported in some cases and the expected benefit could not be obtained [45, 46]. There may be several mechanisms that are effective in the therapeutic benefit of IVIG. IVIG can inhibit the function of many innate immune cells and neutralize active complement components.

It can also affect the acquired immune response by regulating the functions of B and plasma cells, regulator T and T helper cells, and inhibiting inflammatory cytokines.

In addition, it can stimulate the anti-inflammatory response by binding to antiviral antibodies and pro-inflammatory cytokines [47]. In a retrospective study of 58 patients with severe COVID-19 pneumonia, it was observed that IVIG treatment administered within 48 hours after the appearance of clinical findings significantly reduced 28-day mortality compared to the administration of the treatment 48 hours later (23.3%; 57.1%, $p = 0.009$) [48].

In contrast, another retrospective study involving 325 patients reported that IVIG treatment given to severe COVID-19 patients had no positive effect on 28-day or 60-day mortality [49]. Since current IVIGs do not contain antibodies against SARS-Cov-2, IVIG treatment is recommended in COVID-19 treatment guidelines of the National Institute of Health and Surviving Sepsis Campaign [50, 51].

Interferons

Interferons (IFNs) are cytokines that play a key role in reducing viral replication and regulating the immune response against viral infection. The effectiveness of IFN treatment against MERS-CoV and SARS-CoV has been studied. Due to their nonspecific antiviral effects, the effectiveness of combination therapies with other agents has generally been evaluated [52]. In a multi-center, prospective, open-label, randomized, phase II study evaluating 127 patients with COVID-19 disease, it is suggested that the duration of weaning from the mechanical ventilator, hospital stay, and viral carriage time were shorter with lopinavir/ritonavir, ribavirin, and IFNβ-1b combination therapy compared to monotherapies [23]. Clinical studies evaluating the effectiveness of nebular and subcutaneous forms of interferons in the treatment of COVID-19 (NCT04293887, NCT04350281) continues.

Corticosteroids

Corticosteroids have taken their place in the treatment of many diseases such as asthma and other allergic diseases, autoimmune diseases, septic shock, and cancer. On the one hand, they suppress inflammation, on the other hand, they may predispose to infections by causing immunosuppression. It is a class of drugs that have been tried in treatment since the beginning of the COVID-19 pandemic. WHO and CDC did not recommend corticosteroids in the treatment of COVID-19 if there are no comorbidities such as asthma, COPD, and sepsis since their efficacy on SARS and MERS could not be determined and their side effects could be fatal. However, many studies have shown the opposite. Treatment with steroids has been shown to reduce the risk of death in COVID-19 patients who develop ARDS. While the mortality rate is 46% in patients receiving steroid treatment, it is 61.8% in patients who do not [53]. Similarly, the randomized, controlled RECOVERY study showed that dexamethasone reduced the mortality rate in 1/5 of the patients who needed noninvasive oxygen treatment, and in 1/3 of the patients who needed mechanical ventilation [54]. In addition, dexamethasone reduced the length of hospital stay and the need for mechanical ventilation [54].

Important side effects of corticosteroids are avascular necrosis, psychosis, gastrointestinal effects, and diabetes. In the aforementioned RECOVERY study, no side effects were reported in patients given dexamethasone compared to the control group [54]. As a result of the increase in studies supporting the efficacy and safety of corticosteroids, it has been emphasized in the treatment guidelines that short-term (<8 days) and low-dose (0.5 - 1mg/kg/day methylprednisolone and its equivalent) steroid treatment can be administered [55].

Other Pharmacologic Therapies

Convalescent Plasma Therapy

Serum obtained from people who have recovered from an infectious disease, called convalescent plasma, has been used for a long time in the treatment of infectious diseases. Antibodies in plasma show their therapeutic effects by more than one mechanism. The antibodies can act by binding directly to the agent. In a second mechanism, antibodies produce their therapeutic effect by stimulating complement activation, phagocytosis, and antibody-mediated cytotoxicity. Plasma therapy has been used effectively and reliably in the SARS, MERS, and H1N1 pandemics for the last 20 years [56-58]. Since SARS-CoV-2 has similar virological and clinical properties with SARS-CoV-1 and MERS, it is thought that plasma therapy may also be effective in the treatment of this viral infection [59]. In the first studies conducted with COVID-19 patients, it was reported that ARDS symptoms regressed, the duration of mechanical ventilation was shortened, fever decreased, and viral clearance increased [60, 61].

However, these studies are small-scale and single-center studies. Plasma therapy is generally well tolerated; Common side effects are transfusion-related skin reactions, hypervolemia, and lung damage. Recently, an FDA-supported, national, multi-center, open-label EAP study was conducted in 5.000 inpatients with high-risk and very severe COVID-19 findings [62]. Less than 1% of the patients developed serious side effects such as transfusion-related hypervolemia, transfusion-associated lung injury (TRALI), and severe allergic reaction.

On the other hand, a multi-center, randomized controlled study evaluating the efficacy and safety of plasma treatment in 103 COVID-19 patients with severe or life-threatening diseases conducted in China; found recovery time, mortality rate, and length of stay to be similar to the control group [63].

In the same study, no major side effects were reported [63]. The recommended plasma dose for the treatment of COVID-19 varies depending on the neutralizing antibody level and is one or two infusions.

Renin-Angiotensin-Aldosterone System (RAAS) Inhibitors

Besides the protective effects of RAAS inhibitors on the cardiovascular system, they also have anti-inflammatory and immunomodulatory effects.

ACE2 is secreted from all epithelial cells, including lung epithelial cells. ACE2 receptors are the entry point to the host cell for SARS-CoV-2 [64]. The virus binds to ACE2 and inhibits it and the level of angiotensin 2 increases. It has been hypothesized that ACEIs and ARBs exacerbate clinical findings by increasing the number of ACE2 receptors that will allow SARS-CoV2 to bind. However, this hypothesis has not been proven by human studies.

In a large-scale, observational study, SARS-CoV-2 positivity was found in patients using ACEI/ARB at a similar rate to patients not using it [65]. In addition, disease severity was similar in both patient groups [65]. In a case-control study conducted with 6272 COVID-19 patients, it was shown that the use of ACEI/ARB was not associated with the risk of COVID-19 infection, the severity of clinical findings, or the course of infection [66]. Based on these and similar studies, discontinuation of ACEIs/ARBs in the treatment of patients is not recommended unless there is hemodynamic impairment.

Statins

Statins play an important role in the treatment of cardiovascular diseases. They may be useful in the treatment of COVID-19 due to their anti-inflammatory effects and protective effects on the innate immune system [67].

In a multi-center retrospective study aimed at determining the prevalence of myocardial damage in COVID-19 patients, statins have been reported to increase survival in these patients [68]. In another retrospective study, it has been shown that statin use is notably associated with asymptomatic disease [69].

In the same study, the severe disease was observed in 19% of those using statins, while it was observed in 25% of those who did not; but this was not statistically significant [69]. In patients diagnosed with COVID-19, if treatment with a statin is indicated, the drug should be started or continued.

Conclusion

Since the beginning of the SARS-CoV2 pandemic, many different drug groups have been tried for the treatment. However, no specific agent has been developed so far. Drugs act by blocking virus entry into host cells, inhibiting viral replication, and suppressing excessive inflammation. The side effects of the drugs also differ. Treatment protocols should be individualized, taking into account factors such as the patients' clinical conditions, accompanying diseases, and other medications. Treatment protocols will change as the efficacy and safety studies of each drug group are completed.

References

[1] Zhou, P. et al. A pneumonia outbreak associated with a new coronavirus of probable bat origin. *Nature,* 2020. 579(7798): p. 270 - 273.

[2] Yan, R. et al. Structural basis for the recognition of SARS-CoV-2 by full-length human ACE2. *Science,* 2020. 367(6485): p. 1444 - 1448.

[3] Chen, Y., Liu, Q. and Guo, D. Emerging coronaviruses: genome structure, replication, and pathogenesis. *Journal of Medical Virology,* 2020. 92(4): p. 418 - 423.

[4] Fung, T. S. and Liu, D. X. Human coronavirus: Host-pathogen interaction. *Annual Review of Microbiology*, 2019. 73: p. 529 - 557.

[5] Nelemans, T. and Kikkert, M. Viral innate immune evasion and the pathogenesis of emerging RNA virus infections. *Viruses,* 2019. 11(10): p. 961.

[6] Newton, A. H., Cardani, A. and Braciale, T. J. The host immune response in respiratory virus infection: Balancing virus clearance and immunopathology. in *Seminars in Immunopathology*, 2016. Springer.

[7] Fehr, A. R., Channappanavar, R. and Perlman, S. Middle East respiratory syndrome: emergence of a pathogenic human coronavirus. *Annual Review of Medicine,* 2017. 68.

[8] Channappanavar, R. et al. Dysregulated type I interferon and inflammatory monocyte-macrophage responses cause lethal pneumonia in SARS-CoV-infected mice. *Cell Host and Microbe,* 2016. 19(2): p. 181 - 193.

[9] De Wit, E. et al. SARS and MERS: recent insights into emerging coronaviruses. *Nature Reviews Microbiology*, 2016. 14(8): p. 523.

[10] Xiong, Y. et al. Transcriptomic characteristics of bronchoalveolar lavage fluid and peripheral blood mononuclear cells in COVID-19 patients. *Emerging Microbes and Infections*, 2020. 9(1): p. 761 - 770.

[11] Tang, W. et al. Hydroxychloroquine in patients with mainly mild to moderate coronavirus disease 2019: open label, randomised controlled trial. *BMJ,* 2020. 369.

[12] Colson, P. et al. Chloroquine and hydroxychloroquine as available weapons to fight COVID-19. *Int. J. Antimicrob. Agents,* 2020. 105932(10.1016).

[13] Yao, X. et al. In vitro antiviral activity and projection of optimized dosing design of hydroxychloroquine for the treatment of severe acute respiratory syndrome coronavirus 2 (SARS-CoV-2). *Clinical Infectious Diseases,* 2020.

[14] Osadchy, A., Ratnapalan, T. and Koren, G. Ocular toxicity in children exposed in utero to antimalarial drugs: review of the literature. *The Journal of rheumatology*, 2011. 38(12): p. 2504 - 2508.

[15] De Clercq, E. New nucleoside analogues for the treatment of hemorrhagic fever virus infections. *Chemistry–An Asian Journal,* 2019. 14(22): p. 3962 - 3968.

[16] Chen, C. et al. Favipiravir versus arbidol for COVID-19: A randomized clinical trial. *MedRxiv,* 2020.

[17] Cai, Q. et al. Experimental treatment with favipiravir for COVID-19: an open-label control study. *Engineering,* 2020.

[18] Sissoko, D. et al. Experimental treatment with favipiravir for Ebola virus disease (the JIKI Trial): A historically controlled, single-arm proof-of-concept trial in Guinea. *PLoS medicine,* 2016. 13(3): p. e1001967.

[19] Pang, J. et al. Potential rapid diagnostics, vaccine and therapeutics for 2019 novel coronavirus (2019-nCoV): A systematic review. *Journal of clinical medicine,* 2020. 9(3): p. 623.

[20] Young, B. E. et al. Epidemiologic features and clinical course of patients infected with SARS-CoV-2 in Singapore. *JAMA,* 2020. 323(15): p. 1488 - 1494.

[21] Wang, M. et al. Evaluation of current medical approaches for COVID-19: A systematic review and meta-analysis. *BMJ supportive and palliative care*, 2020.

[22] Cao, B. et al. A trial of lopinavir–ritonavir in adults hospitalized with severe Covid-19. *New England Journal of Medicine*, 2020.

[23] Hung, I. F.-N. et al. Triple combination of interferon beta-1b, lopinavir–ritonavir, and ribavirin in the treatment of patients admitted to hospital with COVID-19: An open-label, randomised, phase 2 trial. *The Lancet,* 2020. 395(10238): p. 1695 - 1704.

[24] Stockman, L. J., Bellamy, R. and Garner, P. SARS: systematic review of treatment effects. *PLoS Med.,* 2006. 3(9): p. e343.

[25] Dong, L., Hu, S. and Gao, J. Discovering drugs to treat coronavirus disease 2019 (COVID-19). *Drug Discoveries and Therapeutics*, 2020. 14(1): p. 58 - 60.

[26] Altinbas, S., Holmes, J. A. and Altinbas, A. Hepatitis C Virus Infection in Pregnancy: An Update. *Gastroenterology Nursing,* 2020. 43(1): p. 12 - 21.

[27] Mulangu, S. et al. A randomized, controlled trial of Ebola virus disease therapeutics. *New England Journal of Medicine,* 2019. 381(24): p. 2293 - 2303.

[28] Sheahan, T. P. et al. Broad-spectrum antiviral GS-5734 inhibits both epidemic and zoonotic coronaviruses. *Science translational medicine,* 2017. 9(396).

[29] Wang, Y. et al. Remdesivir in adults with severe COVID-19: A randomised, double-blind, placebo-controlled, multicentre trial. *The Lancet,* 2020.

[30] Beigel, J. H. et al. Remdesivir for the treatment of Covid-19—preliminary report. *The New England Journal of Medicine*, 2020.

[31] Madrid, P. B. et al. Evaluation of Ebola virus inhibitors for drug repurposing. *ACS Infectious Diseases*, 2015. 1(7): p. 317 - 326.

[32] Gautret, P. et al. Hydroxychloroquine and azithromycin as a treatment of COVID-19: Results of an open-label non-randomized clinical trial. *International Journal of Antimicrobial Agents*, 2020: p. 105949.

[33] Wang, Y. et al. Teicoplanin inhibits Ebola pseudovirus infection in cell culture. *Antiviral Research*, 2016. 125: p. 1 - 7.

[34] Xu, X. et al. Effective treatment of severe COVID-19 patients with tocilizumab. *Proceedings of the National Academy of Sciences,* 2020. 117(20): p. 10970 - 10975.

[35] Hon, K. L. et al. Coronavirus disease 2019 (COVID-19): Latest developments in potential treatments. *Drugs in Context,* 2020. 9.

[36] Zhang, X. et al. First case of COVID-19 in a patient with multiple myeloma successfully treated with tocilizumab. *Blood Advances,* 2020. 4(7): p. 1307.

[37] Mazzitelli, M. et al. Use of subcutaneous tocilizumab in patients with COVID-19 pneumonia. *Journal of Medical Virology*, 2020.

[38] Schulert, G. S. and Grom, A. A. Pathogenesis of macrophage activation syndrome and potential for cytokine-directed therapies. *Annual Review of Medicine*, 2015. 66: p. 145 - 159.

[39] Shakoory, B. et al. Interleukin-1 receptor blockade is associated with reduced mortality in sepsis patients with features of the macrophage activation syndrome: Re-analysis of a prior Phase III trial. *Critical Care Medicine,* 2016. 44(2): p. 275.

[40] Aouba, A. et al. Targeting the inflammatory cascade with anakinra in moderate to severe COVID-19 pneumonia: Case series. *Annals of the Rheumatic Diseases,* 2020.

[41] Huet, T. et al. Anakinra for severe forms of COVID-19: A cohort study. *The Lancet Rheumatology*, 2020.

[42] Wang, L. et al. Coronavirus disease 2019 in elderly patients: Characteristics and prognostic factors based on 4-week follow-up. *Journal of Infection*, 2020.

[43] Hussell, T., Pennycook, A. and Openshaw, P. J. Inhibition of tumor necrosis factor reduces the severity of virus-specific lung immunopathology. *European Journal of Immunology*, 2001. 31(9): p. 2566 - 2573.

[44] Feldmann, M. et al. Trials of anti-tumour necrosis factor therapy for COVID-19 are urgently needed. *The Lancet,* 2020. 395(10234): p. 1407 - 1409.

[45] Umapathi, T. et al. Large artery ischaemic stroke in severe acute respiratory syndrome (SARS). *Journal of Neurology*, 2004. 251(10): p. 1227 - 1231.

[46] Ng, K., et al., Pulmonary artery thrombosis in a patient with severe acute respiratory syndrome. *Postgraduate Medical Journal*, 2005. 81(956): p. e3 - e3.

[47] Nguyen, A. A. et al. Immunoglobulins in the treatment of COVID-19 infection: Proceed with caution! *Clinical Immunology*, 2020: p. 108459.

[48] Xie, Y. et al. Effect of regular intravenous immunoglobulin therapy on prognosis of severe pneumonia in patients with COVID-19. *The Journal of Infection,* 2020.

[49] Shao, Z. et al. Clinical Efficacy of Intravenous Immunoglobulin Therapy in Critical Patients with COVID-19: *A multicenter retrospective cohort study*. 2020.

[50] Health, N. I.o. *Coronavirus disease 2019 (COVID-19) treatment Guidelines*. 2020, April.

[51] Alhazzani, W. et al. Surviving Sepsis Campaign: guidelines on the management of critically ill adults with Coronavirus Disease 2019 (COVID-19). *Intensive Care Medicine*, 2020: p. 1 - 34.

[52] Sallard, E. et al. Type 1 interferons as a potential treatment against COVID-19. *Antiviral Research*, 2020: p. 104791.

[53] Wu, C. et al. Risk factors associated with acute respiratory distress syndrome and death in patients with coronavirus disease 2019 pneumonia in Wuhan, China. *JAMA Internal Medicine*, 2020.

[54] Horby, P. et al. Effect of Hydroxychloroquine in Hospitalized Patients with COVID-19: Preliminary results from a multi-centre, randomized, controlled trial. *MedRxiv,* 2020.

[55] Organization, W. H. Clinical management of severe acute respiratory infection (SARI) when COVID-19 disease is suspected. *Interim Guidance V 1.2.* Geneva: WHO; 13 Mar. 2020.

[56] Cheng, Y. et al. Use of convalescent plasma therapy in SARS patients in Hong Kong. *European Journal of Clinical Microbiology and Infectious Diseases,* 2005. 24(1): p. 44 - 46.

[57] Hung, I. F. et al. Convalescent plasma treatment reduced mortality in patients with severe pandemic influenza A (H1N1) 2009 virus infection. *Clinical Infectious Diseases*, 2011. 52(4): p. 447 - 456.

[58] Ko, J.-H. et al. Challenges of convalescent plasma infusion therapy in Middle East respiratory coronavirus infection: A single centre experience. *Antivir. Ther.,* 2018. 23(7): p. 617 - 22.

[59] Lee, P.-I. and Hsueh, P.-R. Emerging threats from zoonotic coronaviruses-from SARS and MERS to 2019-nCoV. *Journal of Microbiology, Immunology and Infection,* 2020.

[60] Shen, C. et al. Treatment of 5 critically ill patients with COVID-19 with convalescent plasma. *JAMA,* 2020. 323(16): p. 1582 - 1589.

[61] Duan, K. et al. Effectiveness of convalescent plasma therapy in severe COVID-19 patients. *Proceedings of the National Academy of Sciences,* 2020. 117(17): p. 9490 - 9496.

[62] Joyner, M. J. et al. Early safety indicators of COVID-19 convalescent plasma in 5,000 patients. *The Journal of Clinical Investigation*, 2020.

[63] Li, L. et al. Effect of Convalescent Plasma Therapy on Time to Clinical Improvement in Patients with Severe and Life-threatening COVID-19: A Randomized Clinical Trial. *JAMA,* 2020.

[64] Lu, R. et al. Genomic characterisation and epidemiology of 2019 novel coronavirus: Implications for virus origins and receptor binding. *The Lancet,* 2020. 395(10224): p. 565 - 574.

[65] Reynolds, H. R. et al. Renin–angiotensin–aldosterone system inhibitors and risk of Covid-19. *New England Journal of Medicine,* 2020.

[66] Mancia, G. et al. Renin–angiotensin–aldosterone system blockers and the risk of Covid-19. *New England Journal of Medicine*, 2020.

[67] Dashti-Khavidaki, S. and Khalili, H. Considerations for statin therapy in patients with COVID-19. Pharmacotherapy: *The Journal of Human Pharmacology and Drug Therapy,* 2020. 40(5): p. 484 - 486.

[68] Lala, A. et al. Prevalence and Impact of Myocardial Injury in Patients Hospitalized with COVID-19 Infection. *Journal of the American College of Cardiology*, 2020.

[69] De Spiegeleer, A. et al. The effects of ARBs, ACEIs and statins on clinical outcomes of COVID-19 infection among nursing home residents. *Medrxiv*, 2020.

In: Coronavirus Disease
Editor: Yildiz Dincer
ISBN: 978-1-53619-296-4

Chapter 6

INTENSIVE CARE MANAGEMENT OF COVID-19 PATIENTS

Olcay Dilken, MD and Yalim Dikmen*, MD
Istanbul University-Cerrahpasa, Cerrahpasa Medical School, Department of Anaesthesiology and Reanimation, Istanbul, Turkey

ABSTRACT

COVID-19 has affected millions of patients and healthcare workers in an unprecedented way. The pandemic took clinicians and hospitals by surprise. Intensive care units should be modified to handle the patient surge. There are few remedies to decrease the burden imposed on the healthcare system. These include management of acute respiratory failure, thrombotic events, cytokine modulating therapies. Only dexamethasone and prone positioning seem to have beneficial effects on oxygenation and need for mechanical ventilation. Nevertheless, tailoring the therapy for specific needs of the patient can decrease adverse effects. In this chapter, we review the current knowledge in the management of the critically ill COVID-19 patients as of September 2020.

Keywords: COVID-19, pneumonia, ARDS, prone position, thrombosis, mechanical ventilation

INTRODUCTION

Since December 2019, a novel coronavirus, named "Severe Acute Respiratory Syndrome Coronavirus 2" (SARS-CoV-2), affected millions of lives. The illness it causes

* Corresponding Author's Email: ydikmen@istanbul.edu.tr.

was termed Coronavirus Disease 2019 (COVID-19). It reached pandemic status by March 2020 and has been putting enormous strain on Intensive Care Units (ICUs) worldwide, both by overwhelming limited ICU capacity and lack of effective treatment options. [1] This new disease showed an unpredictable clinical course, especially in critically ill patients leading to high intensive care mortality exceeding 50% [1, 2].

ICU Organization During COVID-19 Surge

In a recent retrospective cohort of 83,619 patients, mean ICU admission among hospitalized patients with COVID-19 pneumonia was 20.1% [range 4.6-32%). 48.8% of these patients required invasive mechanical ventilation for a mean of 7.8 days or longer [3]. One of the early studies from the Lombardy region in Italy showed that the patients were generally admitted to the intensive care 10 days after the symptom onset, had a median 12 days length of stay. Main risk factors associated with mortality were advanced age, male sex, comorbidities like chronic obstructive respiratory failure and diabetes mellitus, low PaO_2/FiO_2 ratio and need for high positive end-expiratory pressure (PEEP)[1].

There are vast differences in ICU capacity not only among countries but also on the regional level. Thus, it would be impossible to assess the adequacy of all ICU beds for any given pandemic. However, measures to support the ICUs in case of overwhelmed capacity should be taken beforehand. The consequences of not doing so are possible delays in treatment, which is directly associated with mortality [4].

In contrast to a laypersons' belief, ICUs are driven by specialized physicians, skilled nurses, and other healthcare workers, not by medical devices. Insufficiently trained staff may jeopardize patient care. An intensivist-to-patient ratio lower than 1/15 was associated with increased ICU length of stay [5]. The nurse-to-patient ratio is another parameter that assures patient safety. During the peak patient surge in our ICU, we addressed this issue with former ICU nurses and anaesthesiologists to triple our capacity. It should be underlined that unskilled or too much staff may cause problems rather than benefit [6].

Lack of mechanical ventilators led to excess mortality in Northern Italy during early 2020. Strategies should be developed to overcome the shortage. High-flow nasal oxygen (HFNO) and non-invasive ventilation (NIV) can be employed to reduce the need for intubation. However, when intubated, a full-featured ventilator is necessary to manage a COVID-19 patient as opposed to basic volume control resuscitation devices or flow generators [3]. If a shortage occurs, alternative devices such as transport ventilators, anesthesia ventilators can be employed as a last resort. Concomitant use of a single ventilator on multiple patients is nowhere near logical or physiological and never advised.

Although healthcare staff and mechanical ventilators seem to bore the brunt of the surge, many supplies and resources are necessary for an intubated ICU patient. An exhaustive list can be found in [3]. To better deploy sources during a crisis, postponing all elective and medical procedures, providing refresher courses to former critical care staff and transfer of essential healthcare workers from less strained regions should be considered. However, a treatment that has been administered only in an ICU setting before the crisis (such as non-invasive ventilation), should never be transferred to another facility without sufficient experience (like wards).

COVID-19 Related Acute Respiratory Failure

Physicians have been encountering an unprecedented number of acute hypoxemic respiratory failure and ARDS due to COVID-19 for the past 10 months. Acute Respiratory Distress Syndrome (ARDS) occurs in 20-41% of severe COVID-19 patients and they exceedingly require some form of ventilatory support. Non-invasive ventilatory support can be appropriate. However, the failure rate is high and, in some patients, invasive ventilation is inevitable [7].

ARDS is a heterogeneous syndrome that can present as in strikingly different types. Unfortunately, this fact seemed to be forgotten during the start of the pandemic, and patients were termed based on observations. "Happy hypoxemia, Type L and Type H (or high and low elastance), cytokine storm" were proposed in a desperate attempt to clarify a previously unknown disease. Although different treatments for different ARDS types were proposed, emerging evidence shows that respiratory system mechanics of patients with ARDS (with or without COVID-19) are similar [8]. Evidence-based management of "conventional" ARDS includes conservative fluid strategy, early and proper antibiotics for possible bacterial pneumonia, consideration for early invasive ventilation, lung-protective ventilation, use of prone positioning, and considering extracorporeal membrane oxygenation (ECMO) [9]. Additionally, three recent studies proved dexamethasone to be effective in severe COVID-19 patients (see below). Lung protective ventilation, even in patients with relatively conserved lung compliance, can be beneficial [10]. Also, lung-protective ventilation decreases progression to more severe ARDS and pulmonary complications [11]. Furthermore, permissive hypercapnia is mostly well tolerated. However, the acceptable level of carbon dioxide may significantly differ between patients. Thus, before advancing to more liberal tidal volume ventilation, other causes for the hypercarbia should be addressed. PEEP titration remains necessary and complicated for each patient as it possesses the risk of reducing oxygen delivery if the underlying cause leading to hypoxemia is vascular derangement (i.e., pulmonary emboli).

Prone positioning, both in non-intubated and intubated patients, improves oxygenation due to better ventilation-perfusion matching. Prone positioning the patient relieves the dorsal compression of the alveoli by the weight of mediastinum and intraabdominal organs. Subsequently, recruitment occurs and more alveoli are available for gas exchange. Also, continuous alveolar recruitment and derecruitment decrease within tidal volumes [7, 12]. It remains the mainstay of the management of ARDS patients. It can also be performed in awake patients with non-invasive forms of ventilatory support. In a prospective cohort of 56 patients, prone positioning was feasible in 84%. These patients maintained a prone position for at least 3 hours. Oxygenation improved remarkably after prone positioning. However, oxygenation could not be maintained in half of the patients when supine positioning was reinitiated. Early initiation of prone positioning after hospital admission (i.e., 2.7 days vs 4.6 days) was associated with retaining oxygenation [7].

One of the most crucial problems in the management of COVID-19 related ARDS is the timing of intubation and whether to commence invasive mechanical ventilation early. Unfortunately, anecdotal reports and expert opinions are insufficient to answer these questions. In one retrospective study, which analyzed patients from the Wuhan district in China, it was suggested that early intubation and invasive mechanical ventilation were more effective in reducing mortality [13]. However, in this study, invasive mechanical ventilation was initiated only after failed non-invasive respiratory support, and this is hard to consider as an early intervention. Another retrospective multicenter study involving 48 ARDS patients from China had a better methodology, which compared the outcome in patients who were intubated at the time when they fulfilled the ARDS criteria versus the patients intubated after failed noninvasive support [14]. In this study, no difference in mortality was observed in early or late intubation groups. Additionally, 8 patients in the late group never received intubation. A recent survey replied by 1132 ICU physicians from 85 countries showed great heterogeneity in treatment practices regarding admission time, initial oxygenation strategies, ventilator management, etc. In this survey, only 8% of the respondents opted for early intubation in a hypoxaemic patient despite conventional oxygen treatment. Half of the respondents indicated 4 hours of observation before switching to invasive ventilation [15].

Corticosteroids, such as dexamethasone, can reduce the duration of mechanical ventilation and mortality in ARDS patients. In a multicentre randomized controlled trial on 277 patients with (non-COVID) ARDS, patients receiving dexamethasone had more ventilator-free days (12 vs 7, between group difference 4.8 days (95CI% 2,57 to 7,03]. There was a slight increase in newly acquired infections and hyperglycemia [16]. The first major trial to show benefit in COVID-19 patients was the recovery trial that enrolled 6425 patients [17]. Of these, 2104 patients received 6 mg/day dexamethasone for 10 days. The mortality was significantly reduced in patients receiving respiratory support (including supplemental oxygen). However, there was no mortality difference among patients that did not receive respiratory support. Three subsequent RCTs were published in ICU settings to address the use of corticosteroids. In the REMAP-CAP trial, hydrocortisone was likely to be superior to no hydrocortisone (93% probability) [18]. CoDEX trial enrolled 299 moderate and severe ARDS patients to 20 mg/day dexamethasone for 5 days, which was tapered down to 10 mg/day for another 5 days [19]. Patients receiving dexamethasone had more ventilator free-days on day 28 (6.6 vs 4). However, the 28-day mortality was similar between groups (56.3% vs 61.5%). In the CAPE COVID trial, which enrolled 149 patients, severe ARDS patients received 200 mg/day hydrocortisone [20]. There was no significant difference between groups on day 21 in terms of death or respiratory support (42.1 vs 50.7, $p = 0.29$). All of these studies were included in a prospective meta-analysis. 28-day mortality was lower in those receiving corticosteroids (odds ratio 0.66 [95CI% 0.53-0.82]) [21]. However, questions remain regarding side effects, optimal dosing, administration trigger, or illness severity threshold [22]. Nevertheless, corticosteroids remain the only drug that is shown to be beneficial in severe ARDS patients.

Coinfections and secondary respiratory infections also increase in COVID-19 patients and they are associated with decreased survival. Usually, an elevated procalcitonin (PCT) is found in patients with septic shock. Bacterial infections trigger the synthesis of PCT via interferon-γ. On the other hand, viral infections do not stimulate the same response in the host. Thus, PCT remains mostly normal in the uncomplicated COVID-19 cases and an increased PCT may indicate co-infection in the critically ill patients. A PCT $\geq$ 0.5 mg/l indicated a poor outcome in COVID-19 patients with a sensitivity of 88% and specificity of 68% [23].

COVID-19 and Thrombosis

COVID-19 is a hypercoagulable state and it is associated with increased thrombotic events, including pulmonary embolism (PE) [24]. However, the pathophysiology is not fully understood. Very high d-dimer levels may reflect not only systemic inflammation but also thrombosis triggered by the virus [25]. In a retrospective study enrolling 81 COVID-19 pneumonia patients, a D-dimer cut-off value of 1.5 mcg/ml predicted venous thromboembolism (VTE) with 85% sensitivity, 88.5% specificity [26]. In another retrospective study including 127 patients, only D-dimer and CRP levels were found to be associated with VTE. When combined with a D-dimer > 15, a CRP > 280 had a predicted probability of 98% for VTE [27].

The incidence of PE in hospitalized patients is around 1.9%-8.9%. This increases to 26.6% in the critically ill, despite prophylaxis. These numbers are possibly an underestimation of the real incidence as symptoms and findings of PE is nonspecific. For instance, an autopsy of 12 patients revealed deep venous thrombosis (DVT) in 7; none were suspected of having an embolism before death [28]. Nevertheless, routine screening for VTE is currently not recommended [29].

There are several guidelines for laboratory testing in the critically ill with COVID-19. An increase in D-dimer levels (3 to 4-fold (ISTH-IG) or 6-fold (SCC-ISTH) may indicate an embolic event. Regular (not daily) monitoring of platelet count, prothrombin time, and fibrinogen are also recommended [30]. A prophylactic dose of Low Molecular Weight Heparin [LMWH) or subcutaneous unfractionated heparin should be initiated in all suspected or confirmed COVID-19 patients admitted to the hospital [31, 32]. Additionally, mechanical thromboprophylaxis should be considered whenever pharmacological treatment is contraindicated. There is insufficient evidence to suggest mechanical thromboprophylaxis in addition to pharmacological one [30]. Therapeutic anticoagulation should be considered in case of high suspicion of a thromboembolic event. Sudden onset of hypotension or hemodynamic instability should prompt bedside echocardiography. Thrombolytic therapy should be initiated if there is any evidence of right ventricular dilatation or increased pulmonary arterial tension. Other thrombolytic indications include STEMI and acute ischemic stroke [30].

Other Therapies to Mitigate the Effects of COVID-19

Although the term "cytokine storm" is broadly defined, it mostly implies an extreme pro-inflammatory response. Manifestations of the cytokine storm include fever, tachycardia, tachypnoea, and vasoplegia leading to hypotension due to endothelial dysfunction and inflammation [33]. Initial reports on observations of severe COVID -19 infection suggested that cytokines, particularly IL-6, played a key role in propagating lung damage and multiorgan failure. A study found that hyperinflammatory type of COVID-19, defined as CRP greater than 150 mg/dl and ferritin greater than 1500 mcg/l, had increased mortality [34]. Subsequently, cytokine removal therapies and monoclonal antibodies targeting interleukins were administered. As of September, there are over 50 interventional studies listed in the clinical trials database for tocilizumab (an anti-IL-6 drug) alone. However, the presence of a cytokine storm in severe COVID-19 patients is debated. In a healthy volunteer study, plasma IL-6 levels ranged from 1 to 79 pg/ml [35]. On the other hand, patients with ARDS had a median IL-6 concentration of 1618 pg/ml [33], 723 pg/ml [36], 238 pg/ml [37] or 376 pg/ml [38]. Although IL-6 was also increased in patients with COVID-19, the increase is milder compared to ARDS. IL-6 levels of 25, 26 and 64 pg/ml were reported [38]. Furthermore, a single dose of an IL-6 inhibitor can suppress CRP levels and fever for a week and secondary infections can go unnoticed.

Nevertheless, a retrospective observational study in critically ill patients revealed improved mortality among those with baseline CRP levels 15 mg/dl or higher [39]. The authors concluded that tocilizumab may exert its effects in patients progressing to an inflammatory state. It is noteworthy that, tocilizumab was administered on the principal day (a single dose of 400 mg, repeated in case of deterioration) of ICU stay in this study. However, a preprint of the RCT comparing tocilizumab to placebo revealed that tocilizumab failed to improve mortality at day 28. A considerable positive aspect of this study is tocilizumab reduced the duration of ICU stay by 5 days [40].

Extracorporeal cytokine removal therapies have been used for patients with septic shock. The rationale behind the cytokine removal in these patients is to limit the ensuing end-organ damage due to propagated inflammation. Additionally, lung-kidney crosstalk has been proposed recently in ARDS patients [41]. Although the direct mechanism is still not definite, cytokine overproduction and renal medullar hypoxia seem to be relatable [42]. Continuous Renal Replacement Therapy with high and middle cut-off membranes can selectively filter or absorb middleweight molecules, such as IL-6. Subsequently, blood purification therapies were put forward for COVID-19, also. However, only a few case reports reported the benefit of such therapies in this population, and future trials are awaited for definite evidence [43, 44].

Convalescent plasma is collected from the patients who have contracted and recovered from the disease. It has been used for previous pandemics, such as H1N1, SARS, and Ebola, and MERS. Initial case reports showed clinical benefit and reduced mortality in COVID-19 patients, also. Virus load decreased significantly and patients were soon virus negative. A subsequent RCT comparing convalescent plasma to standard treatment showed some clinical improvement in severely ill patients but not in critically ill patients. Likely, pathologic process in those receiving mechanical ventilation and in shock was probably irreversible. Given that the median time between symptom onset and randomization in this study was 30 days, earlier convalescent plasma administration may show better results in the critically ill. Additionally, the study was underpowered to detect significance between the groups. A high-titer antibody may have efficacy against SARS-CoV-2 [45, 46].

Conclusion

COVID -19 has caused tremendous constraints on the healthcare system and workers, as well as the patients. The first wave took the clinicians by surprise as many institutions did not have any structured plan to deal with a pandemic; we should not be surprised twice. However, we are now more prepared for patient surges in the intensive care units albeit lacking evidence-based treatment options for the critically ill COVID-19 patients [2].

REFERENCES

[1] Grasselli G, Zangrillo A, Zanella A, Antonelli M, Cabrini L, Castelli A, et al. Baseline Characteristics and Outcomes of 1591 Patients Infected With SARS-CoV-2 Admitted to ICUs of the Lombardy Region, Italy. *JAMA.* 2020 Apr 28;323(16):1574–81.

[2] Chand S, Kapoor S, Orsi D, Fazzari M J, Tanner T G, Umeh G C, et al. COVID-19-Associated Critical Illness—Report of the First 300 Patients Admitted to Intensive Care Units at a New York City Medical Center. *J. Intensive Care Med.* 2020 Oct 1;35(10):963–70.

[3] Aziz S, Arabi Y M, Alhazzani W, Evans L, Citerio G, Fischkoff K, et al. Managing ICU surge during the COVID-19 crisis: rapid guidelines. *Intensive Care Med.* 2020 Jun 8;1–23.

[4] Harris S, Singer M, Sanderson C, Grieve R, Harrison D, Rowan K. Impact on mortality of prompt admission to critical care for deteriorating ward patients: an instrumental variable analysis using critical care bed strain. *Intensive Care Med.* 2018 May;44(5):606–15.

[5] Dara S I, Afessa B. Intensivist-to-Bed Ratio: Association With Outcomes in the Medical ICU. *Chest.* 2005 Aug 1;128(2):567–72.

[6] Phua J, Weng L, Ling L, Egi M, Lim C-M, Divatia J V, et al. Intensive care management of coronavirus disease 2019 (COVID-19): challenges and recommendations. *The Lancet Respiratory Medicine*. 2020 May 1;8(5):506–17.

[7] Coppo A, Bellani G, Winterton D, Di Pierro M, Soria A, Faverio P, et al. Feasibility and physiological effects of prone positioning in non-intubated patients with acute respiratory failure due to COVID-19 (PRON-COVID): a prospective cohort study. *The Lancet Respiratory Medicine.* 2020 Aug 1;8(8):765–74.

[8] Fan E, Beitler J R, Brochard L, Calfee C S, Ferguson N D, Slutsky AS, et al. COVID-19-associated acute respiratory distress syndrome: is a different approach to management warranted? *The Lancet Respiratory Medicine.* 2020 Aug 1;8(8):816–21.

[9] Murthy S, Gomersall C D, Fowler R A. Care for Critically Ill Patients With COVID-19. *JAMA.* 2020 Apr 21;323(15):1499–500.

[10] Hager D N, Krishnan J A, Hayden D L, Brower R G. Tidal Volume Reduction in Patients with Acute Lung Injury When Plateau Pressures Are Not High. *Am. J. Respir. Crit. Care Med.* 2005 Nov 15;172(10):1241–5.

[11] Neto A S, Cardoso S O, Manetta J A, Pereira V G M, Espósito D C, Pasqualucci M de O P, et al. Association Between Use of Lung-Protective Ventilation With Lower Tidal Volumes and Clinical Outcomes Among Patients Without Acute Respiratory Distress Syndrome: A Meta-analysis. *JAMA.* 2012 Oct 24;308(16):1651–9.

[12] Broccard A F, Shapiro R S, Schmitz L L, Ravenscraft S A, Marini J J. Influence of prone position on the extent and distribution of lung injury in a high tidal volume oleic acid model of acute respiratory distress syndrome. *Critical Care Medicine.* 1997 Jan;25(1):16–27.

[13] Zhang Q, Shen J, Chen L, Li S, Zhang W, Jiang C, et al. Timing of invasive mechanic ventilation in critically ill patients with coronavirus disease 2019. *Journal of Trauma and Acute Care Surgery* [Internet]. 2020 Sep 23 [cited 2020 Sep 29]; Publish Ahead of Print. Available from: https://journals.lww.com/jtrauma/Abstract/9000/Timing_of_invasive_mechanic_ventilation_in.97731.aspx.

[14] Lee Y H, Choi K-J, Choi S H, Lee S Y, Kim K C, Kim E J, et al. Clinical Significance of Timing of Intubation in Critically Ill Patients with COVID-19: A Multi-Center Retrospective Study. *Journal of Clinical Medicine.* 2020 Sep; 9(9):2847.

[15] Azoulay E, de Waele J, Ferrer R, Staudinger T, Borkowska M, Povoa P, et al. International variation in the management of severe COVID-19 patients. *Critical Care.* 2020 Aug 5;24(1):486.

[16] Villar J, Ferrando C, Martínez D, Ambrós A, Muñoz T, Soler J A, et al. Dexamethasone treatment for the acute respiratory distress syndrome: a multicentre, randomised controlled trial. *The Lancet Respiratory Medicine.* 2020 Mar 1;8(3):267–76.

[17] RECOVERY Collaborative Group, Horby P, Lim WS, Emberson JR, Mafham M, Bell JL, et al. Dexamethasone in Hospitalized Patients with Covid-19 - Preliminary Report. *N. Engl. J. Med.* 2020 Jul 17;

[18] Writing Committee for the REMAP-CAP Investigators, Angus D C, Derde L, Al-Beidh F, Annane D, Arabi Y, et al. Effect of Hydrocortisone on Mortality and Organ Support in Patients With Severe COVID-19: The REMAP-CAP COVID-19 Corticosteroid Domain Randomized Clinical Trial. *JAMA.* 2020 Sep 2;

[19] Tomazini B M, Maia I S, Cavalcanti A B, Berwanger O, Rosa R G, Veiga V C, et al. Effect of Dexamethasone on Days Alive and Ventilator-Free in Patients With Moderate or Severe Acute Respiratory Distress Syndrome and COVID-19: The CoDEX Randomized Clinical Trial. *JAMA* [Internet]. 2020 Sep 2 [cited 2020 Sep 24]; Available from: https://jamanetwork.com/journals/jama/ fullarticle/2770277.

[20] Dequin P-F, Heming N, Meziani F, Plantefève G, Voiriot G, Badié J, et al. Effect of Hydrocortisone on 21-Day Mortality or Respiratory Support Among Critically Ill Patients With COVID-19: A Randomized Clinical Trial. *JAMA* [Internet]. 2020 Sep 2 [cited 2020 Sep 24]; Available from: https://jamanetwork.com/journals/jama/fullarticle/2770276.

[21] Group TWREA for C-19 T (REACT) W, Sterne J A C, Murthy S, Diaz J V, Slutsky A S, Villar J, et al. Association Between Administration of Systemic Corticosteroids and Mortality Among Critically Ill Patients With COVID-19: A

Meta-analysis. *JAMA* [Internet]. 2020 Sep 2 [cited 2020 Sep 24]; Available from: https://jamanetwork.com/journals/jama/fullarticle/2770279.

[22] Prescott H C, Rice T W. Corticosteroids in COVID-19 ARDS: Evidence and Hope During the Pandemic. *JAMA* [Internet]. 2020 Sep 2 [cited 2020 Sep 24]; Available from: https://jamanetwork.com/ journals/jama/fullarticle/2770275.

[23] Huang I, Pranata R, Lim M A, Oehadian A, Alisjahbana B. C-reactive protein, procalcitonin, D-dimer, and ferritin in severe coronavirus disease-2019: a meta-analysis: *Therapeutic Advances in Respiratory Disease* [Internet]. 2020 Jul 2 [cited 2020 Sep 29]; Available from: https://journals.sagepub.com/doi/10.1177/175346 6620937175?url_ver=Z39.88-2003&rfr_id=ori%3Arid%3Acrossref. org&rfr_dat=cr_pub++0pubmed.

[24] Rouhezamin M R, Haseli S. Diagnosing Pulmonary Thromboembolism in COVID-19: A Stepwise Clinical and Imaging Approach. *Acad. Radiol.* 2020 Jun; 27(6):896–7.

[25] Oudkerk M, Büller H R, Kuijpers D, van Es N, Oudkerk S F, McLoud T, et al. Diagnosis, Prevention, and Treatment of Thromboembolic Complications in COVID-19: Report of the National Institute for Public Health of the Netherlands. *Radiology.* 2020 Apr 23; 297(1):E216–22.

[26] Cui S, Chen S, Li X, Liu S, Wang F. Prevalence of venous thromboembolism in patients with severe novel coronavirus pneumonia. *Journal of Thrombosis and Haemostasis*. 2020; 18 (6):1421–4.

[27] Dujardin R W G, Hilderink B N, Haksteen W E, Middeldorp S, Vlaar APJ, Thachil J, et al. Biomarkers for the prediction of venous thromboembolism in critically ill COVID-19 patients. *Thrombosis Research*. 2020 Dec 1; 196:308–12.

[28] Wichmann D, Sperhake J-P, Lütgehetmann M, Steurer S, Edler C, Heinemann A, et al. Autopsy Findings and Venous Thromboembolism in Patients With COVID-19. *Annals of Internal Medicine.* 2020 May 6;173(4):268–77.

[29] Thachil J, Tang N, Gando S, Falanga A, Cattaneo M, Levi M, et al. ISTH interim guidance on recognition and management of coagulopathy in COVID-19. *Journal of Thrombosis and Haemostasis.* 2020;18(5):1023–6.

[30] Flaczyk A, Rosovsky R P, Reed C T, Bankhead-Kendall B K, Bittner EA, Chang MG. Comparison of published guidelines for management of coagulopathy and thrombosis in critically ill patients with COVID 19: implications for clinical practice and future investigations. *Critical Care.* 2020 Sep 16;24(1):559.

[31] Sakr Y, Dubois M-J, De Backer D, Creteur J, Vincent J-L. Persistent microcirculatory alterations are associated with organ failure and death in patients with septic shock*. *Critical Care Medicine.* 2004 Sep; 32(9):1825.

[32] Obi A T, Barnes GD, Wakefield T W, Brown S, Eliason J L, Arndt E, et al. Practical diagnosis and treatment of suspected venous thromboembolism during

COVID-19 pandemic. *Journal of Vascular Surgery: Venous and Lymphatic Disorders.* 2020 Jul 1;8(4):526–34.

[33] Sinha P, Matthay M A, Calfee CS. Is a "Cytokine Storm" Relevant to COVID-19? *JAMA Intern. Med.* 2020 Sep 1;180(9):1152–4.

[34] Manson J J, Crooks C, Naja M, Ledlie A, Goulden B, Liddle T, et al. COVID-19-associated hyperinflammation and escalation of patient care: a retrospective longitudinal cohort study. *The Lancet Rheumatology.* 2020 Oct 1; 2(10):e594–602.

[35] Hedrick T L, Murray B P, Hagan R S, Mock J R. COVID-19: Clean up on IL-6. *Am. J. Respir. Cell Mol. Biol.* 2020 Aug 4; rcmb.2020-0277LE.

[36] Maier B, Laurer H-L, Rose S, Buurman W a., Marzi I. Physiological Levels of Pro- and Anti-Inflammatory Mediators in Cerebrospinal Fluid and Plasma: A Normative Study. *Journal of Neurotrauma.* 2005 Jul 1;22(7):822–35.

[37] Bauer T T, Montón C, Torres A, Cabello H, Fillela X, Maldonado A, et al. Comparison of systemic cytokine levels in patients with acute respiratory distress syndrome, severe pneumonia, and controls. *Thorax.* 2000 Jan 1;55(1):46–52.

[38] Kox M, Waalders N J B, Kooistra E J, Gerretsen J, Pickkers P. Cytokine Levels in Critically Ill Patients With COVID-19 and Other Conditions. *JAMA.*

[39] Biran N, Ip A, Ahn J, Go R C, Wang S, Mathura S, et al. Tocilizumab among patients with COVID-19 in the intensive care unit: a multicentre observational study. *The Lancet Rheumatology.* 2020 Oct 1; 2(10):e603–12.

[40] Furlow B. COVACTA trial raises questions about tocilizumab's benefit in COVID-19. *Lancet Rheumatol.* 2020 Oct; 2(10):e592.

[41] Panitchote A, Mehkri O, Hastings A, Hanane T, Demirjian S, Torbic H, et al. Factors associated with acute kidney injury in acute respiratory distress syndrome. *Ann. Intensive Care.* 2019 Jul 1; 9(1):74.

[42] Ronco C, Reis T. Kidney involvement in COVID-19 and rationale for extracorporeal therapies. *Nat Rev Nephrol.* 2020;16(6):308–10.

[43] Padala S A, Vakiti A, White J J, Mulloy L, Mohammed A. First Reported Use of Highly Adsorptive Hemofilter in Critically Ill COVID-19 Patients in the USA. *J. Clin. Med. Res.* 2020 Jul; 12 (7):454–7.

[44] Shareef K A, Bakouri M. Cytokine Blood Filtration Responses in COVID-19. *BPU.* 2020 May 28; 1–9.

[45] Casadevall A, Joyner MJ, Pirofski L-A. A Randomized Trial of Convalescent Plasma for COVID-19—Potentially Hopeful Signals. *JAMA.* 2020 Aug 4; 324(5):455–7.

[46] Li L, Zhang W, Hu Y, Tong X, Zheng S, Yang J, et al. Effect of Convalescent Plasma Therapy on Time to Clinical Improvement in Patients With Severe and Life-threatening COVID-19: A Randomized Clinical Trial. *JAMA.* 2020 Aug 4; 324(5):460–70.

In: Coronavirus Disease
Editor: Yildiz Dincer

ISBN: 978-1-53619-296-4

Chapter 7

ANATOMICAL BASIS OF THE COVID-19

Mehmet Üzel*, MD, PhD and Ö. Alp Taştan, MD
İstanbul University-Cerrahpaşa, Cerrahpaşa Medical Faculty, Department of Anatomy, İstanbul, Turkey

ABSTRACT

The system most affected by the corona virus disease (COVID-19) is the respiratory system. Typical symptoms of the disease and most of the diagnostic and treatment interventions are related to the respiratory system. In this chapter, we address the basic anatomy of the respiratory system, the anatomical background of some of the respiratory-system-related symptoms of the disease, basic clinical anatomy of some of the diagnostic interventions, and to shed some light on the rationale behind some of the clinical interventions applied during the treatment of the disease. In this chapter, readers will find basic clinical anatomy information about of the nasopharyngeal sampling, tracheostomy, pulmonary volumes and capacities, and effects of the prone position on the prognosis of the patients.

Keywords: anatomy, sampling, prone position

INTRODUCTION

Severe acute respiratory syndrome coronavirus 2 (SARS-CoV-2) affects many systems in the body but most of the typical symptoms of its disease (COVID-19) are related to the respiratory system. The typical symptoms of COVID-19 are fever, dry

* Corresponding Author's Email: muzel@istanbul.edu.tr.

cough, fatigue, sputum production, and dyspnea [1-3]. When the clinic of the COVID-19 is considered, microbiology, immunology, biochemistry, internal medicine, pharmacology, intensive care, and radiology are some of the medical areas that come into mind firstly; anatomy is not one of them in general. On the other hand, some diagnostic interventions (such as nasopharyngeal and oropharyngeal samplings, bronchoalveolar lavage), some of the clinical interventions (such as intubation, tracheostomy, prone positioning) necessitates firm anatomical knowledge to apply them properly or to understand the rationale behind them. This chapter aims to give basic clinical anatomy information about the clinic of the COVID-19.

Basic Anatomy of the Upper Respiratory Tract

Coronavirus transmission occurs via respiratory droplets, and the first entry point is mainly the upper respiratory tract [1, 4]. The upper respiratory tract is the first part of the conducting portion of the respiratory system. Nose, pharynx, and larynx are the main parts of the tract [5, 6].

Nose

The nose is the first part of the airway and can be subdivided into external nose and nasal cavity. Air enters through the external nose, which is the pyramidal-shaped portion that projects from the face, via two elliptical openings called nostrils or nares. These openings are separated by the nasal septum and covered laterally by alae (wings) of the nose. Nostril dimensions vary greatly among individuals. They approximately measure 0,5-1 cm horizontally and 1,5-2 cm anteroposteriorly, with a narrowing in front. The supporting skeleton of the external nose is made up of bone and hyaline cartilage. Bony part is composed of two nasal bones, the frontal process and the anterior nasal spine of maxillae, the nasal part of the frontal bone and, the bony parts of nasal septum. Paired lateral nasal cartilage, which is continuous with septal cartilage, and two alar cartilages form the cartilaginous part [6-8].

Nasal Cavity

The nasal cavity is located between the roof of the oral cavity and the cranial base. It is divided into two halves by the nasal septum, which is formed by the perpendicular plate of ethmoid, vomer, and septal cartilage. The anterior part of the cavity, which is covered by alar cartilage, is called the nasal vestibule. Air enters the cavity via nostrils into the nasal vestibule and travels through the cavity until it reaches the choanae or the posterior nasal aperture, where the nasal cavity opens into the nasopharynx. The adult choanae usually measure 2,5 cm and 1,3 cm in height and width, respectively. Each half of the nasal cavity possesses a roof, a medial and lateral wall, and a floor. The roof can be examined in three parts. The anterior (frontonasal) part is formed by the frontal and nasal bones. This part slopes upwards and backward to form the bridge of the nose. The Central (ethmoidal) part is horizontal and is formed by the cribriform plate of the ethmoid bone which separates the anterior cranial fossa from the nasal cavity. The posterior (sphenoidal) part is a downward-sloping segment that is formed by the anterior part of the sphenoid bone. The floor extends from the anterior to the posterior aperture and has a smooth and concave surface. It slopes up from anterior to posterior. The palatine processes of maxillae and horizontal plates of palatine bones form the floor of the nasal cavity. The medial walls of both halves of the nasal cavity are formed by the nasal septum. The lateral wall is the broadest and the most complicated one among the walls of the nasal cavity. From anterior to posterior, the maxilla, the labyrinth of the ethmoid, and the perpendicular plate of the palatine bone from the lateral wall. Besides, this wall contains three scroll-like projections of bone called superior, middle, and inferior conchae (turbinates). The superior and middle conchae are medial processes of the ethmoidal labyrinth, whereas the inferior conchae are independent bones. The space underlying each concha is named meatus. Air passes through these meatuses and becomes turbulent. Turbulence keeps air in the cavity for a longer period, so it helps the inhaled air become warmer and humidified. There are several openings which connect the nasal cavity with other structures. The spheno-ethmoidal recess, located superoposterior to the superior concha, receives the opening of the sphenoidal sinus, and the superior nasal meatus receives the openings of posterior ethmoidal sinuses. Middle ethmoidal cells form a rounded elevation at the middle nasal meatus called ethmoidal bulla, on which they open. Below the ethmoidal bulla lies a semi-circular groove called semilunar hiatus. The maxillary sinus opens into the nasal cavity via semilunar hiatus. This hiatus curves in front of the ethmoidal bulla and forms a funnel-shaped passage called the ethmoidal infundibulum, which drains the frontal sinus. The inferior nasal meatus is the longest nasal meatus and it receives the opening of the nasolacrimal duct, which drains tears from the lacrimal sac [6-9].

Paranasal Sinuses

Frontal bone, ethmoid bone, sphenoid, and maxilla houses air-filled cavities, which are named after the bones they are located in, called paranasal sinuses. These sinuses, lined with respiratory epithelium, help to warm and humidifying the inhaled air, add resonance to the voice, and decrease skull bone weight. Only maxillary and ethmoidal sinus are present at birth. All sinuses enlarge and become fully developed at adolescence [5-8].

Pharynx

Pharynx is a cone-shaped muscular tube which belongs to both alimentary and respiratory systems. It lies between the cranial base and C6 vertebra, posterior to nasal cavities, oral cavity, and larynx. Pharynx has three parts; nasopharynx, oropharynx, and laryngopharynx. Choanae connects the nasal cavities to the nasopharynx, isthmus of fauces (oropharyngeal isthmus) connects the oral cavity to the oropharynx, and the laryngeal inlet connects the laryngeal cavity to laryngopharynx. The nasopharynx is found above the soft palate behind nasal cavities. Mucosa covering the inferior part of the body of the sphenoid and the basilar part of the occipital bone form the roof and the superior portion of the posterior wall of the nasopharynx. In the middle part of the junction of the roof and the posterior wall, a lymphoid tissue called the pharyngeal tonsil (adenoid) is found. The pharyngeal opening of the pharyngotympanic (Eustachian) tube occupies the lateral wall of the nasopharynx on both sides. The opening is located approximately 1 cm posterior and just below the posterior end of the inferior nasal concha. The superoposterior part of the opening has an elevation called torus tubarius. Under the mucosa covering the torus tubarius, a mass of lymphoid tissue, called tubal tonsils (Gerlach's tonsil), can be found. The salpingopharyngeal fold, which covers the salpingopharyngeal muscle, descends posterior to the torus tubarius. A small depression, called pharyngeal recess (fossa of Rosenmüller), which extends posteriorly and laterally, is also located posterior to the torus tubarius. The oropharynx is the middle part of the pharynx and is located posterior to the oral cavity, between the soft palate and the superior border of the epiglottis. It has both digestive and respiratory functions. The anterior part of its lateral wall is bordered by two arches; palatoglossal arch and palatopharyngeal arch. Palatine tonsil is located between these two arches. The inferior part of the anterior wall of the oropharynx is made by the root of the tongue. There is a collection of lymphoid tissue under the mucosa covering the root of the tongue, called lingual tonsil. Single pharyngeal tonsil, bilateral tubal tonsils, bilateral palatine tonsils, and single lingual tonsil form a lymphoid ring at the pharynx. This ring is called the pharyngeal lymphoid ring or Waldeyer's ring. It acts as the first line of defense for infections. Laryngopharynx is the inferior part of the pharynx. It is located between hyoid bone (the level of C3 vertebra) or the upper margin of the epiglottis and the inferior border of the cricoid cartilage (the level of C6 vertebra) or the superior border of the oesophagus. Laryngeal inlet is located on the anterior wall, and has two depressions on each side, called piriform fossa (recess) [5-9].

Larynx

Larynx is a specialized organ that functions as a sphincter for air passage and responsible for voice production. It is located at the anterior part of the neck, between laryngopharynx and trachea. The supporting skeleton of the larynx is composed of hyaline cartilages, which are connected by membranes and ligaments, and moved by muscles. There are nine cartilages that forms the framework; thyroid cartilage (1), cricoid cartilage (1), epiglottis (1), arytenoid cartilage (2), corniculate cartilage (2), and cuneiform cartilage (2). Thyrohyoid membrane is a broad structure that connects the hyoid bone to the superior border of thyroid cartilage. Internal branch of the superior laryngeal nerve and the superior laryngeal vessels pass through this membrane. Cricotracheal ligament attaches the cricoid cartilage to the first ring of the trachea. Quadrangular membrane is stretched between the lateral border of the epiglottis and anterolateral face of the arytenoid cartilage on the same side. The free inferior border of this membrane thickens to form the vestibular ligament which then constitutes the vestibular fold when covered with mucosa. Cricothyroid membrane extends between thyroid cartilage and cricoid cartilage. In cases of emergency (laryngeal obstruction), it is recommended to perform a laryngotomy at the site of this membrane. Conus elasticus (cricovocal membrane) also attaches to the superior border of cricoid cartilage inferiorly but it has a free superior border which forms the vocal ligaments on each side. Vocal ligaments then form the vocal folds when covered by mucosa. The gap between the vocal folds is called rima glottidis. The muscles of larynx can be categorized as extrinsic and intrinsic muscles. Extrinsic muscles (digastric, stylohyoid, mylohyoid, geniohyoid, stylopharyngeus, salpingopharyngeus, palatopharyngeus, sternothyroid, sternohyoid, omohyoid muscles) are mainly responsible for elevation and depression of the larynx whereas the intrinsic muscles (oblique arytenoid, transverse arytenoid, thyroepiglottic, cricothyroid, thyroarytenoid (vocalis), lateral cricoarytenoid, posterior cricoarytenoid muscles) are responsible for phonation and sphincter function of the larynx [5-9].

Anatomy of Olfactory Dysfunction

The lining of the nasal cavities consists mainly of respiratory epithelium, except for the nasal vestibule and the olfactory cleft where the olfactory epithelium is present [6]. The olfactory epithelium (mucosa) contains olfactory receptor nerve cells, which enter through the cribriform plate of the ethmoid bone [8]. Olfactory mucosa lines approximately 5-9 cm^2 of the total 150 cm^2 mucosal area covering the nasal cavities, including structures that are superoposterioly located in the nasal cavity [6, 10]. The spike of SARS-CoV-2 uses the host receptor Angiotensin-Converting Enzyme 2 (ACE2), which is found abundantly in the respiratory epithelium, to enter the cells [1, 3]. The olfactory epithelium and respiratory epithelium are closely related, so it is only natural for COVID-19 to cause olfactory dysfunction due to the neurotropic properties of the virus [10, 11].

Anatomy of Ocular Transmission

Lacrimal gland, which is located in the superolateral portion of the orbit, constantly produces tears [6, 7]. Some tears are absorbed by cornea and conjunctiva or evaporate [6, 12]. Remaining tears are drained by lacrimal canaliculi into the lacrimal sac. Then tears pass through a 12 mm long nasolacrimal duct to reach the upper respiratory tract via an opening located at the inferior nasal meatus [6, 12]. This transport allows pathogens like SARS-CoV-2 from conjunctival or corneal epithelium, which expresses ACE2, to be transferred to the respiratory epithelium [10, 12].

Anatomy for Upper Respiratory Tract Sampling

For diagnostic testing for SARS-CoV-2 in patients who meet the diagnostic criteria, that are put forward by World Health Organization (WHO), Central for Disease Control and Prevention (CDC) recommends collecting upper respiratory system specimens [1, 13]. These samples include nasopharyngeal swaps, oropharyngeal swaps, mid-turbine swap, nasal swab, and nasopharyngeal wash/aspirate or nasal wash/aspirate [1, 13, 14]. Anatomy knowledge of the respiratory system is required to collect these specimens safely and correctly [4, 15]. Nasopharyngeal and oropharyngeal swaps are frequently used [4], therefore anatomic considerations for both will be discussed below.

Nasopharyngeal Swab

Nasopharyngeal swap is recommended by WHO as a reference diagnostic method in COVID-19 [16]. Specimen is collected by inserting a flexible swab stick through the nostril [13]. Tilting the patient's head slightly posterior is recommended to make the nasal passages more accessible [4, 17]. The swap is inserted parallel to the palate along the floor of the nasal cavity until encountering a resistance that indicates contact with the nasopharynx or reaching the estimated distance [4, 13]. The distance between nostrils to the nasopharynx is approximately 9,4 cm in females and 10 cm in males [18]. The required distance can also be estimated by measuring the distance between nostrils (or the philtrum) and tragus, which is roughly 5 cm longer than the distance between nostrils and the nasopharynx in both genders [4, 13, 18]. The swap should not be directed medially, because the nasal septum contains anastomosis of arterioles and veins that are prone to bleeding [4, 6]. The most notable one is the Kiesselbach's plexus (Little's area) which is formed at the anterior part of the nasal septum by the anterior ethmoidal artery (from the ophthalmic artery), the posterior ethmoidal artery (from the ophthalmic artery), the sphenopalatine artery (from the maxillary artery), the greater palatine artery (from the maxillary artery), and the septal branch of the superior labial artery [4, 6, 7].

Oropharyngeal Swab

Oropharyngeal swab shows a lower positive rate than nasopharyngeal swab but has a lower risk of bleeding compared to nasopharyngeal swab [2, 4]. The swab is inserted through the mouth and the specimen is collected from the posterior wall of the oropharynx and over the palatine tonsils.

Basic Anatomy of the Lower Respiratory Tract

The airways below the larynx are collectively called tracheobronchial tree. The tracheobronchial tree is morphologically divided into trachea, bronchi, bronchioli, and alveoli.

Trachea is the first and most superior part of the tracheobronchial tree. The trachea is mobile and has a tubular form. It starts from the lower border of the cricoid cartilage of the larynx at the C6 vertebra level and ends at the tracheal bifurcation at the level of the intervertebral disc between T4 and T5 vertebrae. The tracheal bifurcation may rise about one vertebral level during expiration, and lower to T6 vertebral (or manubriosternal junction, i.e., angle of Louis) level during deep inspiration. The length of the trachea is between 10 and 15 cm [6, 9], and its cross-sectional area is about 3 cm^2 in adults [19]. The size of the trachea is correlated with the size of the person. The general rule is that the width of the trachea is the same as the diameter of the index finger of the same person. The external transverse diameter of the trachea is approximately 2-2,5 cm in adult males, approximately 1,5 cm in adult females, and approximately 0,5 cm in infants [6, 7, 20]. It consists of 16-20 C-shaped hyaline cartilages. These cartilages are oriented horizontally, and their convex surfaces are directed anteriorly. A fibroelastic tissue connects tracheal cartilages. Because the tracheal cartilages are C-shaped and the posterior wall, which is composed of smooth muscle (i.e., tracheal muscle), is flattened, the cross-section of the trachea is D shaped.

The cervical part of the trachea is between the lower border of the cricoid cartilage and the thoracic inlet. This part of the trachea has important relations regarding the tracheostomy. The jugular arch, sternohyoid and sternothyroid muscles, isthmus of the thyroid gland (in front of the 2.-4. tracheal cartilages), an anastomotic branch of the superior thyroid arteries, inferior thyroid veins, thyroid ima artery (variation) are located anteriorly; in children, the brachiocephalic trunk crosses in front of the trachea at or a little above the upper border of the manubrium of the sternum. The oesophagus is posterior to the trachea. The common carotid arteries, inferior thyroid arteries, lobes of the thyroid glands are located lateral to the trachea. The recurrent laryngeal nerves ascend in the tracheoesophageal groove. The cervical part is supplied by inferior thyroid artery, and innervated by the vagal branches and sympathetic trunk [6].

The thoracic part of the trachea is located within the superior mediastinum. It bifurcates at the level of the sternal angle (manubriosternal junction, angle of Louis) into two main bronchi for each lung, passing inferolateral to enter the lungs at their hila. The right main bronchus is wider, shorter, and runs more vertically than the left one as it passes directly to the hilum of the lung. The left main bronchus passes inferolateral, inferior to the arch of the aorta and anterior to the esophagus and thoracic aorta, to reach the hilum of the lung. Because of differences in sizes and directions of the two main bronchi, inhaled foreign bodies tend to enter the right bronchus [6, 7, 20]. The cartilage at the tracheal bifurcation is the carina. If the sharp edge of the carina becomes flattened, this usually indicates enlargement of the hilar lymph nodes or gross distortion of the pulmonary anatomy by fibrosis, tumor, or other pathology [9].

Within the lungs, the bronchi branch to form the rest of the branches of the tracheobronchial tree. Each primary (main) bronchus divides into secondary (lobar) bronchi, each of which supplies a lobe of the lung. Each secondary bronchus divides into tertiary (segmental) bronchi that supply the bronchopulmonary segments. The bronchopulmonary segments are the largest subdivisions of a lobe. They have a pyramidal shape, and their apices are directed towards the root of the lung. They are supplied independently by a segmental bronchus and a tertiary branch of the pulmonary artery. There are usually 10 segments in each lung, but this number is subject to variation. Because each segment has separate bronchial, vascular, lymphatic, and nervous supply, they are surgically resectable [6, 7, 20]. After the tertiary segmental bronchi, bronchioles start. There are 20-25 generations of bronchioles that end as terminal bronchioles. Bronchioles lack cartilage in their walls. Each terminal bronchiole gives rise to several respiratory bronchioles, which have alveoli extending from their lumens. The pulmonary alveolus is the basic structural unit of gas exchange in the lung. Each respiratory bronchiole gives rise to 2-11 alveolar ducts, each of which gives rise to 5-6 alveolar sacs. Alveolar ducts are elongated airways densely lined with alveoli, leading to the alveolar sacs, into which alveoli open. The total number of the alveoli in the adult is between 300-400 million [6, 7, 20, 21], and the total surface area is approximately 140 m^2 [19].

Anatomy of the Tracheostomy

Tracheostomy is the creation of a hole in the anterior aspect of the trachea. This intervention is applied during clinical situations such as upper airways obstructions, laryngeal and craniofacial traumas, laryngeal edema, and laryngeal cancers. The hole can serve independently, or a tube can be inserted through it. After identifying the thyroid and cricoid cartilages, the neck is extended, and a vertical incision is made from the cricothyroid membrane to the suprasternal notch. Superficial fascia and the fibers of the platysma are dissected (anterior jugular veins should be avoided), investing fascia is incised, the pretracheal muscles are split. Depending on the decision of the physician, the second tracheal ring (which is superior to the isthmus of the thyroid gland), third to fifth tracheal rings (after dissecting the isthmus of the thyroid gland), or tracheal rings below the isthmus can be cut. The major structures around the trachea should be avoided during the procedure [6, 20].

Basic Anatomy of the Lungs

Lungs are soft and spongy organs, which are essential for respiration. Each lung consists of lobes, which are two on the left and three on the right side. Each lung is situated in the thoracic cavity on both sides of the mediastinum in their pleural cavities. In adults, right lung weighs approximately 620-625 g, and the left 565-570 g [6, 8, 9].

Each lung has a cone shape and has apex, base, three borders, and two surfaces. The apex of the lung is the part that extends superiorly through the thoracic inlet. It rises 3-4 cm above the first costal cartilage and is in contact with the cervical pleura, which is covered by suprapleural membrane (Sibson's fascia). The tip of the apex is 2,5-4 cm above medial third of the clavicle [6, 8, 9]. Base of the lung is deeply concave and sits on the diaphragm. Because the right half of the diaphragm is higher, the base of the right lung is deeper [6]. The costal surface is smooth and relates to the thoracic wall. The posterior costal surface is vertically longer than the anterior surface [6, 9]. The mediastinal surfaces of the lungs constitute the lateral walls of the mediastinum. The left mediastinal surface is closely related to the left ventricle and auricle, the arch of aorta, the left subclavian and common carotid arteries, left brachiocephalic vein, trachea, oesophagus, the left vagus, and the thoracic duct. The right mediastinal surface is closely related to the right atrium and right ventricle, superior and inferior vena cava, the azygos vein, the trachea, the right vagus, and phrenic nerves [6, 9]. The most peculiar feature of the mediastinal surface is the hilum, which is the site of entry and exit for the principal bronchus, pulmonary artery, pulmonary veins, bronchial vessels, pulmonary autonomic plexus, and lymphatic vessels. All these structures are enveloped by a pleural sleeve and are collectively called pulmonary root.

Cough Reflex

Cough is one of the most important defensive mechanisms of the respiratory system, and one of the most common symptoms of COVID-19 infection [1]. It clears the secretions and particles from the airways and serves protection against foreign material (including inflammation and mediators associated with inflammation) aspiration. The trachea (especially carina) and bronchi are very sensitive to light touch, and the terminal bronchioles and the alveoli are sensitive to corrosive chemical stimuli. Afferent nerve impulses from the airways pass mainly through the vagus nerves (CN X) to the medulla of the brain. There, an automatic sequence of events causes some sequential events: 2,5 L of air is inspired rapidly, the epiglottis and glottis close, abdominal and internal intercostal muscles contract forcefully, the pressure inside the lungs rises to 100 mmHg, the epiglottis and glottis open, air inside the lungs expelled with a very high velocity (75-100 miles/hour) [6, 22].

Pleura

Pleura is the serous membrane covering all the surfaces (except the hilum) of the lung, internal surface of the thoracic wall, and most of the superior surface of the diaphragm. Each lung has its own pleura. The pleura has two layers which are named according to their site of attachment: parietal pleura is attached to the thoracic wall and diaphragm, and the visceral pleura to the lung parenchyma [6, 9].

Muscles of Respiration

Respiration has two phases: inspiration and expiration. While the quiet and forced inspirations are active (accomplished by muscular activity), the expiration is passive (accomplished by elastic recoil of the tissues) in quite respiration but active in forced expiration. The muscles of respiration can be divided into two groups: inspiratory muscles and expiratory muscles. The primary inspiratory muscles are the diaphragm and the external intercostal muscles; secondary inspiratory muscles are sternocleidomastoid, scalene (anterior, middle, and posterior) muscles, and pectoralis major and minor. Primary expiratory muscles are the internal and innermost intercostal muscles; secondary expiratory muscles are transversus thoracis, subcostals, serratus posterior inferior, rectus abdominis, external and internal obliques, transversus abdominis, latissimus dorsi, and quadratus lumborum [6, 23]. Depending on the muscles used during inspiration, breathing can be grouped in two types: abdominal (diaphragmatic) breathing uses the diaphragm as the power generator, while the thoracic breathing uses external intercostal muscles as the power generator. Infants and small babies have ribs lying horizontally and weak intercostal muscles, so the diaphragm and abdomen are the primary means of ventilation [21].

Pulmonary Volumes and Capacities

Pulmonary volume (also known as lung volume or respiratory volume) refers to the volume of air in the lungs at a given phase of the respiratory cycle. A combination of the pulmonary volumes is called pulmonary capacity. There are four pulmonary volumes and four pulmonary capacities. The tidal volume is the volume of air inspired or expired with quiet respiration (~0,5L). The inspiratory reserve volume is the extra volume of air that can be inspired when the person inspires with full force (~3L). The expiratory reserve volume is the maximum extra volume of air that can be expired after the end of the tidal expiration (~1,1L). The residual volume is the volume of air remaining in the lungs after the most forceful expiration (~1,2L) [22]. The inspiratory capacity is the sum of the tidal volume and the inspiratory reserve volume (~3,5L). The functional residual capacity is the sum of the expiratory reserve volume and the residual volume (~2,3L). The vital capacity is the sum of the inspiratory reserve volume, the tidal volume, and the expiratory reserve volume (~4,6L). The total lung capacity is the maximum volume to which the lungs can be expanded with the maximum effort and is the sum of the vital capacity and the residual volume (~5,8L) [22].

Effect of the Prone Position on the Volumes, Perfusion, and Ventilation of the Lungs

During the COVID-19 pandemic, the media shared different images of hospitalized patients lying in prone position (PP) in intensive care units. PP is being used since 1970s to treat hypoxemia in patients who have acute respiratory distress syndrome (ARDS) [19, 24]. Treatment of the ARDS requires tracheal intubation and mechanical ventilation. PP was shown to be beneficial in ARDS patients; it may even postpone or avoid tracheal intubation [25]. PP improves gas exchange [19, 24, 25], provides more even tidal volume distribution in the lungs [24], improves resting lung volume in the dorsocaudal regions of the lungs [24], improves ventilation-perfusion relationship [19, 24, 25], improves peripheral oxygen saturation [25], ameliorates the severity or development of ventilator-induced lung injury [25], improves clearance of lung secretions [26], reduces neutrophil and pro-inflammatory mediator levels (IL-1β, IL-6, and 1 IL-8) in bronchoalveolar lavage fluid [24] and improves mortality in ARDS patients [19, 24, 25]. PP is most effective in improving oxygenation when initiated during the exudative phase of the ARDS [24]. PP improves lung mechanics, which occurs via changes in anatomical relationships.

PP has effects on the transpulmonary pressure (Ptp), and ventrodorsal transpulmonary pressure difference. The Ptp is defined as the difference between the alveolar pressure (Pal) and pleural pressure (Ppl). In supine position (SP), the dorsal Ppl raises (because of the compressive effect of the lung weight on the dorsal parts of the lung) and Ptp diminishes; ventral Ppl diminishes and Ptp increases. The net result is ventral alveoli are overinflated and the dorsal alveoli are underinflated (atelectasis) [19, 25, 27, 28]. PP diminishes the difference between ventral and dorsal Ptp; when the patient is in PP, larger mass of lungs is suspended from a wider posterior chest area and Ppl diminishes at the dorsal parts of the lungs. Because of this, dorsal Ptp increases, dorsal alveoli open, ventilation in the dorsal parts of the lungs improves, difference between ventral and dorsal Ptp decreases, and more uniform ventilation is achieved [19, 24, 27, 29].

The effect of the PP on the perfusion of the lungs is slight [27] and pulmonary perfusion is preferentially distributed to the dorsal lung regions in both SP and PP [24]. Because perfusion is unaffected and ventilation is diminished in the dorsal part of the lungs, V/Q ratio diminishes (V/Q mismatch). This mismatch creates a physiological shunt in the dorsal part of the lungs [29]. In PP, dorsal alveoli are inflated, ventilation is improved, V/Q mismatch improves, intrapulmonary shunt decreases (~50%) and oxygenation improves [24, 29].

When an ARDS patient lies in SP, the heart and diaphragm compress the dorsal lung parenchyma. Because of the compression of the lungs by either structure, hypoxemia increases, and ventilator-associated lung injury worsens [19, 24, 27, 29] and this effect is exacerbated by obesity [19]. In PP, heart lies on the sternum, compression of the heart on the dorsal lung parenchyma decreases, ventilation and oxygenation improves.

PP reduces neutrophil and pro-inflammatory mediators (IL-1β, IL-6, and IL-8) levels in bronchoalveolar lavage fluid. Of particular interest is IL-8, which is a chemo-attractant cytokine for neutrophils and secreted by the alveolar epithelium and macrophages in response to excessive stretch. The result of the neutrophil infiltration is proteolytic enzyme release that causes lung injury. PP creates more homogeneous pleural pressure gradients and more uniform strain-stress relationships throughout the lungs, so the stretch is released, IL-8 is secreted less, neutrophil attraction and lung injury diminishes [24].

In SP, ventral parts of the lungs are overinflated and overdistended, and dorsal parts open and collapse cyclically during mechanical ventilation. These changes cause ventilatory-induced lung injury that increases IL-6 expression. Another cause for increased levels of IL-6 is hyperoxemia during mechanical ventilation. In PP, ventilation becomes uniform in the lungs, need for mechanical ventilation diminishes, and FiO_2 lowers rapidly. As a result, IL-6 levels decrease [30].

CONCLUSION

For a proper and effective treatment of a disease, firm knowledge of pathology and pathophysiology of that disease is necessary. In COVID-19, the anatomy does not seem to be related to the clinic of the disease. However, basic clinical anatomy knowledge is necessary during some diagnostic (nasopharyngeal sampling, oropharyngeal sampling) and therapeutic (tracheostomy, prone positioning) treatments. Physicians applying those treatments should be aware of the potential risks, their prevention, and treatment, as well.

REFERENCES

[1] Harapan, H., Itoh, N., Yufika, A., Winardi, W., Keam, S., Te, H., et al. (2020). Coronavirus disease 2019 (COVID-19): A literature review. *Journal of Infection and Public Health*, 13 (5): 667-673.

[2] Wang, X., Tan, L., Wang, X., Liu, W., Lu, Y., Cheng, L., et al. (2020). Comparison of nasopharyngeal and oropharyngeal swabs for SARS-CoV-2 detection in 353 patients received tests with both specimens simultaneously. *International Journal of Infectious Diseases*, 94 107-109.

[3] Yuki, K., Fujiogi, M., and Koutsogiannaki, S. (2020). COVID-19 pathophysiology: A review. *Clinical Immunology*, 215 (April).

[4] Mawaddah, A., Gendeh, H. S., Lum, S. G., and Marina, M. B. (2020). Upper respiratory tract sampling in COVID-19. *Malaysian Journal of Pathology*, 42 (1): 23-35.

[5] McKinley, M. and O'Loughlin, V. (2012). *Human Anatomy*. 3rd Ed. McGraw-Hill.

[6] Standring, S. (2016). *Gray's Anatomy*. 41st Ed. Elsevier, Churchill Livingstone.

[7] Moore, K. L., Dalley, A. F., and Agur, A. M. R. (2018). *Clinically Oriented Anatomy*. 8th Ed. Lippincott Williams & Wilkins, Philadelphia.

[8] Snell, R. S. (2019). *Clinical Anatomy by Regions*. 10th Ed. Lippincott Williams & Wilkins, Philadelphia.

[9] Ellis, H., Feldman, S., and Harrop-Griffiths, W. (2004). *Anatomy for Anaesthetists.* 8th Ed. Blackwell Publishing, Oxford.

[10] Gengler, I., Wang, J. C., Speth, M. M., and Sedaghat, A. R. (2020). Sinonasal pathophysiology of SARS-CoV-2 and COVID-19: A systematic review of the current evidence. *Laryngoscope Investigative Otolaryngology*, 5 (3): 354-359.

[11] Baig, A. M., Khaleeq, A., Ali, U., and Syeda, H. (2020). Evidence of the COVID-19 Virus Targeting the CNS: Tissue Distribution, Host-Virus Interaction, and Proposed Neurotropic Mechanisms. *ACS Chemical Neuroscience*, 11 (7): 995-998.

[12] Sun, C. Bin, Wang, Y. Y., Liu, G. H., and Liu, Z. (2020). Role of the Eye in Transmitting Human Coronavirus: What We Know and What We Do Not Know. *Frontiers in Public Health*, 8 (April): 1-7.

[13] CDC (2020). Interim guidelines for collecting, handling, and testing clinical specimens from persons for coronavirus disease 2019 (COVID-19). *Centers for Disease Control and Prevention*, Accessed August 1, 2020.

[14] Singhal, T. (2020). A Review of Coronavirus Disease-2019 (COVID-19). *The Indian Journal of Pediatrics*, 87 (April): 281-286.

[15] Hong, K. H., Lee, S. W., Kim, T. S., Huh, H. J., Lee, J., Kim, S. Y., et al. (2020). Guidelines for Laboratory Diagnosis of Coronavirus Disease 2019 (COVID-19) in Korea. *Annals of Laboratory Medicine*, 40 (5): 351-360.

[16] Péré, H., Podglajen, I., Wack, M., Flamarion, E., Mirault, T., Goudot, G., et al. (2020). Nasal swab sampling for SARS-CoV-2: A convenient alternative in times of nasopharyngeal swab shortage. *Journal of Clinical Microbiology*, 58 (6): 2-3.

[17] Marty, F. M., Chen, K., and Verrill, K. A. (2020). How to obtain a nasopharyngeal swab specimen. *New England Journal of Medicine*, 382 (22): 2-3.

[18] Lim, H., Lee, J. H., Son, K. K., Han, Y. J., and Ko, S. (2014). A method for optimal depth of the nasopharyngeal temperature probe: The philtrum to tragus distance. *Korean Journal of Anesthesiology*, 66 (3): 195-198.

[19] Johnson, N. J., Luks, A. M., and Glenny, R. W. (2018). Gas exchange in the prone posture. *Respiratory Care*, 62 (8): 1097-1110.

[20] Snell, R. S. (2006). *Clinical Anatomy by Systems.* 1st Ed. Lippincott Williams & Wilkins, Philadelphia.

[21] MacGregor, J. (2008*). Introduction to the Anatomy and Physiology of Children.* 2nd Ed. Routledge, London.

[22] Guyton, A. C. and Hall, J. E. (2006). *Textbook of Medical Physiology*. Elsevier, Philadelphia.

[23] Palastanga, N. and Soames, R. W. (2012). *Anatomy and Human Movement: Structure and Function.* 6th Ed. Elsevier.

[24] Kallet, R. H. (2015). A comprehensive review of prone position in ARDS. *Respiratory Care*, 60 (11): 1660-1687.

[25] Coppo, A., Bellani, G., Winterton, D., Di Pierro, M., Soria, A., Faverio, P., et al. (2020). Feasibility and physiological effects of prone positioning in non-intubated patients with acute respiratory failure due to COVID-19 (PRON-COVID): a prospective cohort study. *The Lancet Respiratory Medicine*, 8 (8): 765-774.

[26] Valter, C., Christensen, A. M., Tollund, C., and Schønemann, N. K. (2003). Response to the prone position in spontaneously breathing patients with hypoxemic respiratory failure. *Acta Anaesthesiologica Scandinavica*, 47 (4): 416-418.

[27] Malhotra, A. and Kacmarek, R. M. (2020). Prone ventilation for patients with mild or moderate acute respiratory distress syndrome. *Annals of the American Thoracic Society*, 17 (1): 24-29.

[28] Polak, S. B., Van Gool, I. C., Cohen, D., von der Thüsen, J. H., and van Paassen, J. (2020). A systematic review of pathological findings in COVID-19: a pathophysiological timeline and possible mechanisms of disease progression. *Modern Pathology*.

[29] Pelosi, P., Caironi, P., Taccone, P., and Brazzi, L. (2001). Pathophysiology of prone positioning in the healthy lung and in ALI/ARDS. *Minerva Anestesiologica*, 67 (4): 238-247.

[30] Chan, M. C., Hsu, J. Y., Liu, H. H., Lee, Y. L., Pong, S. C., Chang, L. Y., et al. (2007). Effects of prone position on inflammatory markers in patients with ARDS due to community-acquired pneumonia. *Journal of the Formosan Medical Association*, 106 (9): 708-716.

In: Coronavirus Disease
Editor: Yildiz Dincer
ISBN: 978-1-53619-296-4

Chapter 8

GENETIC BACKGROUND OF DIFFERENCES IN THE INCIDENCE OF CORONA VIRUS INFECTION

R. Dilhan Kuru*[*]*, PhD and İlhan Onaran, PhD
Istanbul University- Cerrahpasa, Cerrahpasa Medical Faculty,
Department of Medical Biology, Istanbul, Turkey

ABSTRACT

Variability in susceptibility and disease severity in response to viral exposure is a distinctive feature of infectious diseases. It has also been noted a wide range of inter-individual variations in the infectivity, disease severity, and progression of COVID-19. Furthermore, it has been observed that susceptibility to COVID-19 shows geographical variation. Increasing evidence suggests a major role for host genes that affect viral infectivity and pathogenicity in explaining inter-individual and ethnic differences in susceptibility to coronavirus infections. Comparison of more than half a million genetic variants in individuals with the disease and population controls shows that many genes might be involved in susceptibility to COVID-19 infection. Some hypotheses have been proposed to explain how genes play a role in determining or influencing the efficacy of infection, the immune response to infection, or the severity of COVID-19 symptoms. These hypotheses include several genomic variants in the Angiotensin-Converting Enzyme, TMPRSS2, histocompatibility complex class I, and other few genes, the ABO blood group polymorphism, epigenetic alterations regulating host response, and telomere shortening, Throughout the recently published literature, we will discuss the recently published literature on host genetic factors related to coronaviruses, focusing on human studies in the context of COVID-19 susceptibility, severity, and progression as well as in geographical variation.

Keywords: COVID-19, SARS-CoV-2, genetics, susceptibility, genetic variation, clinical variability, gender difference

[*] Corresponding Author's Email: dilhank@istanbul.edu.tr.

Introduction

One of the most important research questions on the ongoing severe acute respiratory syndrome coronavirus 2 (SARS-CoV-2) pandemic is why some people are more susceptible than others to SARS-CoV-2? Additionally, it is now evident that susceptibility to COVID-19 shows geographical variation. There are enormous clinical variabilities between individuals infected with SARS-CoV-2. This condition is ranged from silent to fatal infections [1]; the reason for this is currently not clear. Hypotheses suggested explaining observed differences include age, biological sex, other prior existing health conditions, and genetic factors. A twin study reported that 50% of the variance of the 'predicted covid-19' phenotype is due to genetic factors [2]. As with many complex diseases, the reality for most individuals most likely involves a complex interaction of genetic (viral and host genetics) and non-genetic variables. As related to hosting genetic factors, multiple in silico and molecular prediction studies show that multiple genes can be crucially involved in infection and progression of COVID-19. The scientific community suggests that single nucleotide polymorphisms (SNPs), or commonly known gene polymor-phisms in the angiotensin-converting enzyme (ACE2), the transmembrane serine protease 2 (TMPRSS2), and other few genes reported, genetic variability in major histocompatibility complex (MHC) class I genes (human leukocyte antigen [HLA] A, B, and C), the ABO blood group polymorphism, epigenetic changes that might affect viral entry and replication, and excessive immune response to the virus, and telomere shortening may influence susceptibility to SARS-CoV-2 infection and the outcome of the COVID-19 disease. The preliminary results from the COVID-19 host genetics consortium which was established to discover and study the human genetic variants that modulate the susceptibility of developing COVID-19 symptoms and severity show several suggestively associated loci. However, very little is understood about the role of gene networks in determining or influencing the efficiency of infection and progression of COVID-19. Understanding these gene networks can situate susceptible individuals/populations, inform personalized treatment, and help vaccine development.

Throughout the recently published literature, we will focus on the most studied genetic variations which play a pivotal role in determining or influencing the efficacy of infection, the immune response to infection, or the severity of COVID-19 in the context of human studies.

Association of Sex Chromosomes with COVID-19

Gender difference has always been interesting in infectious disease research according to the World Health Organization (WHO) (as of April 18th, 2020). The male to female ratio among confirmed cases is 1.03:1 with a median age of 51 (interquartile range, IQR: 36–65) years [https://www.who.int/emergencies/diseases/novelcoronavirus2019/situation reports. Accessed 25 Apr 2020]. Interestingly, the International Organization for gender equality and health equity Global Health reports sex-disaggregated data as 50/50. The gender difference in response to COVID-19 infection may play a larger role in the clinical disparity. Often reported, men are more susceptible to coronavirus infection and severe prognosis of the disease. On the other hand, studies shown that Sry expression on the Y chromosome is related to the reduction of the immune response. As known, the X chromosome has about 3000 different genes and encoding for more than 800 miRNAs. Genes of importance for immune response are encoded on the X chromosome. X chromosome inactivation (XCI) provides an equivalent gene dosage for both sexes [4].

X Linked Genes and X Inactivation

During early female embryogenesis, one of the X chromosomes is inactivated to have an equal dosage in the products of X-linked genes in males and females [5, 6]. The XCI process is formed by a multistep epigenetic mechanism. However, inactivation is not uniform and one-third of X-chromosomal genes escape from inactivation. XCI is incomplete in humans with one-third of X-chromosomal genes been expressed from both active (Xa) and inactive (Xi) X chromosomes in human female cells. These genes that escape X inactivation have been called ‘escapers’. Many of these genes are located at the ends of each arm of the X chromosome in areas known as pseudoautosomal regions (PAR1 and PAR2). These regions are present on both sex chromosomes. The genes that escape from X-chromosome inactivation may transcribe as two working copies [7]. There are other genes escaping from XCI, besides the genes in the PAR regions. These genes are defined as showing >10% expression from the inactive X allele compared to the active X allele [8]. In addition, the evidence was reported that at least 23% of X-linked genes continue to be expressed by the inactive X chromosome, and this condition is leading to a female bias less than two folds in the expression levels [9]. These regions escaping from XCI are including immune-related factors. For example, toll-like receptors (TLRs) [4], and *ACE2* gene are biallelically expressed in females in keeping with their location to Xp22 within a chromosome region prone to escape XCI. The *TIMP1* (tissue inhibitor of metalloproteinase 1) gene encoding proteins involved in response to infections and septic shock, maps to Xp11, within a region enriched in dosage-sensitive genes with a low chance of escaping XCI and is characterized by a variable expression from the inactive X chromosome. However, there are regions with immune-related genes escaping silencing in female lymphocytes, such as *CXCR3* at Xq13, encoding a chemokine receptor and *CD40L* at Xq16 encoding CD40 ligand, a B cell costimulatory molecule member of the tumor necrosis factor (TNF) family, for which biallelic expression is restricted to some mature B and T cells. Because of a functional advantage, these cells become overexpressed in tissues involved in the immune response. In addition, it has been suggested that there are miRNA-223 at Xq12, a fine tuner of granulocyte production and the inflammatory response, and miRNA-424 at Xq26, regulating monocyte/macrophage differentiation [10]. Different females may have different levels of mosaicism according to the percentage of the cell population with the parental X chromosome preferentially inactivated. This process may occur randomly or by selection against the cell population with a pathogenic variant on the active X. But 10% of healthy females over 50 years have haploinsufficiency for X-linked genes in immune-related cells with reduction of variation in their expression, losing their advantage compared to males. It has been shown that females have the capability to stronger and adaptive immune response than males. Likewise, Larissa said that X-linked genes may have a role in the emergence and maintenance of different immune reactions against COVID-19 in women and men, but there is no study on this issue yet [11].

Toll-Like Receptor 7 (TLR7)

Anti-viral immunity includes both innate immune and adaptive immune responses. Innate immune receptors have two main varieties as transmembrane and cytosolic. This situation is important for innate immunity, and thus adaptive for immune responses. Toll-like receptors (TLRs) are a family of sensor proteins that help the immune system to differentiate between "self" and "non-self." TLR 3, 7, 8, and 9 are immune receptor which play role in host survival to viral infection [12]. They can detect the complete viral particles, including viral nucleic acid and viral envelope proteins, and defective viral particles [13]. Upon recognition of a virus, TLR signaling upregulates the expression of pro-inflammatory cytokines and costimulatory molecules, by the accumulation of type I interferons (IFNs) and IFN–stimulated genes (ISGs) [14, 15].

TLR7 activating by synthetic ligands such as imidazoquinolines is an endosomally located sensor. It is also a key component of antibody-mediated immunosuppression against the reactivation of endogenous retroviruses [12]. TLR7 detect single-stranded RNA viruses. It is expressed on variable immune cells such as plasmacytoid dendritic cells, B lymphocytes and myeloid cells, and non-immune cells including hepatocytes, epithelial cells, and keratinocytes [4]. After ligand binding, TLR7 dimerizes and activates signaling pathway involving myeloid differentiation primary response gene 88 (MyD88), mitogen-activated protein kinase (MAPK) cascades, NF-κB activation, as well as IFN regulatory factor (IRF)-7 and IRF-5 activation via IL-1 receptor-associated kinases (IRAK)-1/2/4 and TNF receptor-associated factor-3/6. As a result, pro-inflammatory cytokines (TNF-α, IL-6, IL-1β, IL-12) and IFN-α are produced, and TLR7 may stimulate

B cells to enhance antibody production [12]. It is reported that IL-6 is very important in the dysregulated host immune response of poor prognosis COVID-19 patients [16]. The lower susceptibility to viral infections in females is observed from birth to adulthood. It is accepted that females develop stronger innate and adaptive immune responses than males. The activity of the innate immune response was reported to vary between males and females. Firstly, the TLR7 expression level is increased in women. Biallelic expression of TLR7 has been found in immune cells of women (and Klinefelter syndrome males) and this results in higher TLR7 protein expression in leukocyte populations of females [12]. Secondly, higher IFN-α production in females was demonstrated by several *in vitro* studies using stimulation with synthetic TLR7 ligands. Berghöfer et al. suggested that female peripheral blood lymphocytes produced much higher IFN-α levels than males after TLR7 stimulation by a large cohort study of healthy individuals [16]. TLR7 expression is higher on the immune cells of females after puberty. Also, in XX females IFN-α production was always above than monosomy X (Turner's syndrome) females and XY males [4]. So, males have a relatively reduced antiviral immunity, since they produce a lesser amount of IFNs and inflammatory cytokines and possess a lower number of circulating T cells [11, 13]. Although females have stronger immunity, they also develop more autoimmune diseases than males [4].

HOST GENETIC FACTORS RELATED TO SARS-COV-2 ENTRY INTO HOST CELLS

Host genetic studies using both candidate-gene and genome-wide strategies approaches identified significant associations between SARS-CoV-1 susceptibility or outcome and genetic variations such as single nucleotide polymorphisms in the human genome. Some of these genetic variations are associated with the human genes required for SARS-Cov/CoV-2 entry. The endosomal cysteine protease cathepsin B and L, TMPRSS2, glucose-regulated protein 78 kDa (GRP78), and ACE2 are commonly exploited by SARS-CoV/CoV-2 for cellular entry. Single nucleotide polymorphism variants in the genes for these proteins have significant differences in frequencies among the population groups. Also, several polymorphisms of genes required for SARS-CoV/CoV-2 entry has linkages with diabetes, cardiovascular disease, and hypertension, which, as comorbidities, significantly increase the severity of virus infection.

ACE2 and TMPRSS2

When coronaviruses, as well as influenza viruses, invade the target cells, usually the lungs, they need two proteins in the cell membrane, ACE2 receptor, and TMPRSS2.

Following the surface spike proteins on the viral capsid attach to the ACE2 receptor, the virus initiates non-endosome entry of its genome across the cell membrane with the assistance of TMPRSS2, which catalyzes the cleavage of the bound spike protein. Thus, it causes a conformational change that promotes the fusion of viral and cellular membranes and thereby allows the release of the virus into the cell.

As regards the role of host genetic factors in coronavirus susceptibility or outcome, the human ACE2 has a rich pool of rare variants and is one of the most studied genes. The SARS-CoV-1 and COV-2 genomes shared around 80% of homology and used the same ACE2 to enter the cell [17]. Comparative genetic analyses of data from different databases indicate that several ACE2 variants could reduce the association between ACE2 and S-protein in SARS-CoV [18]. Several studies also suggest that the expression level and expression pattern of human ACE2 in different tissues might be critical for the susceptibility and progression of 2019-nCoV/SARS-CoV-2. Although a study group did not identify genetically supporting the existence of coronavirus S-protein binding-resistant ACE2 mutants in different populations by using the GTEx database [19], another group demonstrated that certain variants in the gene (rs73635825 and rs143936283) result in different intermolecular interactions with SARS-CoV-2 spike protein [20]. Hussain et al. [20] by a comparative modeling and molecular super-imposition study revealed that ACE2 alleles, rs73635825, and rs143936283 have a low binding affinity for SARS-CoV-2 spike protein. Therefore, these alleles may lead to resistance against COVID-19. It has been generally accepted that the ACE2 genetic variants may influence the protein's binding to the virus and its subsequent invasion of the cell. Although the frequencies of allelic variants of the ACE2 varies from one country to another [21], the genetic basis of ACE2 expression and function in different populations is still largely unknown.

Although it has been known that increased TMPRSS2 expression is related to two SNPs (rs2070788 and rs383510) and the susceptibility to H7N9 influenza [22], it has received less attention in genetic association studies to date. An in vitro study showed that a cell line expressing TMPRSS2 is highly susceptible to SARS-CoV-2 infection [23]. Recently, it has been recognized that SARS-Co-V2 uses the cellular protease TMPRSS2 for S protein priming. Russo et al. [24] published that the lung-specific expression quantitative trait loci (eQTL) variants for TMPRSS were associated with increased expression of TMPRSS2. They suggested that the eQTL variants may confer different susceptibility or response to SARS-CoV-2 infection. However, further research is needed to determine if these genetic variants in COVID-19 susceptibility, incidence, and progression.

Interferon (IFN)-Induced Transmembrane (IFITM)

It is generally postulated that RNA virus entry into cells by endocytosis is regulated with interferon (IFN)-induced transmembrane (IFITM) proteins, which confer cellular resistance to many pathogenic viruses by preventing viral fusion with cholesterol depleted. IFITM3, the most potent antiviral IFITM, inhibits an early event after endocytosis of virion particles. Sequence variants of the IFITM3 gene exhibit ethnic differences [25]. Among these variants, the polymorphism rs12252 C allele is considered to produce an alternate spliced transcript that encodes an aberrant truncated protein of IFITM3. Zhang et al. (2013) found a significant association between the IFTM3-rs12252CC genotype and influenza severity and hypothesized that the high frequency of the C allele in Asian populations may influence the epidemiology of influenza since this genotype was the much higher in the Han Chinese population compared with Caucasians [25]. A recent Indian study by a clinical exome data of 103 individuals also identified this genotype as risk inducing for SARSCoV-2 infection [26]. In the same study, one IFTM3 polymorphism, rs34481144 is also proposed as a protective variant for COVID-19 by increased memory Cytotoxic T Lymphocytes (CTLs) survival and more efficient viral clearance from infected airways. Therefore, genetic variations in the genes coding for IFITM proteins can lead to variability in establishing SARSCoV2 infection in the host.

Host Genetic Factors Related to Sars-CoV-2 Replication/Protein Expression for Regulating Coronavirus Infection

Glucose Regulated Protein 78 kDa (GRP78)

Glucose regulated protein 78 kDa (GRP78) or immunoglobulin heavy chain binding protein (BiP) localizes to the lumen of the endoplasmic reticulum (ER) and is involved in the folding and assembly of proteins as an ER stress sensor under reasonable conditions. GRP78 is also found on the cell surface as a signal receptor. During cellular stress, elevated expression of GRP78 increases the chance for GRP78 to escape ER retention and translocate to the cell membrane. Cell surface GRP78 (csGRP78) triggers various downstream cell signaling pathways by interacting with its ligands. Various pro-proliferative, pro-survival ligands, and pro-apoptotic ligands have been discovered. Furthermore, there is evidence that the substrate-binding site of csGRP78 is susceptible to virus recognition and it can be mediate the virus entry into the host cell [27]. Chu et al. (2018) published that GRP78 is capable of facilitating surface attachment of MERS-CoV spike protein. An *insilico* study suggests the existence of a SARSCoV-2 spike protein-

GRP78 binding site. However, it is not yet known whether the expression of GRP78 and its polymorphisms have a role in determining the susceptibility and resistance to coronaviruses.

Cyclophilins

Cyclophilins (CyPA), a subgroup of the large immunophilins protein family, are peptidyl-prolyl isomerases involved in the folding of cellular proteins and cell signaling. They play a pivotal role in the replication of several RNA viruses, including nidoviruses (arteriviruses and coronaviruses), and are necessary for proper viral propagation. Cyclophilin A (CypA) and B have been shown to interact with non-structural protein 1 (nsp1) of SARS-CoV intracellularly [29]. Therefore, cyclophilins and its overexpression are significant in the pathogenesis of viral infection. It has been reported that SNP variants causing amino acid exchanges around enzymatic peptidyl-prolyl cis/trans isomerase in CypA may directly affect the propagation of HCoV-229E [30]. Although polymorphisms in the CypA gene have also been documented to influence susceptibility to HIV-1 infection, whether these variations play a role in COVID-19 susceptibility and progression remains largely undocumented.

Host Genetic Factors in the Immune reSponse to SARS-CoV-2

HLA Loci

Classical human leukocyte antigen (HLA) molecules encoded by MHC genes are a specific group of molecules expressed on the cell surface. They are crucial for the recognition of non-selfmolecules by the acquired immune system. MHC molecules acting as a receptor for viral peptides present the peptides to the virus-specific cytotoxic CD8+ T lymphocytes. These cells recognize the conformational structure of the peptide-binding groove of the MHC class I molecules, bound to viral peptides. Variations within MHC class I genes determine both variation in the conformational structure of the peptide-binding groove and its binding to varied antigen peptides. Therefore, it is generally accepted that HLA genes are critical in the immune response against pathogens and more authors consider them as the leading candidates in conferring susceptibility to infectious diseases. MHC classical class I and class II genes exhibit many variants (alleles) and have several thousand reported polymorphisms. Several genetic variants at HLA genes have been identified that account for inter-individual differences to the immune response against common viruses. Accumu-lating evidence suggests that genetic variability in the HLA-A, -B, and -C genes may also affect susceptibility to and severity of the disease caused by SARS-CoV-2 [31]. However, whether distinct HLA allele distribution in various populations provide distinct protection or vulnerability to COVID-19 is unclear.

A Genome-Wide Association Study (GWAS) demonstrated that HLA may act as a susceptibility factor for several common infectious diseases [32]. Several studies on SARS-CoV-1 reported higher risk allele frequency of HLA-B*46:01, HLA-B*07:03, HLA-C*08:01, and HLA-DRB1*1202 and the increased protective allele frequency of HLA-DRB1*03:01, HLA-C*15:02, and HLA-DRB1*03:01. Contrary to this, some studies have been inconsistent and conflicting. On the other hand, in silico studies predicted that HLA-B*15:03, HLA-A*02:03 and HLA-A*31:01; and HLA-A:02:01 as effective antigen presenters for SARS-CoV-2, implying that these would provide protection, while HLA-A*03:02 and HLA-B*46:01 had fewest predicted binding peptides for the virus, implying that these would increase susceptibility to COVID-19 [31, 33, 34]. These studies also suggested that HLA-A*02:02, HLA-B*15:03, HLA-C*12:03 haplotypes exhibited the highest and HLA-A*25:01, HLA-B*46:01, HLA-C*01:02 haplotypes displayed the lowest predicted repertoire of epitopes from SARS-CoV-2. Based on bioinformatic prediction and molecular modeling studies with reporting positive findings, HLA molecules could be considered as a genetic gateway for SARS-CoV-2 infection.

Taking into account spatial variation of COVID-19 positive cases, it is becoming increasingly apparent that population-specific HLA alleles or haplotypes could act as a critical intrinsic determinant of protective immunity against SARS-CoV-2 and make population groups and some individuals resistant or susceptible to COVID-19 infection. Results from the studies investigating the geographical pattern in COVID-19, the risk of virus infection, and its clinical outcome in African and Indian populations have been comparatively less than European and other world populations. Based on their comprehensive in silico analyses, HLA-A*02 subtypes that are predicted to be protective exhibit higher frequency in Indian and several African populations, which are comparatively less than among populations for the risk and severity of COVID-19. HLA-C*12:03 as the susceptibility allele appears to be the most frequent in the European population. However, whether distinct HLA allele distribution in various populations confers protection or vulnerability to COVID-19 is a topic of debate and discussion.

Inflammatory Factors and IL-6

Cytokine storm and then an exacerbated inflammatory response have been proposed as the basis of the pathophysiological process of SARS-CoV-2 infection. The severity of the disease has been demonstrated to be correlated with high serum levels of IL-2 receptor (IL-2R) and IL-6 (≥80 pg/mL) in patients with COVID-19.

Variations in the production and activity of cytokines are associated with SNPs in various regions of cytokine genes, such as IL12RB1 and IFN-γ +874A allele, and influence the susceptibility and/or resistance to various infectious pathogens. It is now well-established that ethnicity greatly influences cytokine gene polymorphism distribution. Although there is evidence supporting the associations between several cytokine gene polymorphisms and SARS-CoV, there are no studies on the impact of cytokine gene polymorphisms on the risk of SARS-CoV-2. But, taking into account a critical role of cytokines in influencing the severity of COVID-19 and an important role of genetic background in determining the pattern of the inflammatory response, allelic variations in cytokine genes look like to play an underlying role in COVID-19.

Some other Possible Candidate Immune Genes to COVID-19 Susceptibility

As known, there are various upstream regulators, such as the Toll-like receptor (TLR) involved in the control of cytokine expression. Additionally, components of the innate immune system such as complement components have also close interactions for cytokine responses. Therefore, host genetic factors concerning these components may affect disease susceptibility and pathogenesis.

Few other genetic factors in the immune response to SARSCoV-2 about these components were suggested or reported. One of them is Ticam2, codes for an adaptor protein in the activation of the TLR signaling pathways. A mice study revealed that allelic variation in the Ticam2 influences susceptibility to SARS-CoV infection [35]. Also, researchers demonstrated that TRIF which is another adaptor protein of TLR signaling pathways, required for initiating the innate immune response to severe SARS-CoV infection and it protects mice from coronavirus infection [36]. Although, there are no studies on the role of the TLR pathway in SARS-CoV-2 infection, given the genetic variation within the TLR genes or components of the TLR pathway and its distinct distribution pattern in various ethnic populations, the genes involved in TLR signaling could emerge as a major host determinant of differential susceptibility to SARS-CoV-2 infection and severity. However, this assumption needs to be tested empirically for SARS-CoV-2.

TLR pathway genes reported concerning COVD 19 susceptibility or outcome are also discussed in Section "sex chromosomes and COVID-19".

The complement system efficiently recognizes and eliminates viral pathogens by opsonizing viruses and virus-infected cells. Some writers note that coronaviruses activate multiple complement pathways; There are *in vitro* and *in vivo* evidence indicating that complement activation plays a critical role in pathogenesis and disease progression of

SARS-CoV and SARS-CoV-2. For example, a recent study demonstrated that highly pathogenicN proteins of SARS-CoV, MERS-CoV, and SARS-CoV-2 aggravated inflammatory lung injury by aberrant complement activation [37]. Considering that polymorphisms of complement genes are associated with the risk of various infectious diseases as well as various diseases, perhaps complement gene variations in ethnic populations modulate the risk and severity of SARS-CoV-2 infection.

Epigenetic Modifications and COVID 19

Epigenetic changes that regulate chromatin structure have a major impact on genome stabilization and maintenance of cellular homeostasis. They have been implicated in the pathophysiology of the virus infection. The epigenetic regulation of gene expression relies on post-translational chemical changes. These changes occur at the level of chromatin as well as on RNA and DNA, are including primary methylation, but also acetylation, phosphorylation, ubiquitination, and sumoylation. These modifications bridge between genotype and phenotype by changing the function of the gene locus without changing the DNA sequence. DNA methylation is the inheritable epigenetic process by which methyl groups are added to the C-5 position of the cytosine ring of DNAby DNA methyltransferases (DNMTs). In addition, more than 98% of DNA methylation occurs in a CpG dinucleotide context in somatic cells, while as much as a quarter of all methylation appears in a non-CpG context in embryonic stem cells (ESCs). DNA methylation is erased during zygote formation and then reestablished in the embryo at approximately the time of implantation. Most DNA methylation is essential for cell development, and it plays a key role in several processes including the packing of DNA in the nucleus genomic imprinting, X-chromosome inactivation, and suppression of repetitive element transcription and transposition and, when dysregulated, causes to diseases like cancer. DNA methylation is regulated by a family of DNMTs. These family members have been determined as DNMT1, DNMT2, DNMT3A, DNMT3B, and DNMT3L [38]. In recent years, 110 types of RNA nucleotide modifications have been reported, spanning RNA types including messenger RNA (mRNA), transfer RNA (tRNA), ribosomal RNA (rRNA), transfer-messenger RNA (tmRNA), small nuclear RNA (snRNA), and chromosomal RNA, many of which are currently well cataloged at the RNA Modification Database (http://mods.rna. albany.edu/mods). RNA modifications not only mark and regulate mentioned these transcripts but also diversify and extend the protein's functionality from the annotated genes [40]. Recent work in this area showed that chemical modifications at the RNA level play a role in gene transcription, translational efficiency, and RNA stability [41]. These modifications of coding and non-coding RNA are including, adenosine methylations, cytosine modifications, isomerization of uridine, and ribose modification [42]. Mass Spec technologies have discovered a series of RNA modifications that are not only non-coding RNAs, including tRNA) and rRNA but are also commonly found within functional mRNAs. Thus, some of the mapped modifications showed dynamic patterns and tissue-specific distribution explaining to the new field of RNA-epigenetics or epitranscriptomics domains. Transcriptomic and epitranscriptomic analyses have primary importance in the study of viruses by determining their structure and function. So, it is provided important information about host infection [41]. Likewise, new data from the Centre for RNA Research and their collaborators at the Korean National Institute of Health (KNHI) within the Korea Centers for Disease Control and Prevention (KCDC) have presented a high-resolution map of SARS-CoV-2. As known, each RNA viral transcript has 5'-cap structure and a 3' poly(A) tail. Nanopore-based direct RNA sequencing was observed motif being the AAGAA present throughout the viral genome. The poly(A) tail plays an important role in RNA turnover and this internal modification may contribute to viral RNA stability and translation efficiency. When the virus enters the host cell, it replicates a genomic RNA that consists of nine open reading frames (ORFs). Thus, the genomic RNA is translated to produce proteins. There are nine subgenomic RNAs transcribed from the genomic RNA. They are encoding conserved structural proteins, namely, the spike protein (S), an envelope protein (E), membrane protein (M), and nucleocapsid protein (N) that synthesize the viral particle [41, 43]. Generally, the virus entering point at the host cell is the ACE2 type I membrane receptor. These receptors are present in arterial and venous endothelial cells, lung type II alveolar cells, enterocytes of the small intestine, and arterial smooth muscle cells in the cerebral cortex and brainstem. According to obtained the data, during SARS-CoV-2 enters into cells, it is using the receptor-binding domain (RBD) of the spike (S1) protein that contains a core structure and a receptor-binding motif (RBM) to bind the outer surface of the receptor.

Previous studies have shown a strong association between SARS- Cov infection and ACE2 expression levels. Also, a series of comorbidities have been reported in patients who died of COVID-19 infection, including chronic diseases. As known, the *ACE2* gene is located on the X chromosome and is closely related to XCI [41]. XCI is an epigenetic regulation and explained in more detail above. Zylicz et al. mapped the X chromosome inactivation in several human tissues. Male and female differences were investigated in the expression of X-chromosomal protein-coding and long non-coding RNA (lncRNA) genes and single-cell transcriptomes, along with genomics in Genotype Tissue Expression (GTEx) project. It was detected that although XCI is essentially uniform across human tissues, some heterogeneity can also occur between cells, tissues, and individuals. The data have shown that escaper genes were caused to result in sex biases in gene expression and so in phenotypic diversity. *ACE2* was found among one of these genes in female lung tissue, showing a more heterogeneous sex bias. Moreover, *ACE2* expression was slightly higher in males than in female tissues. This condition may be the reason for higher respiratory infection severity in male than in female patients [9, 44].

Recently research studies in the regulation of the ACE2 gene by DNA methylation indicated that the host epigenome may represent a risk factor for COVID-19 infection [41]. Moreover, age-dependent DNA methylation was detected close to the transcription start site of the ACE2 gene by the techniques of DNA methylation analysis in airway epithelial cells. Corley et al. using Illumina DNA methylation sequence data from samples of different biological ages, they found that a CpG near the ACE2 transcription start site showed a decreased level of methylation during aging. Previous studies had suggested that DNA methylation levels are reduced during aging. Thus, differential methylation patterns of genes involved in inflammation, aging, and immunity response were obtained. These data could explain the higher morbidity rates of the virus infection in older individuals and patients with underlying medical conditions [45]. Additionally, the *ACE2* promoter has been found hypomethylated in endometrial carcinoma and renal papillary cell carcinoma tissues. Thus, ACE2 expression levels increase in these patients. When these patients were affected by SARS-CoV-2, their prognosis may worsen [46].

It was reported that epigenomic alterations play a basic role in distinguishing immune cell phenotypes and regulating inflammatory responses to intrinsic or extrinsic stressors with aging. Specific epigenetic modifications such as histone acetylation/ methylation in chromatin play essential roles in response to viral infection. Epigenomic patterns of aging result in decreases in naive T cells and increases in monocytes and cytotoxic cell functions. Whereas, the size of alterations is more significant in men than in women, with an accompanied loci specific methylation decline in the B cells. Thus, it is thought that gender and age differences in epigenetic patterns of immune cells may partially explain the diversity in the severity of COVID-19. However, the epigenetic changes in CpG-sites located in subtelomeric regions which control innate immunity can mediate inflammatory responses to COVID-19 [47].

Epigenetic and Possible Treatment/Vaccine Options for SARS-CoV-2

As is known, the epigenetic regulation of multiple genes can be intervened by natural factors and named as epi-drug. Inhibition of *ACE2* and furin expression with the use of drugs such as vitamin D and quercetin for the treatment of SARS CoV-2 is recommended [48]. Other candidate epi-drugs for epigenetic silencing of ACE2 and interferon genes are curcumin, deferasirox, 8-hydroxyquinolones (8HQ), and sulforaphane (from broccoli) [49 - 51]. It is suggested that all of these substances are natural medicines and could help to reduce disease severity and susceptibility. Ferritin values in severe SARS-CoV-2 patients increase and accordingly their clinical results worsen [48]. Curcumin is especially important as it has ferritin-lowering effects [52].

TELOMERE LENGHT AND COVID 19

Telomeres are repetitive nucleotides (TTAGGG)n at the ends of each chromosome. They play a role in maintaining genome stability and regulate immunity in response to viral infection. Subtelomere regions contain CG-enriched genes that regulate immunity. These genes are influenced by telomere length and regulate telomere repeat-containing RNA (TERRA) transcription. Their expression can be upregulated in response to viral infection by activation of interferon-stimulated genes. Thus, telomere shortening, coupled with dysregulated innate and adaptive immune responses to viral infection, can cause severe outcomes in older adults with COVID-19 [47, 53]. Earlier studies reported that telomeres play a major role in influencing the process of cellular senescence and can be associated with maintaining lung health. In addition, telomere dysfunction was also associated with smoking and chronic obstructive pulmonary disease [54 - 56]. Some agents in smoke may activate DNA damage response by influencing telomere function and the level of CD4+ and CD8+ T cells significantly is reduced. Furthermore, viral replication activates interferon regulatory factors (IRFs) and TLR-3-induced NF-κB pathway; which towards the increase in the production of proinflammatory cytokines and cytokine storm. There is evidence that the NK cells are significantly increased in older adults while the percentages of type T of cells decreased. In aged individuals, APCs secretion of pro-inflammatory cytokines increased while they secrete reduced levels of anti-inflammatory and immune-regulatory cytokines. One of the especially differences at the DNA level between old age persons and children is their telomere length. The immune system is extremely sensitive to the shortening of telomeres. Because the immune system depends on cell renewal and clonal expansion of T and B types of cells [57]. Lymphopenia which a decline in the number and exhaustion of T lymphocytes characterizes severe acute respiratory syndrome by betacoronaviruses. It is thought that the short leukocyte telomere length (LTL) may partially explain the lymphopenia associated with COVID-19. As known, within every person, hematopoietic cells show age-dependent telomere shortening. Lymphopoiesis is linked to telomere length and telomerase, whose activity varies in different lymphocyte lineages [58]. There is a marked variation in LTL between humans. This difference is dependent on the effects of gender, paternal age at conception, and environmental exposures. Various research showed that short LTL was associated with a high risk of hospitalization due to pneumonia and a significant risk of death related to infections. Another study on immunity after flu vaccination documented that, individuals with long telomere length in B-lymphocytes produced a more strong antibody response when compared to individuals with short B-lymphocyte telomere length [57]. According to authors, inter-individual differences in telomere length and the concomitant propensity of T cells to undergo senescence due to aging might play a critical role in severe lymphopenia associated with

COVID-19 and its often fatal outcome. Older people and those with pre-existing conditions are very much affected by COVID-19 and are more susceptible to poor clinical prognosis. The aging-related decreases in NAD+ with a reduction in telomeres length negatively influence the immune response and COVID-19 outcome. In addition, the use of NAD+ as an immunomodulator in older patients with COVID-19 could decrease the severity of immune reaction in those patients and improve their clinical condition [57, 58].

Relationship between ABO Blood Group Distribution and COVID-19

The ABO blood group consists of two antigens (A and B antigens), which are the ABO gene product and includes 4 blood types, namely, A, AB, B, and O. Blood typing are performed as ABO, Rh with standard antibody-based methods. Blood group antigens present at least 300,1 on red blood cells (RBCs), since the discovery of the ABO system [59, 60]. The human ABO blood group is located on chromosome 9 (9q34.1–34.2) [61]. Many studies have reported that the ABO blood group plays an important role in various human diseases, such as cardiovascular, oncological, and some infectious and non-infectious diseases. Human histo-blood group antigens (HBGAs) are some of the important antigens on the surface of human red blood cells. These antigens are highly expressed in a wide variety of cells and tissues, including epithelia, platelets, vascular endothelia, and neurons, and also important as receptors for immune responses. The ABO blood types have polymorphic traits within the *ABO* gene, and blood types have considerably different distributions across ancestry groups. Differences in blood group antigen expression can affect a different level to host susceptibility to many infections. A series of studies shown that the ABO blood group has been previously found to relate to the risk of multiple infectious diseases such as hepatitis B, malaria, rota, dengue viruses, and SARS coronavirus. Furthermore, many blood group antigens have the effect of facilitating intracellular uptake, signal transduction, or cell adhesion through the organization of membrane micro-domains. Blood group antigens can modify the innate immune response to infection [61 - 65]. In addition, an association was shown between variants within ABO and activity of ACE which modulating sensitivity to SARS-COVID 2 by genome-wide association studies. The numerous association studies between blood type and COVID-19 present reasons to believe true associations may exist between blood type with morbidity and mortality due to COVID-19 [64]. In recent data, the results of studies demonstrated that there was a significant association between the A blood group and COVID-19. They reported that females with blood type A are more susceptible to COVID-19 infection [60, 63]. Similarly, Li et al., determined that the rate of patients with

SARS-CoV-2-infected A blood group was significantly higher than healthy controls, while the proportion of patients with SARS-CoV-2-infected O blood group was lower. Also, they suggested that blood group A patients were at higher risk of hospitalization than blood group O patients following SARS-CoV-2 infection [66]. As known, blood type O individual expresses the H antigen, the biosynthetic precursor to A and B antigens. In addition to red blood cells, numerous tissues and secretions such as the endothelium, intestinal mucosa, heart, kidney, and other organs express ABH antigens. This antigen is a carbohydrate antigen and expressed on glycoproteins and glycosphingolipids (GSLs). Earlier, glycan analysis of SARSCoV S protein shown that SARSCoV S protein has a broad range of structures, such as complex Nglycans with 2–4 antennae able to support ABH epitopes. This is highly probable for the virus targeted to respiratory and gastrointestinal mucosa [60]. Several different study groups, reported a possible association between blood type A and a higher risk for COVID-19 infection and mortality while blood group O was associated with a lower risk of infection and mortality. However, there is still a lack of data on the relationship between ABO blood typing and the severity of COVID-19 disease [64, 67, 68]. There are also opinions against these data. For example, Latz et al. performed a study using a large multi-institutional cohort of patients. According to this study, there was no association noted between ABO blood type and COVID-19 disease severity defined as intubation or death, but blood type O had the lowest frequency of disease positivity, similar to other groups [62]. Conversely, Ellinghaus et al. suggested that there is also a lower probability of intubation for all non-O blood types [68].

Cheng et al. suggested that patients with blood group O had decreased susceptibility to SARS-CoV infection [69]. It has been reported that anti-A antibodies found in individuals with blood group O might block the interaction between SARS-CoV and its receptor, thus protecting against SARS-CoV infection. Based on these results, it can be speculated that the susceptibility to COVID 19 decreased in individuals with blood type O, while increased in individuals with blood type A may be related to the presence of anti-A antibody in the blood. Because anti-A antibodies can block the interaction between the virus and its receptor. This condition may explain why blood group A is sensitive to the virus while blood group O is not. In addition, Wu et al. indicated that blood type might have some influence on the clinical characteristics of patients with COVID-19 in their study. They observed that the clinical features of people with different blood types after infection with COVID-19 were different. As a result, it is thought that the blood type of individuals may not be one of the risk factors for COVID-19, but may be related to the clinical characteristics of COVID-19 patients [61, 70].

Table 1. Host Genetic Factors related to COVID-19 disease reported from previous studies as protective and permissive genes

Gene(s) or Locus	Genetic variation/alteration	Effect of genetic alteration	Association/ Possible mechanism (s) -process influenced by host genetic factor/variation	Ref (s)
ACE2	Escaping from XCI	Two dose expressed in females	Excessive Immune response	[4, 10, 11]
	Epigenetic modifications	Hypomethylation during aging	Susceptibility to infections	[9, 41, 44, 45]
	SNPs: rs73635825 rs143936283		Protection/ low binding affinity with SARS-CoV-2 spike protein	[20]
TMPRSS2	eQTL	Increased expression of TMPRSS2	Different susceptibility or response to SARS-CoV-2	[24]
IFTM3	rs34481144		Protection/increased memory CTLs survival and more efficient viral clearance	[26]
TLRs	Escaping from XCI	Two dose expressed in females	Protection/relatively reduced antiviral immunity	[4, 11, 12]
HLA	HLA-B*15:03, HLA-A*02:03 and A*31:01; and HLA-A:02:01		Protection/ effective antigen presentation for SARS-CoV-2	[31, 33, 34].
	Haplotype: HLA-A*02:02, HLA-B*15:03, HLA-C*12:03		Susceptibility/ fewest predicted binding peptides for virus-increased susceptibility to COVID-19	
	HLA-A*03:02 and HLA-B*46:01			
	Haplotype: HLA-A*25:01, HLA-B*46:01, HLA-C*01:02			
CG-enriched genes in sub telomere which are regulated TERRA transcription	Short telomere length		Susceptibility dysregulated innate and adaptive immune responses/Lynphopenia -T lymphocytes	[47, 57, 58]
The ABO blood group	Blood type O		Protection/ blocking the interaction between the virus and its receptor	[61, 69, 70]

There is also evidence for the relationship between Rh type and very few diseases compared to ABO. Similarly, Rh(D) phenotypes (positive and negative Rh blood types) are important for immune response. Zietz et al. found that there were greater risk differences between Rh blood than between ABO strains, and in particular Rh-negative individuals had a lower risk [62, 64].

Conclusion

Some human genetic variants have previously been identified that influence susceptibility or resistance to infection with various virus pathogens. Even though many questions remain unresolved, there is also a growing consensus among the scientific community that some genetic variants in genomes of individuals might confer differential susceptibility and influence the severity and progression of SARS-CoV-2 infection, as well as age, biological sex, and major comorbidity factors such as cardiovascular disease and metabolic disorders. Taking into account the general findings in the literature (Table 1), we discussed the expression level or mutation and variation in some host genetic factors such as ACE2, TMPRSS2, GRP78, TLR7, HLA, ABO blood group, as well as epigenetic changes regulating host response and inter-individual variation in leukocyte telomere length. Many of these host genetic factors also exhibit population-specific variation and is associated with susceptibility and/or resistance to various viral diseases.

There are multiple limitations to our summaries for each identified genetic variations concerning COVID-19 susceptibility. Firstly, the studies and information on SARS-CoV-2 infection continue to increase very rapidly since its emergence. Therefore, we can't cover them all here. Secondly, some studies that have been conducted may not have reported relevant data because of publication biases. Thirdly, most studies, including a large patient population, were conducted in China, and the study of asymptomatic carriers was limited. Lastly, the potential impact of previous exposure to other coronavirus species in influencing population discrepancy and severity of SARS-CoV-2 is also uncertain. Moreover, it should be kept in mind that the large majority of studies reporting positive findings may be affected by a strong risk of bias or confounding. More research findings with a larger dataset are needed to help to understand the role of gene networks in determining or influencing the efficiency of infection and progression of COVID-19.

References

[1] Casanova J-L., Helen C-S., and The COVID Human Genetic Effort (2020). A Global Effort to Define the Human Genetics of Protective Immunity to SARS-CoV-2 Infection. *Cell*, 181, June 11:1194-99, doi: 10.1016/j.cell.2020.05.016 2020.

[2] Williams, F-M., Freydin, M., Mangino, M., Couvreur, S., Visconti, A., Bowyer, R-C., Roy, CI -L., Falchi, M., Sudre, C., Davies, R., Hammond, C., Menni, C., Steves, C., Spector, T. (2020). Self-reported symptoms of covid-19 including symptoms most predictive of SARS-CoV-2 infection, are heritable. *medRxiv [Preprint]*, doi: 10.1101/2020.04.22.20072124.

[3] World Health Organization. WHO Website. *Coronavirus disease (COVID-2019) situation reports*. Situation Report 89. https://www.who.int/emergencie s/disea ses/novel -coron aviru s-2019/situa tion-repor ts. Accessed 25 Apr 2020.

[4] Salvati L., Biagioni B., Vivarelli E. and Parronchi P. (2020) A gendered magnifying glass on COVID-19. *Clinical and Molecular Allergy*, 18, 1:1-11, doi: 10.1186/s12948-020-0012.

[5] Lyon, M.F. (1961). Gene action in the X-chromosome of the mouse (Mus musculus L). *Nature*, 190, 372-373. doi: 10.1038/190372a0.

[6] Lyon, M. F. (1962). Sex chromatin and gene action in the mammalian X-chromosome. *American journal of human genetics*, Jun; 14(2):135-48.

[7] Galupa R and Heard E. X-chromosome inactivation: A crossroads between chromosome architecture and gene regulation. *Annual Review of Genetics,* 52, 535-566, 2018, doi: 10.1146/annurev-genet-120116-024611.

[8] Carrel, L.; Willard, H.F. X-inactivation profile reveals extensive variability in X-linked gene expression in females. *Nature* 2005;434: 400-404. doi: 10.1038/ nature03479.

[9] Tukiainen, T., Villani, A-C., Yen, A., Rivas, M-A., Marshall, J-L., Satija, R., Aguirre, M., Gauthier, L., Fleharty, M., Kirby, A., Cummings, B-B., Castel, S-E., Karczewski, K-J., Aguet, F., Byrnes, A., GTEx Consortium, Lappalainen, T., Regev, A., Ardlie, K-G., Hacohen, N., MacArthur, D-G. (2017). Landscape of X chromosome inactivation across human tissues. *Nature*, October 11, 550(7675): 244–248, doi: 10.1038/nature24265.

[10] Schurz, H., Salie, M., Tromp, G., Hoal, E-G., Kinnear, C-J., Möller, M. (2019). The X chromosome and sex-specific effects in infectious disease susceptibility. *Human genomics*,13, 2:1-12, doi: 10.1186/s40246-018-0185-z.

[11] Larizza L.(2020). Sex-bias in COVID-19 disease: when one more X chromosome makes the difference. *E.C.A. - European Cytogeneticists Association, Newsletter*, 46: 2-8.

[12] Souyris, M-C., Azar, C., Daviaud, P., Canivet, D.,Grunenwald, A., Pienkowski, S., Chaumeil, C., Mejía, J., Guéry, J-E., Charles, J. (2018). TLR7 escapes X chromosome inactivation in immune cells. *Science Immunology*, 3, 19:1-11, doi: 1126/sciimmunol.aap8855.

[13] Saghazadeh A., Rezaei N. (2020). Immune-epidemiological parameters of the novel coronavirus–a perspective. *Expert Review of Clinical Immunology*, 16, 5: 465-470, doi: 10.1080/1744666X.2020.1750954.

[14] Karnam, G., Rygiel, T-P., Raaben, M., Grinwis, GC-M., Coenjaerts, F-E., Ressing, M-E., Rottier, PJM., Haan, C A- MDe, Meyaard, L. (2012). CD200 Receptor Controls Sex-Specific TLR7 Responses to Viral Infection. *PLoS Pathogens*, 8, 5:1-8, doi: 10.1371/journal.ppat.1002710

[15] Mihm, S. (2020). COVID-19: Possible Impact of the Genetic Background in IFNL Genes on Disease Outcomes. *Journal of Innate Immunity*, 12, 3: 273-274, doi: 10.1159/000508076.

[16] Berghöfer, B., Frommer, T., Gabriela, H., Fink, L., Bein, G., Hackstein, H. (2006). TLR7 Ligands Induce Higher IFN-α Production in Females. *The Journal of Immunology*, 177, 4: 2088-2096, doi: 10.4049/jimmunol.177.4.2088.

[17] Zhou, P., Yang, X-L., Wang, X-G., Hu, B., Zhang, L., Zhang, W., Si, H-R., Zhu, Y., Li, B., Huang, C-L., Chen, H-D., Chen, J., Luo, Y., Guo, H., Jiang, R-D., Liu, M-Q., Chen, Y., Shen, X-R., Wang, X., Zheng, X-S., Zhao, K., Chen, Q-J., Deng, F., Liu, L-L., Yan, B., Zhan, F-X., Wang, Y-Y., Xiao, G-F., Shi, Z-L. (2020). A pneumonia outbreak associated with a new coronavirus of probable bat origin. *Nature*, 579, (7798):270–273, doi: 10.1038/s41586-020-2012-7.

[18] Li, W., Zhang, C., Sui, J., Kuhn, J. H., Moore, M. J., Luo, S.,Wong, S-K.,Huang, Keming, X.,Vasilieva, N., Murakami, A., He, Y., Marasco, W-A., Guan, Y., Choe, H., Farzan, M. (2005). Receptor and viral determinants of SARS-coronavirus adaptation to human ACE2. *The EMBO journal*, 24, 8: 1634-1643, doi: 10.1038/ sj.emboj.7600640.

[19] Cao, Y., Li, L., Feng, Z., Wan, S., Huang, P., Sun, X., Wen, F., Huang, X., Ning, G., Wang, W. (2020). Comparative genetic analysis of the novel coronavirus (2019-nCoV/SARS- CoV-2) receptor ACE2 in different populations. *Cell Discov.* 6: 1–4, doi: 10.1038/s41421-020-0147-1.

[20] Hussain, M., Jabeen, N., Raza, F., Shabbir, S., Baig, A-A., Amanullah, A., Aziz, B. (2020). Structural variations in human ACE2 may influence its binding with SARS-CoV-2 spike protein. *J. Med. Virol.*, Published online April 6, doi: 10.1002/ jmv.25832.

[21] Asselta, R., Paraboschi, E-M., Mantovani, A., Duga, S. (2020). ACE2 and TMPRSS2 variants and expression as candidates to sex and country differences in COVID-19 severity in Italy. *medRxiv.*, April 11:1-20, doi: 10.1101/2020.03.30. 20047878.

[22] Cheng, Z., Zhou, J., To, KK-W., Chu, H., Li, C., Wang, D., Yang, D., Zheng, S., Hao, K., Bossé, Y., Obeidat, M., Brandsma, C-A., Song, Y-Q., Chen, Y., Zheng, B-J., Li, L., Yuen, K-Y.(2015). Identification of TMPRSS2 as a susceptibility gene for severe 2009 pandemic A (H1N1) influenza and A (H7N9) influenza. *Journal of Infectious Diseases*, 212, (8):1214-1221, doi: 10.1093/infdis/jiv246.

[23] Matsuyama, S., Nao, N., Shirato, K., Kawase, M., Saito, S., Takayama, I., Nagatac, N., Sekizukad, T., Katoha, H., Kato, F., Sakataa, M., Taharaa, M., Kutsunae, S., Ohmagarie, N., Kurodad, M., Suzukic, T., Kageyama, T., Takedaa, M. (2020). Enhanced isolation of SARS - CoV - 2 by TMPRSS2- expressing cells. *Proceedings of the National Academy of Sciences of the United States of America (PNAS)*, 117(13): 7001–7003, doi: 10.1073/pnas. 2002589117.

[24] Russo, R., Andolfo, I., Lasorsa, V-A., Iolascon, A., Capasso, M. (2020). Genetic analysis of the novel SARS-CoV-2 host receptor TMPRSS2 in different populations. *bioRxiv.*, April 20: 1-15, doi: 10.1101/2020.04.23.057190.

[25] Zhang, Y-H., Zhao, Y., Li, N., Peng, Y-C., Giannoulatou, E., Jin, R-H., Yan, H-P., Wu, H., Liu, J-H., Liu, N., Wang, D-Y., Shu, Y-L., Ho, L-P., Kellam, P., McMichael, A., Dong, T. (2013). Interferon-induced transmembrane protein-3 genetic variant rs12252-C is associated with severe influenza in Chinese individuals. *Nat. Commun.*, 4:1–6. doi: 10.1038/ncomms2433.

[26] Iyer, G-R., Samajder, S., Zubeda, S., Narayana S, D-S., Mali, V., PV, S- K., Sharma, A., Abbas, N-Z., Bora, N-S., Narravula, A., Hasan, Q. (2020). Infectivity and progression of COVID19 based on selected host candidate gene variants. *Frontiers in Genetics*, 11, 861:1-13.

[27] Ibrahim, I-M., Abdelmalek, D-H., Elshahat, M-E., Elfiky, A-A. (2020). COVID - 19 Spike - host cell receptor GRP78 binding site prediction. *Journal of Infection*, 80:554-562, doi: 10.1016/j.jinf.2020.02.026 0163-4453.

[28] Chu, H., Chan, C-M., Zhang, X., Wang, Y., Yuan, S., Zhou, J., Au-Yeung, RK-H., Sze, K-H., Yang, D., Shuai, H., Houb, Y., Lib, C., Zhaob, X., Poonb, VK-M., Leungb, S-P., Yeunga, M-L., Yanf, J., Lug, G., Jinh, D-Y., Gaof, G-F., Chana, JF-W., Yuen, K-Y. (2018). Middle East respiratory syndrome coronavirus and bat coronavirus HKU9 both can utilize GRP78 for attachment onto host cells. *J. Biol. Chem.*, 293: 11709-11726, doi: 10.1074/jbc.RA118.001897.

[29] Tanaka, Y., Sato, Y., Sasaki, T. (2013). Suppression of coronavirus replication by cyclophilin inhibitors. *Viruses, 5,* (5):1250-1260, doi: 10.3390/v5051250.

[30] von Brunn, A., Ciesek, S., von Brunn, B., Carbajo-Lozoya, J. (2015). Genetic deficiency and polymorphisms of cyclophilin A reveal its essential role for Human Coronavirus 229E replication. *Curr Opin Virol.*, 14:56-61, doi: 10.1016/j.coviro. 2015.08.004.

[31] Nguyen, A., David, J-K., Maden, S-K., Wood, M-A., Weeder, B-R., Nellore, A., Thompson, R-F. (2020). Human leukocyte antigen susceptibility map for severe acute respiratory syndrome coronavirus 2. *Journal of Virology*, 94: e00510-20. doi: org/10.1128/JVI.00510-20.

[32] Tian, C., Hromatka, B-S., Kiefer, A-K., Eriksson, N., Noble, S-M., Tung, J-Y., Hinds, D-A. (2017). Genome-wide association and HLA region fine-mapping studies identify susceptibility loci for multiple common infections. *Nat Commun.*, 8, 599:1-13, doi: 10.1038/s41467-017-00257-5.

[33] Ahmed, S-F., Quadeer, A-A., McKay, M-R.(2020). Preliminary identification of potential vaccine targets for the COVID-19 coronavirus (SARS- CoV-2) based on SARS-CoV immunological studies. *Viruses*, 12, (3), 254: 1-15, doi: 10.3390/ v12030254.

[34] Campbell, K-M., Steiner, G., Wells, D-K., Ribas, A., Kalbasi, A. (2020). Prediction of SARS-CoV-2 epitopes across 9360 HLA class I alleles. *BioRxiv.*, doi: 10.1101/2020.03.30.016931.

[35] Gralinski, L-E., Menachery, V-D., Morgan, A-P., Totura, A-L., Beall, A., Kocher, J., Plante, J., Harrison-Shostak, D-C., Schäfer, A., Pardo-Manuel de Villena, F., Ferris, M-T., Baric, R-S. (2017) Allelic variation in the Toll-like receptor adaptor protein Ticam2 contributes to SARS-coronavirus pathogenesis in mice. *G3 (Bethesda)*,7:1653-1663, doi: 10.1534/g3.117.041434.

[36] Totura, A-L., Whitmore, A., Agnihothram, S., Schäfer, A., Katze, M-G., Heise, M-T., Barica, R-S. (2015). Toll-like receptor 3 signaling via TRIF contributes to a protective innate immune response to severe acute respiratory syndrome coronavirus infection. *mBio.*, May 26; 6(3): e00638-15: 1-14, doi: 10.1128/mBio. 00638-15.

[37] Gao, T., Hu, M., Zhang, X., Li, H., Zhu, L., Liu, H., Dong, Q., Zhang, Z., Wang, Z., Hu, Y., Fu, Y., Jin, Y., Li, K., Zhao, S., Xiao, Y., Luo, S., Li, L., Zhao, L., Liu, J., Zhao, H., Liu, Y., Yang, W., Peng, Ji., Chen, X., Li, P., Liu, Y., Xie, Y., Song, J., Zhang, L., Ma, Q., Bian, X., Chen, W., Liu, X., Mao, Q., Cao, C. (2020). Highly pathogenic coronavirus N protein aggravates lung injury by MASP-2-mediated complement over-activation. *MedRxiv.*, doi: org/10.1101/2020.03.29.20041962.

[38] Jin, B., Li, Y., Robertson K-D. (2011). DNA methylation: Superior or subordinate in the epigenetic hierarchy? *Genes and Cancer*, 2, 6:607-617, doi: 10.1177/ 1947601910393957.

[39] *RNA Modification Database* (http://mods.rna. albany.edu/mods).

[40] Li, S., Mason, C-E. (2014). The pivotal regulatory landscape of RNA modifications. *Annual Review of Genomics and Human Genetics*, 15:127-150, doi: 10.1146/annurev-genom-090413-025405.

[41] Chlamydas, S., Papavassiliou, A-G. and Piperi C. (2020). Epigenetic mechanisms regulating COVID-19 infection. *Epigenetics*, 00, 00:1-9, doi: 10.1080/15592294. 2020.1796896.

[42] Roundtree, I-A.,Evans, M-E., Pan, T., He, C. (2017). Dynamic RNA modifications in gene expression regulation. *Cell*, June 15, 169(7): 1187–1200. doi: 10.1016/j. cell.2017.05.045.

[43] Kim, D., Lee, J-Y., Yang, J-S., Kim, J-W., Kim, V-N.,Chang, H. (2020). The Architecture of SARS-CoV-2 Transcriptome. *Cell*, 181, 4: 914-921.e10, doi: 10. 1016/j.cell.2020.04.011.

[44] Żylicz, J-J., Bousard, A., Žumer, K., Francois, D., Eusra, M., Rocha, S-T., Schwalb, B., Syx, L., Dingli, F., Loew, D., Cramer, P., Heard, E. (2019). The Implication of Early Chromatin Changes in X Chromosome Inactivation. *Cell*, 176,1-2:182-197.e23, doi: 10.1016/j.cell.2018.11.041.

[45] Corley. M., Ndhlovu, L-C. (2020). DNA Methylation Analysis of the COVID-19 host cell receptor, Angiotensin I Converting Enzyme 2 gene (ACE2) in the Respiratory System Reveal Age and Gender Differences. *Medicine and Pharmacology*, March, 19:1-29, doi: 10.20944/preprints201810.0478.v1.

[46] Yang, J., Li, H., Hu, S., Zhou, Y. (2020). ACE2 correlated with immune infiltration serves as a prognostic biomarker in endometrial carcinoma and renal papillary cell carcinoma: implication for COVID-19. *AGING*, 12, (8): 6518-6535.

[47] Salimi, S., Hamlyn, J-M. (2020). COVID-19 and Crosstalk With the Hallmarks of Aging. *The Journals of Gerontology*, Series A:1-8, doi: 10.1093/gerona/glaa149.

[48] Pruimboom L. (2020). Methylation Pathways and SARS-CoV-2 Lung Infiltration and Cell Membrane-Virus Fusion Are Both Subject to Epigenetics. *Frontiers in Cellular and Infection Microbiology*, 10, May:1-5, doi: 10.3389/fcimb.2020.00290.

[49] Sfera, A., Fayard, L., Osorio, C., Price, A. (2018). Epigenetic interventions for brain rejuvenation: anchoring age-related transposons. *Neural Regeneration Research*, 13:635-636, doi: 10.4103/1673-5374.230283.

[50] Hassan, F, Rehman, M-S., Khan, M-S., Ali, M-A., Javed, A., Nawaz, A., Yang, C. (2019). Curcumin as an alternative epigenetic modulator: mechanism of action and potentialeffects. *Front. Gene*, 10:1–16. doi: 10.3389/fgene.2019.00514.

[51] Kaufman-Szymczyk, A., Majewski, G., Lubecka-Pietruszewska, K., Fabianowska-Majewska, K. (2015). The role of sulforaphane in epigenetic mechanisms, including interdependence between histone modification and DNA methylation. *Int. J. Mol. Sci.*, 16:29732–29743. doi: 10.3390/ijms161226195.

[52] Sfera, A., Bullock, K., Price, A., Inderias, L., Osorio, C. (2017). Ferrosenescence: the iron age of neurodegeneration? *Mech. Ageing Dev.*, 174:63–75. doi: 10.1016/ j.mad.2017.11.012.

[53] Wang, Z., Deng, Z., Tutton, S., Lieberman, P-M. (2017). The telomeric response to viral infection. *Viruses*, 9(8):218:1-15, doi: 10.3390/v9080218.

[54] Birch, J., Barnes, P-J., Passos, J-F. (2018). Mitochondria, telomeres and cell senescence: Implications for lung ageing and disease. *Pharmacology and Therapeutics*, 183: 34-49, doi: 10.1016/j.pharmthera.2017.10.005.

[55] Busquets, X., Pons, J., Sauleda, J., Macnee, W., Agustı, AG-N. (2006). Telomere shortening in smokers with and without COPD. *Eur Respir J*, 27: 525–528, doi: 0.1183/09031936.06.00087005.

[56] Passos, J-F,. Von Zglinicki, T. (2005). Mitochondria, telomeres and cell senescence. *Experimental Gerontology*, 40, 6:466-472, doi: 10.1016/j.exger. 2005.04.006.

[57] Omran, H-M., Almaliki, M-S. (2020). Influence of NAD+ as an ageing-related immunomodulator on COVID 19 infection: A hypothesis. *Journal of Infection and Public Health*, 13: 1196–1201, doi: 13 (2020) 1196–1201.

[58] Aviv A. (2020). Telomeres and COVID-19. *The FASEB Journal*, 00:1–6, doi: 10.1096/fj.202001025.

[59] Westhoff, C-M. (2019). Blood group genotyping. *Blood*, 133, 17:1814-1820, doi: 10.1182/blood-2018-11-833954.

[60] Mohammadpour, S., Torshizi Esfahani, A., Halaji, M., Lak, M., Ranjbar, R. (2020). An updated review of the association of host genetic factors with susceptibility and resistance to COVID-19. *Journal of Cellular Physiology*, May:1-6, doi: 10.1002/jcp.29868.

[61] Wu, Y., Feng, Z., Li, P., Yu, Q. (2020). Relationship between ABO blood group distribution and clinical characteristics in patients with COVID-19. *Clinica Chimica Acta*, 509, June: 220-223, doi: 10.1016/j.cca.2020.06.026.

[62] Latz, C-A., DeCarlo, C., Boitano, L., Png, CY-M., Patell, R., Conrad, M-F., Eagleton, M., Dua, A. (2020). Blood type and outcomes in patients with COVID-19. *Annals of Hematology*, 99, 9: 2113-2118, doi: 10.1007/s00277-020-04169-1.

[63] Fan, Q., Zhang, W., Li, B., Li, D-J., Zhang, J., Zhao, F. (2020). Association Between ABO Blood Group System and COVID-19 Susceptibility in Wuhan. *Frontiers in Cellular and Infection Microbiology*, 10:1-7, doi: 10.3389/fcimb.2020. 00404.

[64] Zietz, M., Zucker, J., Tatonetti, N. (2020). Testing the association between blood type and COVID-19 infection, intubation, and death. *medRxiv: the preprint server for health sciences*: 1-27, doi: 10.1101/2020.04.08.20058073.

[65] Garratty, G., Glynn, S-A., McEntire, R. (2004). ABO and Rh(D) phenotype frequencies of different racial/ ethnic groups in the United States. *Transfusıon*, 44:703-706, doi: 10.1111/j.1537-2995.2004.03338.x.

[66] Li, J., Wang, X., Chen, J., Cai, Y., Deng, A., Yang, M. (2020). Association between ABO blood groups and risk of SARS-CoV-2 pneumonia. *British Journal of Haematology*, 190, 1:24-27, doi: 10.1111/bjh.16797.

[67] Zhao, J., Yang, Y., Huang, H., Li, D., Gu, D., Lu, X., Zhang, Z., Liu, L., Liu, T., Liu, Y., He, Y., Sun, B., Wei, M., Yang, G., Wang, X., Zhang, L., Zhou, X., Xing, M., Wang P -G. (2020). Relationship between the ABO Blood Group and the COVID-19 Susceptibility. *medRxiv: the preprint server for health sciences*:1-18, doi: 10.1101/2020.03.11.20031096.

[68] Ellinghaus, D., Degenhardt, F., Bujanda, L., Buti, M., Albillos, A., Invernizzi, P., Fernández, J., Prati, D., Baselli, G., Asselta, R., Grimsrud, M-M., Milani, C., Aziz, F., Kässens, J., May, S., Wendorff, M., Wienbrandt, L., Uellendahl-Werth, F., Zheng, T., Yi, X., de Pablo, R., Chercoles, A-G., Palom, A., Garcia-Fernandez, A-E., Rodriguez-Frias, F., Zanella, A.,Bandera, A., Protti, A., Aghemo, A., Lleo, A., Biondi, A., Caballero-Garralda, A., Gori, A., Tanck, A., Carreras Nolla, A., Latiano, A., Fracanzani, A-L., Peschuck, A., Julià, A., Pesenti, A.,Voza, A., Jiménez, D., Mateos, B., Nafria Jimenez, B., Quereda, C., Paccapelo, C., Gassner,

C., Angelini, C., Cea, C., Solier, A., Pestaña, D., Muñiz-Diaz, E., Sandoval, E., Paraboschi, E-M., Navas, E., García Sánchez, F., Ceriotti, F.,Martinelli-Boneschi, F., Peyvandi, F., Blasi, F., Téllez, L., Blanco-Grau, A., Hemmrich-Stanisak, G., Grasselli, G., Costantino, G., Cardamone, G., Foti, G., Aneli, S., Kurihara, H., ElAbd, H., My, I., Galván-Femenia, I., Martín, J., Erdmann, J., Ferrusquía-Acosta, J., Garcia-Etxebarria, K., Izquierdo-Sanchez, L., Bettini, L-R. et al. (2020). Genomewide Association Study of Severe Covid-19 with Respiratory Failure. *N Engl J Med.*, Jun 17:1-13, doi: 10.1056/NEJMoa2020283.

[69] Cheng, Y., Cheng, G., Chui, C., Lau, F-Y., Chan, P-K., Ng, M-H., Sung, J-J., Wong, R-S. (2005). ABO blood group and susceptibility to severe acute respiratory syndrome. *JAMA,* Mar 23, 293(12):1450-1. doi: 10.1001/jama.293.12.1450-c.

[70] Guillon, P., Clément, M., Sébille, V., Rivain, J-G., Chou, C-F., Ruvoën-Clouet, N., Le Pendu, J. (2008). Inhibition of the interaction between the SARS-CoV Spike protein and its cellular receptor by anti-histo-blood group antibodies. *Glycobiology*, 18, 12:1085-1093, doi: 10.1093/glycob/cwn093.

In: Coronavirus Disease
Editor: Yildiz Dincer

ISBN: 978-1-53619-296-4

Chapter 9

The Clinical Course of COVID-19 in Elderly Patients

Hakan Yavuzer**, *MD and Rabia Bag Soytas, MD
Istanbul University - Cerrahpasa, Cerrahpasa Medical Faculty,
Department of Internal Medicine, Division of Geriatrics, Istanbul Turkey

Abstract

COVID-19 disease, which affects the whole world and is declared as a pandemic by the world health organization, affects the elderly mostly due to both physiological changes because of aging and its comorbidities. Studies have reported that mortality and morbidity are higher in the elderly than young people. Like other infections, COVID-19 disease can manifest itself with different symptoms, as the immune response decreases with aging. Also, they have difficulties in describing and expressing the symptoms because of the decrease in their cognitive functions, which leads to a delay in hospital admissions. Although there are no findings specific to the elderly in laboratory values and radiological imaging, some findings were found to be more common in the elderly. Among the treatment options, a different treatment protocol specific to the elderly is not applied. However, since the comorbidities of geriatric patients and the number of medicine they use are high, care should be taken in terms of medicine side effects and drug-drug interactions during treatment. The COVID-19 epidemic affects the elderly not only physically, but also socially and psychologically. All these situations lead to a more severe course of COVID-19 disease by causing increased malnutrition and sarcopenia in the elderly and making them frailer. During the COVID-19 pandemic process, elderly patients should be evaluated considering all these conditions and necessary medical, psychological, and social support should be provided.

Keywords: COVID-19, clinic, elderly, SARS-CoV-2

* Corresponding Author's Email: drhakanyavuzer@gmail.com.

INTRODUCTION

The Coronavirus disease 2019 (COVID-19) outbreak, which occurred due to the new coronavirus (SARS-CoV-2) and spread rapidly all over the world, was declared as a pandemic by the World Health Organization (WHO) on March 11, 2020 [1]. The pathogen has been identified as a novel enveloped RNA beta-coronavirus called acute respiratory syndrome coronavirus 2 (SARS-Cov-2). It can cause a wide range of diseases ranging from mild illness like flu to critical illness such as sepsis, multiple organ failure, and severe respiratory failure. The disease is transmitted from person to person by droplets and by touching mouth, nose, and eye mucosa with dirty hands after touching surfaces containing viruses. Symptoms of the disease; the first symptoms appear within an average of 5-6 days (may extend from 2-14 days) after the virus enters the body [2].

The elderly population in the world is gradually increasing. While the population aged 65 and over was 6% in 1990, it increased to 9% in 2019. In 2050, it is expected to be 16% [3]. It is known that patients over the age of 65 are frailer due to comorbidities and age-related physiological changes and they are more affected by many diseases than young people [4]. It has been reported that the majority of those who were hospitalized and died among patients infected with COVID-19 consisted of elderly patients causing higher mortality rates, especially in the elderly with cardiovascular disease, chronic respiratory disease, diabetes, or another health problem such as cancer [5]. The Centers for Disease Control and Prevention (CDC) reported that 17% of the total population in the United States is over 65 years. However, 65 years and older patients were responsible for 31% of COVID-19 infections, 45% of hospitalizations, 53% of intensive care unit admissions, and 80% of deaths caused by COVID-19 [6]. Also, many studies have shown that mortality increases with an increasing age [7]. In a study with 72.314 cases, it was shown that the overall mortality rate was 2.3% but increased to 8% between the ages of 70-79 and 14.5% in patients over 80 years old [5]. Therefore, it is important to know the clinical, laboratory, and radiological characteristics and treatment options of elderly patients infected with COVID-19.

CLINICAL CHARACTERISTICS

Older individuals are more prone to infections due to multiple chronic diseases, weak immune systems and their recovery are slower than younger people. As a result of natural changes that occur in the body with aging, the symptoms and clinical course of COVID-19 may be different from young individuals.

According to the CDC, 63.1% of adults aged 60 and older have hypertension, 38% of people aged 65 and older have chronic kidney disease (CKD), and 26.8% of adults aged

65 and older have diabetes [8-10]. In a study in which 312 patients infected with COVID-19 aged 65 and older were included, 77.2% of the patients were reported to have comorbidity. Like the general population, the most common comorbidity in these patients (57.1%) was hypertension, followed by diabetes mellitus (38.8%), cardiovascular disease (29.8%), chronic lung disease (8.65%), cerebrovascular disease (6.4%) [11]. In another study, 69.5% of geriatric patients had comorbidity, and the most common comorbidities included hypertension (43.8%), diabetes (25.7%), and cardiac disease (16.2%) [12]. Older patients with comorbidities were more likely to progress to severe disease [13]. Therefore, it is vital to know and control chronic diseases in elderly patients with COVID-19. For example, when we consider the most common comorbidities, it is very important to keep blood pressure and glucose under control.

The risk and severity of developing an infection depend on the relationship between the pathogen's virulence, its inoculum, and the host's defense system. Virulence of a pathogen is determined by the ability to attach and replicate in a host environment. With the physiological changes brought about by aging, macrophage function changes, mucocutaneous defenses are compromised, cytokine production decreases, and T cell function is insufficient. Comorbid conditions such as diabetes, congestive heart failure, kidney failure, chronic lung disease, and malnutrition deteriorate the immune system. For these reasons, infections may show an atypical course in geriatric patients. Current data show that COVID-19 infections may also start with atypical presentations in a significant portion of the elderly [14]. Geriatric patients with COVID-19 may only have fatigue, myalgia, headache, or vomiting without fever or cough. It should be kept in mind that this situation may cause patients to apply to the hospital later, to be diagnosed later, and to start treatment later, and therefore to be more fatal. For example, traditionally, fever is defined as the body temperature above 38°C, but one-third of the elderly with acute infection usually does not have a fever at these values. A previous report noted that fever may be reduced or even absent in elderly patients with bacterial or viral infections due to low basal temperature, impaired thermal homeostasis due to aging, and frequently-used medicine such as aspirin [15]. In addition, healthy elderly people tend to have lower body temperatures compared to young people. The Infectious Diseases Practice Guidelines Committee of America has defined fever in the elderly as:

1. A single oral temperature> 100°F (37.8°C)
2. Repeated oral temperatures> 99°F (37.2°C) or rectal temperatures > 99.5°F (37.5°C)
3. Temperature increase> 2°F (1.1°C) relative to baseline temperature

The most common symptoms in the general population are fever (98%), cough (76%), shortness of breath (55%), and myalgia or fatigue (up to 44%) [16]. Although these symptoms are the most common in elderly patients, their incidence is different compared to young people. In studies of elderly individuals with COVID-19 infection, the most common symptoms were reported to be shortness of breath (76%), high fever (52%), and cough (48%) [7]. In another study; 66.7% of elderly patients had a fever, 64.8% cough, and 33.3% fatigue on admission. Other symptoms include shortness of breath (29.5%), diarrhea (9.5%), anorexia (8.6%), headache (8.6%), myalgia (7.6%), and vomiting (5.7%). In the same study, the median incubation period in elderly patients was 8 days, and the time from the onset of symptoms to hospitalization was 5 days. The atypical course of the disease in the elderly and the delayed perception of the symptoms due to the decrease in the cognitive functions of the elderly cause late admissions to the hospital. This causes the late initiation of treatment and a more serious and mortal course of the disease.

Cough and shortness of breath symptoms can be misleading in older individuals. The cough reflexes in the elderly are weakened and differential diagnosis should be made well in the elderly who present with dyspnoea due to the prevalence of chronic respiratory failure and heart failure causing dyspnoea. It was observed that the complaints of cough and sputum were similar among the elderly and young people, while the complaints of shortness of breath were more common in the elderly [17].

In a study in which 214 patients were evaluated, neurological findings were detected in 36.4% of the patients. In this study, neurological symptoms were classified into three categories. CNS symptoms or signs (headache, dizziness, impaired consciousness, ataxia, acute cerebrovascular disorder or epilepsy) were detected in 24.8% patients, neuropathy symptoms (hypogeusia, hyposmia, or neuropathic pain) were detected in 8.9% patients, skeletal muscle symptoms were detected in 10.7% patients [18].

In a review in the literature, the smell changes were reported as 60.7%, and the frequency of taste changes was reported as 56.4% [19]. Fatigue, weakness, headache, and gastrointestinal system findings in elderly patients are similar to those in young people. Along with these, elderly patients may present with confusion and impaired oral intake. In addition, it has been reported that cardiac complications such as myocarditis, pericardial effusion, and arrhythmia can be seen in cases with a severe course of the disease [20]. The pre-diagnosis of COVID-19 infection should be kept in mind in patients presenting with these complaints.

While trying to control the infection in elderly patients, we should also consider the complications we encounter frequently. Delirium is a common complication of infections, especially in older adults. In the first studies, it was shown that 20-30% of COVID-19 patients develop delirium on admission to the hospital or during the disease [21]. In all age groups, this rate has been reported to be 60-70% in those with severe disease. Although the exact cause of this relationship is unknown, it is thought that there may be multiple factors such as direct neurological invasion, cerebrovascular involvement or indirect high fever, hypoxia, dehydration, inflammation, medications, or metabolic disorders.

COVID-19 disease has been reported to increase the risk of thrombotic events, including stroke. In some studies, the incidence of ischaemic stroke in patients infected with COVID-19 is approximately 2.5%. In a study, the rate of hemorrhagic stroke was found to be 0.9%, and it was reported that 88% of these patients were using anticoagulants [22]. Although the mechanisms of cerebrovascular events in COVID-19 have not been clarified, it has been reported that coronavirus directly infects endothelial cells and causes widespread endothelial inflammation in cases with severe respiratory syndrome. This may be a mechanism leading to ischaemic stroke or hemorrhagic stroke.

Laboratory Characteristics

In available studies in the literature, it has been reported that lymphopenia is common in patients with SARS-CoV-2 infection. It has been observed to occur in 32.5-75.4% of COVID-19 patients in different studies [23]. Lymphopenia was also a common finding in severe acute respiratory syndrome coronavirus (SARS CoV) and Middle East respiratory syndrome coronavirus (MERS-CoV). Also, one study reported that severe cases of COVID-19 were reported to have lower lymphocyte count and higher neutrophil count than non-severe cases; therefore Neutrophil/lymphocyte ratio (NLR) tends to be higher in patients with severe infection [24].

Commonly, the studies reported that D-dimer, lactate dehydrogenase (LDH), and C-reactive protein (CRP) levels increased, and albumin level decreased among elderly patients with COVID-19 [12]. In a study comparing elderly people with middle-aged and younger individuals, it was shown that elderly patients had lower lymphocyte counts and higher CRP levels [25]. CRP is an acute-phase protein produced by the liver that can be elevated in a variety of conditions such as inflammation, cardiovascular disease, and infection. Some studies reported that CRP height is related to COVID-19 mortality [26]. Although D-Dimer is a specific marker of fibrinolysis used to predict venous thromboembolism, it may also increase inflammation and indicate a poor prognosis. As a matter of fact, there are investigations in the literature that show that high D-dimer levels predict COVID-19 mortality [27]. The decreased albumin and increased LDH suggest that SARS-CoV-2 infection is associated with extrapulmonary organ injury, such as hepatic or myocardia injury. In addition, there is reliable evidence that increasing LDH values reflect the degree of pulmonary damage in Acute Respiratory Distress Syndrome (ARDS) patients [28]. High procalcitonin levels have been reported in moderate-to-severe cases [29]. In a meta-analysis, it was reported that troponin, CK-MB, and NT-proBNP were significantly higher in severe COVID-19 cases than in mild cases and mortality was higher in patients with acute cardiac injury [30].

Ferritin is a protein that contributes to cytokine storm with its immunosuppressive and proinflammatory effects. In some studies, it has been reported that the ferritin level correlates with the severity of the COVID-19 disease [31]. Publications are showing that it predicts mortality. Therefore, it may be important to check the ferritin level on admission to the hospital and follow-up of the disease ints, including elderly patients, to be more controlled against the disease.

Especially in elderly patients with COVID-19, it is important to monitor the course of the disease and its response to treatment with laboratory tests, as patients may have difficulty in identifying symptoms and the disease may be atypical.

RADIOLOGICAL CHARACTERISTICS

The most important involvement site of Coronavirus Disease 2019 (COVID-19) is the lung [32]. Therefore, it is very important to demonstrate lung involvement radiologically. Although the gold standard in the diagnosis of the disease is the Real-Time Polymerase Chain Reaction (RT-PCR) test, radiological imaging has started to be used extensively due to the inadequacy of the test in some places and its early false-negative results [33]. However, radiological methods are not screening tests in the diagnosis of COVID-19; It should not be forgotten that it should be used as a method to help diagnose and monitor the disease. In imaging, chest radiography, thoracic computed tomography (CT), and in some limited centers, thoracic ultrasonography (US) is used for this purpose. Chest radiography is the first-choice imaging method for demonstrating COVID-19 pneumonia. However, it should be kept in mind that the limited ground-glass opacification (GGO) in the lungs, especially in the early phase of the disease, cannot be seen on radiography. The sensitivity of chest radiography in demonstrating disease involvement has been reported to be 30-60% [34]. Typical findings on CT related to COVID-19 pneumonia are GGO, flagstone appearance, consolidation, air bronchogram, vascular enlargement, bronchial dilatation, halo sign, inverted halo sign, nodules, air-bubble sign, subpleural - parenchymal bands, and pleural changes [35]. In a study evaluating 919 COVID-19 patients, it was found that 88% of patients had ground-glass opacification (GGO), 87.5% had bilateral involvement, 76% had peripheral distribution, and 78.8% had multilobar involvement. Isolated GGO or GGO and consolidations were found to be the most common CT findings [36]. In the studies comparing the elderly and middle-aged groups, it was observed that multilobar and widespread involvement were more common in elderly individuals [27]. In the chest imaging of older adults; bilateral reticular-nodular opacities (58%), GGOs (48%), pleural effusions (about 33%), peribronchial thickening (about 25%), and focal consolidations (20%) have been reported [37].

TREATMENT

There is currently no specific treatment for COVID-19 infection with proven efficacy. Over 100 randomized controlled trials are being conducted for effective treatment trials against COVID-19. Since there is no treatment specific to COVID-19, medicines such as hydroxychloroquine, favipiravir, remdesivir, lopinavir-ritonavir, which were licensed for the treatment of other diseases in humans before, has been recommended and used during the current pandemic in our country and other countries. Numerous studies are still going on for the effectiveness and safety of these medicines in COVID-19. There is no difference between elderly patients and younger patients in terms of treatment options.

Chloroquine (CQ) and hydroxychloroquine (HCQ) have been used for more than 70 years to treat malaria and some autoimmune diseases. These medicines have become the candidate medicines for the treatment of COVID-19 infection because of their immunomodulatory effects and the effects that prevent viruses from entering the cell. It has been reported that at the beginning of the pandemic process, the use of CQ shortens the duration of the disease and slows its progression [38]. In addition, there are studies in the literature that suggest the use of HCQ reduces viral load in COVID-19 infection [39]. There are also studies on the negative effects of CQ and HCQ treatment. Despite their conflicting results, CQ and HCQ are included in COVID-19 treatment guidelines around the world. HCQ therapy is known to prolong the QT interval. Risk factors for QT prolongation include advanced age, female gender, history of heart disease, hypokalaemia, the use of furosemide and thiazide diuretics, kidney and liver failure, and the use of other medicines that prolong the QT interval. Elderly individuals are particularly at risk for QT prolongation and Torsades de Pointes. There is a risk of QT prolongation due to the high risk of hypertension in many elderly people, history of using antihypertensive medicines combined with diuretics, concomitant heart failure, polypharmacy, and inappropriate medicine use, and care should be taken in the use of HCQ in these patients. In patients without risk, the corrected QT (QTc) should be calculated by taking a basal electrocardiogram (ECG) before starting the medicine. If basal QTc is > 500 ms, HCQ therapy should be avoided. If the QTc length is normal, treatment is started and daily ECG monitoring is recommended [40]. Care should be taken in this regard especially in elderly patients, and they should be evaluated in detail regarding drug interactions during the treatment of COVID-19 infection. In addition, the combined use of azithromycin-HCQ, which was previously included in the guideline, is no longer recommended due to the high number of side effects.

It has been shown in animal studies and in vitro studies that Lopinavir inhibits the protease activity of coronaviruses. Additionally, in SARS and MERS outbreaks, lopinavir/ritonavir treatment is effective and reduces mortality, so it has been a candidate medicine for COVID-19 treatment [41]. In a lopinavir/ritonavir versus arbidol comparative study of individuals with mild to moderate COVID-19 infection, no significant difference was found between treatments [42]. In severe cases of COVID-19, the addition of lopinavir/ritonavir therapy to standard therapy has been reported to provide no additional benefit in terms of clinical improvement but rather increase the frequency of side effects [43]. The results of other studies in the literature were similar. In summary, lopinavir/ritonavir monotherapy or combination therapy has not been shown to contribute to the standard therapy.

Remdesivir, which has a broad antiviral activity and works by targeting viral RNA-dependent RNA polymerase (RdRp), has also been shown to be effective against coronaviruses [44]. In a randomized study involving 1059 patients (538 assigned to remdesivir and 521 assigned to placebo), it was shown that the mean recovery time for those who used the placebo was 15 days while it was 11 days for those who used remdesivir. In addition, remdesivir was found to be sufficiently tolerated and safe. It was found that serious side effects were lower in those who used remdesivir compared to those using a placebo. However, adverse events such as gastrointestinal symptoms (anorexia, nausea, and vomiting), increased liver enzymes, and worsening of cardiopulmonary status were seen at a higher rate in remdesivir users than in placebo users [45]. There is no different data on the use of remdesivir in the elderly.

Favipiravir acts by inhibiting RNA-dependent RNA polymerase. Vitro studies have shown that favipiravir is effective against coronaviruses. In a study of 120 patients with mild to moderate infections, when favipiravir and arbidol therapies were compared, clinical improvement at day 7 was better in patients using favipiravir [46]. In another study, favipiravir and lopinavir/ritonavir treatments were compared; it has been shown that viral clearance is faster (4 vs 11 days) and radiological lung recovery is better (91% vs 62% in 14 days) using favipiravir [47].

In patients with severe COVID-19 pneumonia, macrophage activation syndrome (MAS) and secondary lymphocytic lymphohistiocytosis may develop due to excessive hyperstokinemia (IL-1, IL-6, IFN-gamma, etc.). In the MAS table of COVID-19 patients, especially the elevation of IL-6 is remarkable. For this reason, cytokine suppression treatments have come into question in the treatment of these patients. Tocilizumab is an agent that functions as an IL-6 monoclonal antagonist. Tocilizumab has recently come to the fore as a medicine that has shown serious benefits in clinical improvement in severe COVID-19 pneumonia. Some studies have shown that administration of tocilizumab (4 mg/kg/d) given through intravenous infusion at 24-hour intervals at the beginning of the patient's SARS is effective in reducing the need for ventilator support and improving lung functions in patients with severe COVID-19 [48].

Corticosteroids have been shown to shorten the intensive care period in COVID-19 patients with severe persistent shock. In one study, it has been shown that 10-day oral or intravenous 6 mg dexamethasone treatment reduces 28-day mortality in patients who need oxygen or require ventilator support [49]. It has been reported to be beneficial only to patients with COVID-19 with respiratory failure [50]. Its effect has not been demonstrated in patients who do not need respiratory support.

Studies on convalescent plasma therapy continue, and the studies so far have shown that it is useful in the treatment of severe and life-threatening COVID-19 infection. It has been reported to be more beneficial especially when administered before intubation [51].

In addition to all these treatments, the medicines used by the elderly infected with COVID-19 should be evaluated and necessary recommendations should be made due to their comorbidities. For example; Angiotensin-converting enzyme 2 (ACE2) is a co-receptor for viral entry into SARS-CoV-2; this suggests that it has a role in the pathogenesis of COVID-19. Therefore, angiotensin-converting enzyme inhibitors (ACEIs) and Angiotensin II receptor blockers (ARBs) use are thought to increase COVID-19 mortality and morbidity. However, some studies have shown that ACEIs prescribed at the clinic do not inhibit ACE2, which acts as a carboxypeptidase [52]. As a result, no evidence was found regarding the benefit or harm of ACEI/ARB use in observational studies. Elderly patients who are currently using ACEI/ARB as antihypertensive do not need to discontinue the medicine unless they have a different indication. Although studies are reporting that the use of statins is more likely to increase liver enzymes in patients with COVID-19 infection, there are also studies suggesting that COVID-19 infection increases the risk of acute cardiac damage and therefore the use of statins should be continued. Therefore, evaluation of the use of statin on an individual basis was decided. The ESC guidelines recommended that statins be continued in patients who use them because of their immunomodulatory and cardioprotective effects [53]. Also, when using antipyretic in elderly patients; considering the renal failure, toxicity, and gastrointestinal bleeding side effects, nonsteroidal anti-inflammatory medicines (NSAIDs) should be avoided as much as possible, and paracetamol should be preferred primarily.

During the pandemic period, elderly patients without COVID-19 infection who remain at home and immobile for a long time should be evaluated in terms of sarcopenia and malnutrition, which are important geriatric syndromes, and necessary supportive treatments and recommendations should be made. Also, malnutrition and sarcopenia may increase the frailty of patients, causing them to have a more serious COVID-19 infection.

Another important point that should not be ignored during the pandemic process is that the elderly are undoubtedly affected psychologically. The curfew imposed on people aged 65 and over in many countries and their relatives' not visiting them to protect the elderly from COVID-19 infection caused social isolation and some psychological problems. Psychological problems may also cause more malnutrition and frailty in the elderly, leading to a decrease in immune responses and a more serious COVID-19 infection, and increased morbidity and mortality. For this reason, it is very important to evaluate the elderly psychologically and to provide the necessary support during the pandemic process.

Conclusion

It is known that the elderly are the most affected group by the COVID-19 epidemic that affects the whole world. The initial symptoms and course of the disease in the elderly may differ from other age groups. Therefore, these differences should be taken into consideration when evaluating geriatric patients. Although there is no difference in the treatment protocol, the comorbidities of the elderly and multiple medicine use should be considered, and alert should be made in terms of medicine side effects and drug-drug interactions. In addition, it should not be forgotten that elderly patients are affected by the epidemic not only physically, but also socially and psychologically, and the necessary support should be provided in these areas.

References

[1] WHO (2020). *WHO Timeline- COVID-19*. Available at: https://www.who.int/news-room/detail/08-04-2020-who-timeline- covid-19. Accessed September 7, 2020.

[2] Zhu, N., Zhang, D., Wang, W., Li, X., Yang, B., Song, J., Zhao, X., Huang, B., Shi, W., Lu, R., Niu, P., Zhan, F., Ma, X., Wang, D., Xu, W., Wu, G., Gao, G. F., Tan, W., & China Novel Coronavirus Investigating and Research Team. 2020. "A Novel Coronavirus from Patients with Pneumonia in China, 2019." *The New England journal of medicine*. 382(8), 727–733.

[3] United Nations (UN), Department of Economic and Social Affairs, Population Division (2019). *World Population Ageing 2019*.

[4] Dent, E., Morley, J. E., Cruz-Jentoft, A. J., Woodhouse, L., Rodríguez-Mañas, L., Fried, L. P., Woo, J., Aprahamian, I., Sanford, A., Lundy, J., Landi, F., Beilby, J., Martin, F. C., Bauer, J. M., Ferrucci, L., Merchant, R. A., Dong, B., Arai, H., Hoogendijk, E. O., Won, C. W., Vellas, B. 2019. "Physical Frailty: ICFSR International Clinical Practice Guidelines for Identification and Management." *The journal of nutrition, health & aging*. 23(9), 771–787.

[5] Wu, Z., & McGoogan, J. M. 2020. "Characteristics of and Important Lessons from the Coronavirus Disease 2019 (COVID-19) Outbreak in China: Summary of a Report of 72 314 Cases from the Chinese Center for Disease Control and Prevention." *JAMA*. 323(13), 1239–1242.

[6] CDC COVID-19 Response Team 2020. "Severe Outcomes among Patients with Coronavirus Disease 2019 (COVID-19) - United States, February 12-March 16, 2020." *MMWR. Morbidity and mortality weekly report*, 69(12), 343–346.

[7] Shahid, Z., Kalayanamitra, R., McClafferty, B., Kepko, D., Ramgobin, D., Patel, R., Aggarwal, C. S., Vunnam, R., Sahu, N., Bhatt, D., Jones, K., Golamari, R., &

Jain, R. 2020. "COVID-19 and Older Adults: What We Know." *Journal of the American Geriatrics Society*, 68(5), 926–929.

[8] Centers for Disease Control and Prevention (CDC). *National Diabetes Statistics Report 2020*. https://www.cdc.gov/diabetes/pdfs/data/statistics/nationaldiabetes-statistics-report.pdf. Accessed September 4, 2020.

[9] Fryar, C. D., Ostchega, Y., Hales, C. M., Zhang, G., & Kruszon-Moran, D. 2017. "Hypertension Prevalence and Control Among Adults: United States, 2015-2016." *NCHS data brief*. (289), 1–8.

[10] Centers for Disease Control and Prevention (CDC). *Chronic Kidney Disease in the United States, 2019*. https://www.cdc.gov/kidneydisease/publications-resources/2019-national-facts.html Accessed September 4, 2020.

[11] Li, T., Lu, L., Zhang, W., Tao, Y., Wang, L., Bao, J., Liu, B., & Duan, J. 2020. "Clinical characteristics of 312 hospitalized older patients with COVID-19 in Wuhan, China." *Archives of gerontology and geriatrics*. 91, 104185.

[12] Guo, T., Shen, Q., Guo, W., He, W., Li, J., Zhang, Y., Wang, Y., Zhou, Z., Deng, D., Ouyang, X., Xiang, Z., Jiang, M., Liang, M., Huang, P., Peng, Z., Xiang, X., Liu, W., Luo, H., Chen, P., & Peng, H. 2020. "Clinical Characteristics of Elderly Patients with COVID-19 in Hunan Province, China: A Multicenter, Retrospective Study." *Gerontology*. 1–9.

[13] Yang, X., Yu, Y., Xu, J., Shu, H., Xia, J., Liu, H., Wu, Y., Zhang, L., Yu, Z., Fang, M., Yu, T., Wang, Y., Pan, S., Zou, X., Yuan, S., & Shang, Y. 2020. "Clinical course and outcomes of critically ill patients with SARS-CoV-2 pneumonia in Wuhan, China: a single-centered, retrospective, observational study." *The Lancet. Respiratory medicine*. 8(5), 475–481.

[14] Zhou, F., Yu, T., Du, R., Fan, G., Liu, Y., Liu, Z., Xiang, J., Wang, Y., Song, B., Gu, X., Guan, L., Wei, Y., Li, H., Wu, X., Xu, J., Tu, S., Zhang, Y., Chen, H., & Cao, B. 2020. "Clinical course and risk factors for mortality of adult inpatients with COVID-19 in Wuhan, China: a retrospective cohort study." *Lancet (London, England)*. 395(10229), 1054–1062.

[15] Norman, D. C., & Yoshikawa, T. T. 1996. "Fever in the elderly." *Infectious disease clinics of North America*. 10(1), 93–99.

[16] Huang, C., Wang, Y., Li, X., Ren, L., Zhao, J., Hu, Y., Zhang, L., Fan, G., Xu, J., Gu, X., Cheng, Z., Yu, T., Xia, J., Wei, Y., Wu, W., Xie, X., Yin, W., Li, H., Liu, M., Xiao, Y., Cao, B. 2020. "Clinical features of patients infected with 2019 novel coronavirus in Wuhan, China." *Lancet (London, England)*. 395(10223), 497–506.

[17] Lian, J., Jin, X., Hao, S., Cai, H., Zhang, S., Zheng, L., Jia, H., Hu, J., Gao, J., Zhang, Y., Zhang, X., Yu, G., Wang, X., Gu, J., Ye, C., Jin, C., Lu, Y., Yu, X., Yu, X., Ren, Y., Yang, Y. 2020. "Analysis of Epidemiological and Clinical Features in Older Patients with Coronavirus Disease 2019 (COVID-19) Outside Wuhan."

Clinical infectious diseases: an official publication of the Infectious Diseases Society of America. 71(15), 740–747.

[18] Özdağ Acarli, A. N., Samanci, B., Ekizoğlu, E., Çakar, A., Şirin, N. G., Gündüz, T., Parman, Y., & Baykan, B. 2020. "Coronavirus Disease 2019 (COVID-19) From the Point of View of Neurologists: Observation of Neurological Findings and Symptoms During the Combat Against a Pandemic." *Noro psikiyatri arşivi*. 57(2), 154–159.

[19] Costa, K., Carnaúba, A., Rocha, K. W., Andrade, K., Ferreira, S., & Menezes, P. L. 2020. "Olfactory and taste disorders in COVID-19: a systematic review." *Brazilian journal of otorhinolaryngology*. S1808-8694(20)30066-5.

[20] Zeng, J. H., Liu, Y. X., Yuan, J., Wang, F. X., Wu, W. B., Li, J. X., Wang, L. F., Gao, H., Wang, Y., Dong, C. F., Li, Y. J., Xie, X. J., Feng, C., & Liu, L. 2020. "First case of COVID-19 complicated with fulminant myocarditis: a case report and insights." *Infection*. 1–5.

[21] Mao, L., Jin, H., Wang, M., Hu, Y., Chen, S., He, Q., Chang, J., Hong, C., Zhou, Y., Wang, D., Miao, X., Li, Y., & Hu, B. 2020. "Neurologic Manifestations of Hospitalized Patients with Coronavirus Disease 2019 in Wuhan, China." *JAMA neurology*. 77(6), 683–690.

[22] Rothstein, A., Oldridge, O., Schwennesen, H., Do, D., & Cucchiara, B. L. 2020. "Acute Cerebrovascular Events in Hospitalized COVID-19 Patients." *Stroke*, 51(9), e219–e222.

[23] Wu, J., Liu, J., Zhao, X., Liu, C., Wang, W., Wang, D., Xu, W., Zhang, C., Yu, J., Jiang, B., Cao, H., & Li, L. 2020. "Clinical Characteristics of Imported Cases of Coronavirus Disease 2019 (COVID-19) in Jiangsu Province: A Multicenter Descriptive Study." *Clinical infectious diseases: an official publication of the Infectious Diseases Society of America*. 71(15), 706–712.

[24] Qin, C., Zhou, L., Hu, Z., Zhang, S., Yang, S., Tao, Y., Xie, C., Ma, K., Shang, K., Wang, W., & Tian, D. S. 2020. "Dysregulation of Immune Response in Patients with Coronavirus 2019 (COVID-19) in Wuhan, China." *Clinical infectious diseases: an official publication of the Infectious Diseases Society of America*. 71(15), 762–768.

[25] Liu, K., Chen, Y., Lin, R., & Han, K. 2020. "Clinical features of COVID-19 in elderly patients: A comparison with young and middle-aged patients." *The Journal of infection*, 80(6), e14–e18.

[26] Wang, K., Zuo, P., Liu, Y., Zhang, M., Zhao, X., Xie, S., Zhang, H., Chen, X., & Liu, C. 2020. "Clinical and laboratory predictors of in-hospital mortality in patients with COVID-19: a cohort study in Wuhan, China." *Clinical infectious diseases: an official publication of the Infectious Diseases Society of America*. ciaa538.

[27] Zhang, L., Yan, X., Fan, Q., Liu, H., Liu, X., Liu, Z., & Zhang, Z. 2020. D-dimer levels on admission to predict in-hospital mortality in patients with Covid-19. *Journal of thrombosis and haemostasis: JTH.* 18(6), 1324–1329.

[28] Chiang, C. H., Shih, J. F., Su, W. J., & Perng, R. P. 2004. "Eight-month prospective study of 14 patients with hospital-acquired severe acute respiratory syndrome." *Mayo Clinic proceedings*. 79(11), 1372–1379.

[29] Li, K., Wu, J., Wu, F., Guo, D., Chen, L., Fang, Z., & Li, C. 2020. "The Clinical and Chest CT Features Associated With Severe and Critical COVID-19 Pneumonia." *Investigative radiology*. 55(6), 327–331.

[30] Li, J. W., Han, T. W., Woodward, M., Anderson, C. S., Zhou, H., Chen, Y. D., & Neal, B. 2020. "The impact of 2019 novel coronavirus on heart injury: A Systematic review and Meta-analysis." *Progress in cardiovascular diseases*. S0033-0620(20)30080-3.

[31] Dahan, S., Segal, G., Katz, I., Hellou, T., Tietel, M., Bryk, G., Amital, H., Shoenfeld, Y., & Dagan, A. 2020. "Ferritin as a Marker of Severity in COVID-19 Patients: A Fatal Correlation." *The Israel Medical Association journal: IMAJ*, 8(22), 429–434.

[32] Zhu, N., Zhang, D., Wang, W., Li, X., Yang, B., Song, J., Zhao, X., Huang, B., Shi, W., Lu, R., Niu, P., Zhan, F., Ma, X., Wang, D., Xu, W., Wu, G., Gao, G. F., Tan, W., & China Novel Coronavirus Investigating and Research Team 2020. "A Novel Coronavirus from Patients with Pneumonia in China, 2019." *The New England journal of medicine.* 382(8), 727–733.

[33] Huang, P., Liu, T., Huang, L., Liu, H., Lei, M., Xu, W., Hu, X., Chen, J., & Liu, B. 2020. "Use of Chest CT in Combination with Negative RT-PCR Assay for the 2019 Novel Coronavirus but High Clinical Suspicion." *Radiology*. 295(1), 22–23.

[34] Kong W, Agarwal PP. 2020. "Chest imaging appearance of COVID-19 infection." *Radiology: Cardiothoracic Imaging*. 2(1):e200028.

[35] Bernheim, A., Mei, X., Huang, M., Yang, Y., Fayad, Z. A., Zhang, N., Diao, K., Lin, B., Zhu, X., Li, K., Li, S., Shan, H., Jacobi, A., & Chung, M. 2020. "Chest CT Findings in Coronavirus Disease-19 (COVID-19): Relationship to Duration of Infection." *Radiology*. 295(3), 200463.

[36] Salehi, S., Abedi, A., Balakrishnan, S., & Gholamrezanezhad, A. 2020. "Coronavirus Disease 2019 (COVID-19): A Systematic Review of Imaging Findings in 919 Patients." *AJR. American journal of roentgenology*. 215(1), 87–93.

[37] Arentz, M., Yim, E., Klaff, L., Lokhandwala, S., Riedo, F. X., Chong, M., & Lee, M. 2020. "Characteristics and Outcomes of 21 Critically Ill Patients with COVID-19 in Washington State." *JAMA*. 323(16), 1612–1614.

[38] Gao, J., Tian, Z., & Yang, X. 2020. "Breakthrough: Chloroquine phosphate has shown apparent efficacy in treatment of COVID-19 associated pneumonia in clinical studies." *Bioscience trends*. 14(1), 72–73.

[39] Gautret, P., Lagier, J. C., Parola, P., Hoang, V. T., Meddeb, L., Mailhe, M., Doudier, B., Courjon, J., Giordanengo, V., Vieira, V. E., Tissot Dupont, H., Honoré, S., Colson, P., Chabrière, E., La Scola, B., Rolain, J. M., Brouqui, P., & Raoult, D. 2020. "Hydroxychloroquine and azithromycin as a treatment of COVID-19: results of an open-label non-randomized clinical trial." *International journal of antimicrobial agents*. 56(1), 105949.

[40] *American College of Cardiology* (*ACC*). https://www.acc.org/latest-in-cardiology/articles/2020/03/27/14/00/ventricular-arrhythmia-risk-due-to-hydroxychloroquine-azithromycin-treatment-for-covid-19 Accessed September 4, 2020.

[41] Yao, T. T., Qian, J. D., Zhu, W. Y., Wang, Y., & Wang, G. Q. 2020. "A systematic review of lopinavir therapy for SARS coronavirus and MERS coronavirus-A possible reference for coronavirus disease-19 treatment option." *Journal of medical virology*. 92(6), 556–563.

[42] Li, Y., Xie, Z., Lin, W., Cai, W., Wen, C., Guan, Y., Mo, X., Wang, J., Wang, Y., Peng, P., Chen, X., Hong, W., Xiao, G., Liu, J., Zhang, L., Hu, F., Li, F., Zhang, F., Deng, X., & Li, L. 2020. "Efficacy and Safety of Lopinavir/Ritonavir or Arbidol in Adult Patients with Mild/Moderate COVID-19: An Exploratory Randomized Controlled Trial." *Med (New York, N.Y.)*. 10.1016/j.medj.2020.04.001.

[43] Cao, B., Wang, Y., Wen, D., Liu, W., Wang, J., Fan, G., Ruan, L., Song, B., Cai, Y., Wei, M., Li, X., Xia, J., Chen, N., Xiang, J., Yu, T., Bai, T., Xie, X., Zhang, L., Li, C., Yuan, Y., Wang, C. 2020. "A Trial of Lopinavir-Ritonavir in Adults Hospitalized with Severe Covid-19." *The New England journal of medicine*. 382(19), 1787–1799.

[44] Agostini, M. L., Andres, E. L., Sims, A. C., Graham, R. L., Sheahan, T. P., Lu, X., Smith, E. C., Case, J. B., Feng, J. Y., Jordan, R., Ray, A. S., Cihlar, T., Siegel, D., Mackman, R. L., Clarke, M. O., Baric, R. S., & Denison, M. R. 2018. "Coronavirus Susceptibility to the Antiviral Remdesivir (GS-5734) Is Mediated by the Viral Polymerase and the Proofreading Exoribonuclease." *mBio*. 9(2), e00221-18.

[45] Beigel, J. H., Tomashek, K. M., Dodd, L. E., Mehta, A. K., Zingman, B. S., Kalil, A. C., Hohmann, E., Chu, H. Y., Luetkemeyer, A., Kline, S., Lopez de Castilla, D., Finberg, R. W., Dierberg, K., Tapson, V., Hsieh, L., Patterson, T. F., Paredes, R., Sweeney, D. A., Short, W. R., Touloumi, G., ACTT-1 Study Group Members 2020. "Remdesivir for the Treatment of Covid-19 - Preliminary Report." *The New England journal of medicine*. NEJMoa2007764.

[46] Chen C, Zhang Y, Huang J, Yin P, Cheng Z, Wu J, Chen S, Zhang Y, Chen B, Lu M, Luo Y, Ju L, Zhang J, Wang X. 2020. "Favipiravir versus Arbidol for COVID-19: A Randomized Clinical Trial." *MedRxiv*. doi: 10.1101/2020.03.17.20037432.

[47] Cai, Q., Yang, M., Liu, D., Chen, J., Shu, D., Xia, J., Liao, X., Gu, Y., Cai, Q., Yang, Y., Shen, C., Li, X., Peng, L., Huang, D., Zhang, J., Zhang, S., Wang, F., Liu, J., Chen, L., Chen, S., Liu, L. (2020). "Experimental Treatment with

Favipiravir for COVID-19: An Open-Label Control Study." *Engineering (Beijing, China)*, 10.1016/j.eng.2020.03.007.

[48] Xu, X., Han, M., Li, T., Sun, W., Wang, D., Fu, B., Zhou, Y., Zheng, X., Yang, Y., Li, X., Zhang, X., Pan, A., & Wei, H. 2020. "Effective treatment of severe COVID-19 patients with tocilizumab." *Proceedings of the National Academy of Sciences of the United States of America*. 117 (20), 10970–10975.

[49] "*Oxford university news Release. Low-cost dexamethasone reduces death by up to one third in hospitalised patients with severe respiratory complications of COVID-19.*" https://www.recoverytrial.net/files/recovery_dexamethasone_statement_160620_v2final.pdf (Accessed on September 11, 2020).

[50] Alhazzani, W., Møller, M. H., Arabi, Y. M., Loeb, M., Gong, M. N., Fan, E., Oczkowski, S., Levy, M. M., Derde, L., Dzierba, A., Du, B., Aboodi, M., Wunsch, H., Cecconi, M., Koh, Y., Chertow, D. S., Maitland, K., Alshamsi, F., Belley-Cote, E., Greco, M., Rhodes, A. 2020. "Surviving Sepsis Campaign: Guidelines on the Management of Critically Ill Adults with Coronavirus Disease 2019 (COVID-19)." *Critical care medicine*. 48(6), e440–e469.

[51] Li, L., Zhang, W., Hu, Y., Tong, X., Zheng, S., Yang, J., Kong, Y., Ren, L., Wei, Q., Mei, H., Hu, C., Tao, C., Yang, R., Wang, J., Yu, Y., Guo, Y., Wu, X., Xu, Z., Zeng, L., Xiong, N., Liu, Z. 2020. "Effect of Convalescent Plasma Therapy on Time to Clinical Improvement in Patients with Severe and Life-threatening COVID-19: A Randomized Clinical Trial. *JAMA*. 324(5), 460–470.

[52] Rice, G. I., Thomas, D. A., Grant, P. J., Turner, A. J., & Hooper, N. M. 2004. "Evaluation of angiotensin-converting enzyme (ACE), its homologue ACE2 and neprilysin in angiotensin peptide metabolism." *The Biochemical journal*. 383(Pt 1), 45–51.

[53] Castiglione, V., Chiriacò, M., Emdin, M., Taddei, S., & Vergaro, G. 2020. "Statin therapy in COVID-19 infection." *European heart journal. Cardiovascular pharmacotherapy*. 6(4), 258–259.

In: Coronavirus Disease
Editor: Yildiz Dincer

ISBN: 978-1-53619-296-4

Chapter 10

SARS COV-2 IN PEDIATRIC PATIENTS: HEMATOLOGICAL FACE OF THE DISEASE

Tulin Tiraje Celkan * ***and Ayşe Gonca Kacar***
Istanbul University- Cerrahpasa, Cerrahpasa Medical Faculty,
Department of Pediatric Hematology and Oncology Istanbul Turkey

ABSTRACT

The COVID-19 pandemic is the biggest health problem of our last 10 months, Pediatricians were more fortunate than internal medicine specialists due to the low number of pediatric cases with COVID 19. As the disease spread rapidly throughout the world, the experience with the diagnosis, follow-up, and treatment are collected. There is no clear-cut data for an effective drug against the SARS-CoV2 virus or an effective vaccine to prevent infection. On the other hand, epidemiological data from infected people are promising for the strategy for future. Unlike other infectious diseases, the incidence of the infection and mortality rate is significantly higher in developed countries. COVID 19 is generally mild in children, some might not show any symptoms at all. In this paper, we tried to share latest data about childhood COV-2 infection, especially focused on hematological signs and symptoms and their physiopathology.

Keywords: COVID 19 pandemic, pediatric cases, hematological signs

INTRODUCTION

Coronaviruses are a group of RNA viruses with a roughly 30 kb genome surrounded by a protein envelope belonging to the *Coronaviridae* family, *Nidovirales* order [1]. The

* Corresponding Author's Email: tirajecelkan@yahoo.com.

exact origin of the virus is unknown but current studies have revealed that 2019-nCoV has a zoonotic origin, it emerged from a bat-borne virüs. It can easily spread between persons through respiratory droplets [2]. It has resulted in a worldwide outbreak and is classified as a pandemic by the World Health Organization on March 11, 2020 [3]. By March 1, 2020, SARS-CoV-2 had led to 80 981 confirmed cases of COVID-19 in China, and 44 067 cases in 117 countries. In Korea, the ratio of patients younger than 19 years is 6.7% of total cases, and no child deaths have been reported [4].

Italy, having the second-highest number of Covid-19 infections and the greatest number of deaths after China, reported that children younger than 18 years of age who had Covid-19 composed only 1% of the total patients; and only 11% of these children were hospitalized, and none died [5]. Recent reports on pediatric cases of COVID-19 suggest that COVID 19 is less common in children and they usually have mild illnesses. However, the full spectrum of illness in children is not clearly understood because many pediatric patients might not have been subject to viral testing. Furthermore, there is limited information regarding the duration of SARS-CoV-2 RNA detection in children's respiratory tracts [4]. Thus far, all pediatric cases with laboratory-confirmed 2019-nCoV infection were mild cases, and no deaths had been reported.

Transmission

Respiratory droplets and contact are the main transmission routes in COVID 19 [6]. The incubation period is about 1 to 14 days, and that can last up to 24 days. The virulence of the virus could peak 2 to 3 days before symptom starts, and transmission during the presymptomatic stage is estimated to make up 44% of secondary infections [4]. At the beginning of the Sars COV- 2 outbreak, the infection is transmitted by adults in the community. Then the virus spread to the family and children via infected adults. The first pediatric case was identified in the familial cluster [7]. Close contact with symptomatic or asymptomatic cases with silent infection are the main transmission routes of 2019-nCoV infection in children [6]. Children tend to have no or milder symptoms, so they can easily spread infection to their household. Therefore understanding infectious burden and potential for transmissibility within the pediatric population is critical for developing both short- and long-term responses, including public health policies, to the current pandemic [8]. There is an urgent need for further investigation of the role of children who have an important role in the chain of transmission.

Perinatal transmission of COVID 19 is also not known exactly. There are several reported cases of neonatal infection suggesting a possible neonatal and vertical transmission. In a study by Chen et al., nine neonates born to COVID 19 positive mothers tested negative after cesarean delivery [7]. Breastmilk and placental pathological specimens from COVID 19 positive mothers remained negative for the viruses. Like other coronaviruses (SARS and MERS) it is thought that vertical transmission during third trimester is very rare. But the consequences of SARS COV-2 in early pregnancy like abortion, premature delivery, malformations, organ development is not well known. Also, Dong et al. emphasize that the proportion of severe and critical cases were higher in neonates when compared to the other childhood age group [9]. Breastmilk of the mother with suspected or confirmed COVID 19 is still the first choice in newborns feeding. Secretory IGA in breastmilk can be protective against COVİD 19. Also, breastmilk improves the neurocognitive and immunologic development of the newborn.

Clinical Presentation

Children infected with COVID 19 might be asymptomatic or generally presented with fever, dry cough, fatigue, and have mild upper respiratory symptoms. Gastrointestinal complaints like abdominal discomfort, nausea, vomiting, diarrhea and are rarer clinical symptoms of pediatric COVID 19 [6]. ACE2 the receptor for SARS-COV-2 in human cells is highly expressed in olfactory neuroepithelium lead to the infection in this site, resulting as a typical symptom, anosmia. The severity of COVID-19 was defined based on the clinical features, laboratory testing, and chest X-ray imaging, including asymptomatic infection, mild, moderate, severe, and critical cases. The diagnostic criteria were as follows [10]:

1. **Asymptomatic infection:** Patient has no clinical symptoms and signs and the chest imaging is normal, while the 2019-nCoV nucleic acid test is positive.
2. **Mild:** Patient is presented with acute upper respiratory tracts infection symptoms like fever, fatigue, myalgia, cough, sore throat, coryza Some cases may have no fever, or have only digestive symptoms such as nausea, vomiting, abdominal pain, and diarrhea.
3. **Moderate:** Pneumonia occurs, frequent fever and cough, mostly dry/productive cough, some may have wheezing, but no obvious hypoxemia such as shortness of breath, and dry snoring, and/or wet snoring. Some cases may have no clinical signs and symptoms, but chest CT shows subclinical lung lesions.
4. **Severe:** The disease usually progresses and dyspnea occurs, with central cyanosis. Oxygen saturation is less than 92%, with other hypoxia manifestations.
5. **Critical:** Children can quickly progress to acute respiratory distress syndrome (ARDS) or respiratory failure, and may also have shock, encephalopathy, myocardial injury or heart failure, coagulation dysfunction, and acute kidney injury.

In Dong's study, 94.1% of all patients were confirmed as asymptomatic, mild, or moderate cases, 5.9% of them were severe. Severe cases and their proportion was 10.6%, 7.3%, 4.2%, 4.1%, and 3.0% for the age group of <1, 1-5, 6-10, 11-15, and ≥16 years, respectively [10]. This study revealed that children under 5 years old, especially infants with COVID-19 had more severe disease than the others.

A study suggests that children are just as likely as adults to become infected with SARS-CoV-2 but are less likely to be symptomatic or develop severe symptoms [11]. In several studies, it is reported that children and younger adults who do not have underlying conditions, such as impaired lung function or ımmunsupression, have a much lower risk for severe forms of COVID-19 [12].

There are some suggested hypotheses for this viewpoint:

1. The immune system of children and adults is different from composition and responsiveness. Also immune system's function and component developed with the age of the children (infant, preschool, adolescent)
2. Presence of other simultaneous viruses in the mucosa of lungs and airways, which are common in young children, could limit the growth of SARS-CoV2 by direct virus-to-virus interactions and competition [8]. As the amount of viral copy is diminished; the severity of COVID 19 is reduced.
3. The angiotensin-converting enzyme (ACE) 2 receptor is necessary for SARS-Cov2 binding and infection. These receptors in children are relatively less than adults. ACE2 expression did not correlate with viral load, suggesting that although increased ACE2 expression increased susceptibility for infection, once infected, children could carry high viral loads regardless of level of ACE2 expression.
4. In severe COVID-19 infection; the viral and pulmonary phases are followed by the final hyperinflammatory phase, which can lead to severe acute respiratory distress syndrome (ARDS), impaired cardiac function, and death. Children are less inclined to develop ARDS during respiratory tract infections than adults.

Although children tend to have mild clinical forms of COVID 19 or they are asymptomatic, they can have a large number of viruses and transmit to the other people easily. Also, viruses can persist in feces long after they are absent from nasopharyngeal secretions. For coping with this pandemic, we must protect the children from COVID 19 infection [12].

While acute SARS-CoV-2 infection tends to be mild or symptom-free in most pediatric cases, some children develop a multisystem inflammatory syndrome (MIS-C). Several weeks after possible SARS-CoV-2 infection or exposure, with severe cardiac complications, including hypotension, shock, and acute heart failure. MIS-C criteria, defined by Centers for Disease Control and Prevention (CDC): fever >38°C for >24 hours, laboratory evidence of inflammation, at least two organs involved, and no alternative possible diagnoses and a positive SARS-CoV-2 test by RT-PCR, serology or antigen test, or exposure to a COVID-19 positive patient within 3-4 weeks before the onset of symptoms. In Yonker's et al. study although 11-16 years of group children were mostly affected by COVID 19, the children ages 1-4 years and males are the most highly presented with MIS-C. In addition to fever, MIS-C complained more often about nausea/vomiting and rash and few symptoms of an upper respiratory tract infection. Co-morbidities like asthma, heart disease, hypertension, and diabetes do not differ between MIS-C positive/negative COVID 19 children. Children with severe MIS-C (with hypotension or cardiac abnormalities requiring therapeutic intervention such as steroids, IVIG, and/or anakinra) have more elevated IgM and IgG. Children with MIS-C do not have high levels of viral load on nasopharyngeal or oropharyngeal viral testing, nor do they have detectable viremia, however, they do have hyperactive antibody responses. Children with severe MIS-C have elevated SARS-CoV-2 IgM and IgG levels, showing T and B cell over-reactivity, or auto-antibodies that may be driving an inflammatory process causing MIS-C [8].

IMAGING

Like other types of pediatric pneumonia, chest plain film (CXR) is not indicated for most pediatric patients with known or suspected COVID-19 with mild clinical symptoms that do not require hospitalization; although CXR is usually indicated in neonates with fever and respiratory symptoms[13]. Sequential CXRs may be helpful to assess pediatric patients with COVID-19 who demonstrate worsening clinical symptoms or to assess response to supportive therapy. However, routine daily chest radiographs for stable pediatric COVID-19 patients in the intensive care unit (ICU) are not recommended as they have not been shown to impact adverse outcomes, pediatric ICU or hospital length of stay, or duration of ventilator requirements.

Chest CT imaging is not recommended as a first imaging modality because of the increased radiation sensitivity of pediatric patients. In some clinic situation, for example, the pediatric patients presenting with acute symptoms (i.e., hypoxia, dyspnea, tachycardia), worrisome abnormal laboratory findings (such as an elevated D-dimer), or to evaluate a patient demonstrating clinical deterioration or not responding as expected to supportive treatment, chest CT can be the appropriate diagnostic method [13].

Although CXR is the first imaging study recommended for evaluation of pediatric COVID-19 disease, most of the SARS- COV2 pediatric patients were not severe, plain chest X-ray could not identify all the pulmonary lesions, so Chest CTs were obtained to provide supportive information for diagnosis and management. CXR sensitivity for detection of COVID-19 pneumonia in adult patients has been reported ranging from 69%

to 89%. A single pediatric COVID-19 study reported observing patchy unilateral opacities in 40% of patients. In some suspected pediatric patients with a negative nucleic acid of COVID-19 virus, chest CT findings revealed the diagnosis, which could provide the early treatment of the children and also isolation of the source of infection [14].

CT images of pediatric COVID 19 are similar to those in adults. The typical radiologic findings are unilateral or bilateral subpleural ground-glass opacities, and consolidations with surrounding halo sign. Pleural effusion was not seen. The absorption of lesions on chest CT lagged behind clinical symptoms and nucleic acid detection. Lesions could be still visible on chest CT when two consecutive nucleic acid tests were negative.

Bacterial coinfection and other viral infections are more common in pediatric COVID, so the CT imaging of COVID-19 infection should be differentiated with other virus pneumonia. Adenovirus pneumonia lesions had a higher density, more consolidations, and fewer subpleural lesions. Respiratory syncytial virus and parainfluenza virus pneumonia lesions were mostly distributed along the bronchial tree with a thickened bronchial wall. Influenza viruses could cause grid-like changes in the lungs. In addition, it should be differentiated from bacterial pneumonia, mycoplasma pneumonia, and chlamydia pneumonia, and the density of pneumonia lesions caused by the latter pathogens is relatively higher. COVID-19 pneumonia can be superimposed with pneumonia caused by other types of pathogens, presenting more serious and complex imaging manifestations, so epidemiological and etiological examination should be combined.

Imaging findings in post-COVID 19 Multisystem Inflammatory Syndrome in Children (MIS-C), including airway inflammation, rapidly progressive pulmonary edema, coronary artery aneurysms, and extensive abdominal inflammatory change within the right iliac fossa, with lymphadenopathy and bowel wall thickening. In Hameed et al. study, central bronchial wall thickening is commonly seen in these children (34%) and with none exhibiting lower respiratory tract symptoms. These findings are more likely attributable to airway inflammation and pulmonary arteritis. Echocardiography must be done in MIS-C because it has more aggressive cardiovascular findings than that in Kawasaki disease. Abdominal USG/CT showed features of right iliac fossa mesenteric inflammation and lymphadenopathy. The clinical findings of MIS-C overlap with Kawasaki disease and ischemic stroke as a complication of vasculitis seen in both diseases [15].

Furthermore, as no long-term data is yet available, future studies investigating post-recovery sequelae of disease including alterations of pulmonary function tests and risk for development of permanent lung injury such as pulmonary fibrosis will be important [13].

LABORATORY FINDINGS

In SARS-COV2, some of the inflammatory biomarkers are associated with poor prognosis. C-reactive protein (CRP) elevation was seen in up to 40% of patients and associated with ARDS, cardiac injury, and mortality. Elevated LDH and serum ferritin levels have also been linked in multiple retrospective analyses with a higher risk of ARDS and death. Interleukin-6 (IL-6) was elevated at admission in 52% of patients in a study by Chen et al. and linked to increased mortality [16, 17]. Blood counts and coagulation parameters are deteriorated in severe COVID 19. Lymphopenia, thrombocytopenia, and coagulopathy indicate severe illness and often progress to the disseminated intravascular coagulation (DIC). COVID-19 has also been associated with an increased risk of venous thromboembolic events (VTE).

Lymphopenia

In a retrospective analysis of patients in Hong Kong and Singapore, lymphopenia was first described with SARS-CoV in 2003. It has been associated with adverse outcomes and ıntensive care unit (ICU) stay. Severe lymphopenia (< 0.6 × 109/L) can be considered as one of the indicators of early admission to ICU. Li and Wang et al. reported that there was no correlation between WBC count and severity of the disease. It was also shown that lymphopenia can develop when the leukocyte count was normal [18]. Patients with severe infection were observed to have a significantly lower lymphocyte count and the lymphocyte/WBC ratio. Guan et al. obtained clinical data and showed that on admission, 83.2% of patients had lymphopenia and 33.7% had leukopenia. Thrombocytopenia was also seen in 36.2% of cases, as discussed later. On the other hand, anemia was usually not present with hemoglobin values at normal to very mildly decreased. Hematologic abnormalities were more prominent in patients with severe disease when compared to non-severe presentations. [16]. Wu et al. described similar findings with 64% of patients having lymphopenia at presentation. Decreased lymphocyte counts were associated with poor prognosis and an increased risk of ARDS [19]. Lymphopenia was again documented in 70.3% of patients in Wuhan, with lymphocyte count, >1100/mL were significantly less likely to have a severe illness than those in the 0–500/ mL and 500–1100/mL ranges [20]. Tan et al. emphasized that blood lymphocyte percentage (LYM%) showed the most significant and reliable trend in predicting disease progression [21]. Days 10–12 and 17–19, patients whose lymphocyte percentage was less than 20% and 5%, had the worst clinical outcomes.

The pathophysiology of the association between lymphopenia and clinical course and prognosis is multifactorial. In the incubation period, lymphocyte count is in the normal range. As the virus spreads and concentrates in tissues (lungs, heart, gastrointestinal tract via cell receptor for the SARS COV2 (the angiotensin-converting enzyme 2 (ACE2)), symptoms worsen and radiographic findings become more evident. At this point, both T- and B- cell lymphocyte counts decrease in conjunction with a significant rise in inflammatory markers [22]. Excessive increase in cytokines causes exaggerated inflammatory response named as a cytokine storm. That is characterized by increases in levels of IL-2, IL-6, IL-7, tumor necrosis factor (TNF)- alpha and granulocyte colony-stimulating factor, promoting lymphocyte apoptosis. The ACE receptor is also expressed on the surface of a lymphocyte that was infiltrating various organs of the oral mucosa and the lungs etc. Thus, this can be the other mechanism of the observed lymphopenia, involving direct cytotoxic effects of the virus and cell membrane lysis. Inhibitory effects of lactic acidemia on lymphocytes can be the other potential contributing factors to the development of lymphopenia [23].

Thrombocytopenia

Thrombocytopenia is one of the pathologic laboratory findings that can be seen in SARS COV2 positive patients. Contrary to these findings, some authors reported that patients with significantly higher platelets during treatment have longer average hospitalization periods, and patients with higher platelet lymphocyte ratio (PLR) during treatment prolong their average hospital stay [24]. We thought that thrombocytosis, being an acute phase reactant, might be a good marker for infection at the beginning of COVID 19 infection. It has been interpreted that the PLR of the patients could provide a new indicator in the follow-up of patients with COVID-19 and could indicate the degree of the cytokine storm. Liu et al. also looked into the association between platelet parameters and mortality from COVID-19: In a series of 383 patients, thrombocytopenia at admission was linked to a three-fold increase in mortality compared to patients with normal platelet counts. An increase of 50X109/L of platelets was found to be associated with a 40% decrease in mortality [25]. During the infection period thrombocytopenia is not generally severe enough to cause bleeding complications.

Thrombocytopenia is likely multifactorial and several contributory mechanisms have been postulated. Viral epitopes circulating in the bloodstream would mimic antigens present on platelet surfaces and lead to the formation of antibodies and the platelet-antibody complexes would be destroyed through a complement independent immune-mediated response, just like ITP [26]. Furthermore; multiorgan failure, disseminated intravascular coagulation (DIC) is a common risk for thrombocytopenia. Endothelial damage triggered by a systemic inflammatory response and mechanical ventilation leads to hyperactivation of platelets and thrombosis causing disseminated platelet consumption.

Eosinopenia

Eosinophils are the type of white blood cells that are usually linked with allergic and parasitic diseases. Now they have been demonstrated to possess antiviral capacities and enhance the immune response and reduce the inflammation. It is currently not known whether COVID-19 patients with eosinopenia are also more likely to develop into critical illness. In Zhang's study, 35.3% of patients showed a decrease in eosinophil absolute number ($<0.02 \times 10^{9)}$. Compared with normal eosinophil groups, eosinopenic patients showed serious vital signs on admission, with faster heart rate and relatively higher temperature and a greater proportion of eosinopenic patients were fell into severe conditions. Eosinopenic patients tended to have a lower lymphocyte count and monocyte absolute number. Following the inflammatory markers, eosinopenic patients have higher high sensitive C-reactive protein and procalcitonin. These findings revealed that eosinophils play an important role in maintaining immune regulatory system, by producing inflammatory and homeostatic mediators. Eosinophils were responsible for local immunity and tissue repair. The pathophysiology for eosinopenia in COVID-19 could be multifactorial, involving the suppressed eosinophil egress from the bone marrow, inhibition of eosinophilopoiesis, reduced eosinophil-driving cytokines, or direct interferon-induced apoptosis. IL -33 is responsible for eosinophil activation in the airways, bone marrow, and ciliated epithelial cells which are the main target of coronavirus. Also, IL -33 activates the innate lymphoid cells that produce IL-5 which is important for eosinophil cumulation in the airways. Eosinopenia was very frequent in COVID-19 and could be used in the early prediction of severity before clinical symptoms have significantly worsened, which may help clinicians in identifying potentially severe cases with COVID-19 [2].

Coagulation Disorders in COVID-19

SARS-CoV-2 infection is often associated with hypercoagulability and disseminated intravascular coagulation (DIC). This hypercoagulability is manifested as progressive lung and kidney disease, pulmonary emboli (PE), venous thrombotic events (VTE), recurrent line obstruction, and stroke in adults (SARS-CoV-2) infection.

It is thought that SARS-CoV-2 virus was diffusely present in endothelial cells and the virus uses the ACE2 receptor to directly infect the endothelium and recruit immune cells. Inflammation of the endothelium leads to microvascular dysfunction, vasoconstriction, organ ischemia, and a hypercoagulable state [27].

Although many authors recommend anticoagulation of hospitalized symptomatic adults with COVID-19, guidelines regarding the thrombotic evaluation and anticoagulation management of hospitalized children with COVID-19 remain lacking.

Pediatric hematologists developed pediatric recommendations for children hospitalized due to SARS-CoV-2 infection after revision of anticoagulation recommendations for adults [28]. Fibrinogen and D-dimer are elevated and correlated with acute inflammatory markers such as C-reactive protein. Prothrombin time prolongation is often seen. Unlike classic DIC laboratory findings, a platelet count that is only mildly decreased, a partial thromboplastin time that is normal-to-mildly prolonged, and no signs of microangiopathy and bleeding in contrast to DIC. While an elevated D-dimer may also reflect underlying inflammation, immobility, or liver disease, patients with COVID-19 infection with markedly raised D-dimers are significantly at risk of mortality, and a raised level also implies increased thrombin generation [29].

In the coagulation cascade, activated factor V interacts with activated factor X to form the prothrombinase complex, which catalyzes formation of thrombin and leads to fibrin clot formation. Dysregulation of factor V due to factor V Leiden is a well-known cause of a prothrombotic state. Concurrent elevations of factor V activity and factor VIII activity have also been linked to increased VTE risk. In Stefely's study actor V was significantly elevated in the COVID-19 cases (median 150 IU/dL) compared to both control cases on ventilators and the non-ventilated ones. These findings suggest that the elevation of factor V in severe COVID-19 cannot be simply explained by a general state of severe illness or by ventilator use. Together with the rarity of factor V elevations before the COVID-19 pandemic, these findings suggest a more specific relationship between COVID-19 and factor V elevation. High factor V levels in COVID 19 can be explained by the high amount of megakaryocytes in patient's organs which contain 20-25% of the factor V. While patients with severe COVID-19 might initially present with markedly elevated factor V activity, a subsequent decline in factor V activity could be associated with clinical decompensation. For these reasons factor V can be a candidate biomarker for future clinical trials investigating VTE and anticoagulation therapies in patients with COVID-19 [30].

As there are no clear-cut definitions for anticoagulation for pediatric hospitalized VTE patients, prophylactic anticoagulation may be considered for children with the following risk factors: (a) strong personal or family history of VTE, or (b) an indwelling central venous line and two or more additional risk factors, or (c) four or more risk factors. Prophylactic anticoagulation therapy in children must be done by considering bleeding risk. Confirmation of VTE by imaging may not be needed prior to treatment with anticoagulation if clinical suspicion is high. Therapeutic anticoagulation is considered for the children who used anticoagulation prior to admission and those who are receiving extracorporeal organ support. Catheter-directed alteplase and mechanical thrombolysis can be used for hemodynamically unstable PE or limb-threatening deep vein thrombosis. Use of systemic alteplase for progressive respiratory failure is still investigating. As the pediatric experience in COVID-19 increases, new recommendations for laboratory and imaging evaluation, assessment of thrombotic risk, and anticoagulation therapy in the pediatric patient will be improved [28].

TREATMENT

Although (COVID-19) is mild in nearly all children, a small proportion of pediatric patients develop a severe or critical illness. The four main principles for adequate therapeutic management are early identification, isolation, diagnosis, and treatment [31]. If there is a suspicion about COVID 19 the patient must be isolated in a single room to prevent the possible transmission of disease before laboratory confirmation. Mild cases should be isolated and treated with symptomatic relief medication, preferably paracetamol or dipyrone, to control fever.

The majority of children with COVID-19 experience a mild, self-limited illness, and there is a lack of evidence of efficacy for any antiviral, and due to the possible harms of these medications, the risk-to-benefit ratio must be considered for pediatric patients. Our experience in a hematology-oncology ward also supports the therapy which is tailored for each patient for beginning anticoagulation, antiviral regimens besides supportive therapy. Therefore supportive care is the mainstay of the management strategy [32].

The clinical presentation of COVID-19 in children overlaps significantly with other infections. No clinical, radiographic, or laboratory criteria are sufficiently specific to distinguish COVID-19 from these other pediatric conditions. So that antiviral drug therapy must be started after confirmation of SARS COV 2 infection. A rare exception might be made for critically ill patients with a high suspicion for COVID-19 [32].

Children with mild or moderate disease (there is no need for O2 therapy) recover with supportive care alone. Administration of antivirals early in the disease course to prevent progression thus does not seem warranted because of the possible harms of these drugs. Most children with severe infection will recover with supportive care alone. Use of potentially active antivirals could be considered on a case-by-case basis, taking into account underlying medical conditions and health status that may confer risk for progression to more serious illness.

Antiviral Treatment

Supportive care is the suggested approach for nearly all children. Antivirals may be considered on a case-by-case basis according to underlying conditions. (Table 1)

If an antiviral is used, the panel suggests remdesivir as the preferred agent. Remdesivir is a nucleoside analog prodrug that, when activated, binds to viral RNA-dependent RNA polymerase, resulting in premature RNA chain termination. A recent case series of 53 patients with severe COVID-19 pneumonia who received remdesivir under a compassionate-use protocol reported clinical improvement in 68% after a median follow-up of 18 days, with 13% mortality and a generally acceptable toxicity profile [33]. Efficacy in pediatric patients and optimal dosing, duration of therapy is not established yet.

The Infectious Disease Society of America (IDSA) guideline panel for COVID-19 treatment, recommends hydroxychloroquine/chloroquine in the context of a clinical trial [33]. The antiviral activity is inhibition of viral entry into human cells by increasing the pH of the endosomes required for cell entry, broad anti-inflammatory and immunomodulatory effects, and inhibition of glycosylation of the ACE-2 receptor, the binding site for SARS-CoV-2 [34]. The recommended dose is 3–5 mg/kg/day (max dose 400 mg) hydroxychloroquine sulfate iv, in pediatric patients, twice daily for five days. The use of azithromycin in combination with hydroxychloroquine was associated with a more rapid resolution of virus detection than hydroxychloroquine alone [35]. But combined use of these drugs potentiate QTc prolongation.

According to Chen's review in pediatric patients, interferon-α2b nebulization (100,000–200,000 IU/kg for mild cases, and 200,000–400,000 IU/kg for severe cases, two times/day for 5–7 days.) can be applied [36].

Favipravir is an RNA polymerase inhibitor. It is thought to have potential antiviral action on SARS-CoV-2. In February, a clinical trial on favipiravir for the treatment of COVID-19 was initiated, and results were promising. The preliminary results from a total of 80 patients indicated that favipiravir had more potent antiviral action than lopinavir/ritonavir which were protease inhibitors approved by the FDA for treatment of pediatric HIV [33].

Immunomodulatuar Treatment

Pediatric COVID-19 patients with hyper inflammation whose illness progress to critical COVID-19 may be considered for immunomodulatory treatment. Small subset of pediatric patients is severely affected by COVID-19 with a presentation ARDS, hypercoagulability, hyper inflammation, and multiorgan failure [37]. There are no immunomodulators with proven efficacy for the treatment of COVID-19 in pediatric patients as of July 24, 2020. Therefore, no guidance can be provided to support the use of one immunomodulatory therapy over another. If immunomodulators are used in the treatment of COVID-19, patients should be monitored for adverse effects [38].

IL-6 and IL-1 inhibition may be considered in the care of pediatric patients with critical COVID-19 with priority given to clinical trial enrollment if available. Anakinra can be used as an IL-1 inhibitor based on its safety profile and favorable pharmacokinetics. Glucocorticoid therapy may be considered for pediatric patients with critical COVID-19 with a preference for use in the setting of clinical trials, if available. Steroid is indicated like asthma or catecholamine-refractory shock in COVID 19 pediatric patients.

Convalescent plasma in pediatric COVID-19 may be considered as part of the recently established FDA emergency investigational new drug program if in the United States or as part of a clinical trial. The efficacy of passive transfer of convalescent plasma (CP) is thought to be mediated primarily through viral neutralization, although other mechanisms such as stimulation of antibody-dependent cellular cytotoxicity and enhanced phagocytosis have also been postulated. While the passive transfer of polyclonal antibodies via convalescent plasma may be of benefit, no SARS-CoV-2–specific monoclonal antibody therapies have yet been clinically tested. It is recommended that children >40 kg be dosed with 200–500 mL and children <40 kg be dosed with 10–15 mL/kg, while being aware of volume overload, especially in children with cardiac dysfunction.

The use of IVIG for treatment of acute COVID-19 in pediatric patients is not recommended except for (ya da sadece except) specific clinical situations in which IVIG is typically used and treatment of MIS-C.

JAK inhibitors and Type I or type III IFN should not be used for pediatric COVID-19 patients outside of a clinical trial.

Severe cases with respiratory distress and/or hypoxia (SaO2 < 94%) should be admitted to the hospital. Indications for ICU admission are respiratory failure requiring mechanical ventilation, shock, or other organ dysfunction requiring treatment. The main treatment principles of ARDS are as follows [39] :

1. Early tracheal intubation – rapid sequence intubation is the best practice in this situation. Preoxygenation should be performed using a flexible nasal cannula (up to flows of 4 L/min) or a reservoir mask with a lower flux to maintain a SaO2 >93%. Positive pressure ventilation with a bag-valve-mask or other s imilar apparatus should be avoided not to generate aerosols.
2. Non-invasive ventilation (NIV) should be avoided because of the high risk of aerosol dispersion and contamination among health practitioners.
3. The patient should be maintained in a prone position at least 18 hours per day
4. Protective mechanical ventilation and closed tracheal aspiration systems should be used.
5. Antibiotics should be used only in patients with secondary bacterial infections based on the culture and antibiogram results. Corticosteroids can suppress lung inflammation but also inhibit immune responses and pathogen clearance, and should be avoided except for those with a specific indication (e.g., bronchospasm or some cases of septic shock) Intravenous ımmunglobulin can be used in critically ill child [40].

6. Fluid therapy or vasoactive/inotropic drugs and renal replacement therapy may be needed.
7. Anticoagulation is required in presence of high D-dimers or evidence of thromboembolism [33].

VACCINATION TRIAL

NVX-CoV2373 contains Matrix-M1 adjuvant and a recombinant SARS-CoV-2 (rSARS-CoV-2) nanoparticle vaccine, constructed from the full-length (i.e., including the transmembrane domain), wild-type SARS-CoV-2 spike glycoprotein, which mediates attachment of the virus to the human angiotensin-converting enzyme 2 (hACE2) receptor of host cells for cellular entry and serves as a key target for the development of antibodies and vaccines. The spike protein of vaccine induces high titers of antibodies that blocked hACE2 receptor binding and achieved neutralization of wild-type virüs. The magnitude of response is higher than that is measured in human convalescent serum. Polyfunctional CD4+ and CD8+ T-cell responses were induced with a T helper 1 (Th1) dominant phenotype. Keech et al. initiated a randomized, placebo-controlled, phase 1–2 trial to evaluate the safety and immunogenicity of the rSARS-CoV-2 vaccine in 131 healthy adults [41]. In phase 1, vaccination comprised two intramuscular injections, 21 days apart. At 35 days, NVX-CoV2373 appeared to be safe, and it elicited immune responses that exceeded levels in Covid-19 convalescent serum. The Matrix-M1 adjuvant-induced CD4+ T-cell responses that were biased toward a Thl phenotype. Phase 2 has commenced based on the safety results of the day 35 primary analysis, and phase 3 is in preparatory stages.

Mycobacteria is previously reported to be potent Th1 stimulants [42]. Such an antigen stimulation may increase proliferation in favor of Th1 cells, Bacillus Calmette-Guerin (BCG), a live attenuated vaccine, is being administered routinely against Mycobacterium. BCG can induce sustained nonspecific reactions to infections at the level of trained immunity and heterologous Th1/Th17 responses by prolonged production of IFN-γ, IL-17, and IL-22. In Ozdemir et al. study, the mean of cases per population ratio is statistically significantly lower in BCG-vaccinated countries than in BCG-non-vaccinated countries [42]. The mean of deaths per case ratio is also significantly lower in BCG-vaccinated countries In the Northern Hemisphere, the mean of deaths per population ratio is also found to be significantly lower in BCG-vaccinated countries than in BCG-non-vaccinated countries. Therefore ıt is thought that BCG vaccination has a protective role against COVID 19 ınfection by its ımmunmodulatuar effect. There are also many kinds of vaccines trial (inactive, recombinant) whose phase 3 trials are ongoing.

Conclusion

Recent studies about pediatric COVID 19 revealed that this disease is less common and mild in children. Full-spectrum of illness in children is not clearly understood because many patients might have not been subject to viral testing. At the beginning of SARS COV-2 outbreak, the children are isolated so the virüs are transmitted by adults in the community. Therefore, at the beginning of the pandemic, disease was mostly seen in adults. Although ACE receptor that increased susceptibility for infection is relatively less than adults, once the children are infected, they could carry high viral loads. As the pandemic progressed, more children infected, transmission rate of virüs is increased.

For coping with this outbreak, we must protect the children from SARS COV-2 by social distancing and using facial masks. The decision to open up schools and daycare centers should be reconsidered until the severity of the pandemic subsides.

References

[1] Qiu, H., Wu, J., Hong, L., Luo, Y., Song, Q. & Chen, D. (2020). Clinical and epidemiological features of 36 children with coronavirus disease 2019 (COVID-19) in Zhejiang, China: an observational cohort study. *The Lancet Infectious Diseases*, 20(6), 689–696. https://doi.org/10.1016/S1473-3099(20)30198-5.

[2] Zhang, J. jin, Dong, X., Cao, Y. yuan., Yuan, Y. dong, Yang, Y. bin, Yan, Y. qin, Akdis, C. A. & Gao, Y. dong. (2020). Clinical characteristics of 140 patients infected with SARS-CoV-2 in Wuhan, China. *Allergy: European Journal of Allergy and Clinical Immunology*, 75(7), 1730–1741. https://doi.org/10.1111/all.14238.

[3] Hoang, A., Chorath, K., Moreira, A., Evans, M., Burmeister-Morton, F., Burmeister, F., Naqvi, R., Petershack, M. & Moreira, A. (2020). COVID-19 in 7780 pediatric patients: A systematic review. *EClinicalMedicine*, 24. https://doi.org/10.1016/j.eclinm.2020.100433.

[4] Han, M. S., Choi, E. H., Chang, S. H., Jin, B. Lo, Lee, E. J., Kim, B. N., Kim, M. K., Doo, K., Seo, J. H., Kim, Y. J., Kim, Y. J., Park, J. Y., Suh, S. B., Lee, H., Cho, E. Y., Kim, D. H., Kim, J. M., Kim, H. Y., Park, S. E. & Kim, J. H. (2020). Clinical Characteristics and Viral RNA Detection in Children with Coronavirus Disease 2019 in the Republic of Korea. *JAMA Pediatrics, 03080*, 1–8. https://doi.org/10.1001/jamapediatrics.2020.3988.

[5] Andrianou, X., Bella, A., Manso, M. Del, Urdiales, A. M., Fabiani, M., Bellino, S., Boros, S., Rota, M. C., Filia, A., Punzo, O., Siddu, A., Benedetto, C. Di, Tallon, M., Ciervo, A., Castrucci, M. R., Pezzotti, P., Stefanelli, P., Rezza, G. & Scondotto, S. (2020). *Epidemia COVID-19.*, 1–13.

[6] Shen, K., Yang, Y., Wang, T., Zhao, D., Jiang, Y., Jin, R., Zheng, Y., Xu, B., Xie, Z., Lin, L., Shang, Y., Lu, X., Shu, S., Bai, Y., Deng, J., Lu, M., Ye, L., Wang, X., Wang, Y. & Gao, L. (2020). Diagnosis, treatment, and prevention of 2019 novel coronavirus infection in children: experts' consensus statement. In *World Journal of Pediatrics*, (Vol. *16*, Issue 3, pp. 223–231). Institute of Pediatrics of Zhejiang University. https://doi.org/10.1007/s12519-020-00343-7.

[7] Cao, Q., Chen, Y. C., Chen, C. L. & Chiu, C. H. (2020). SARS-CoV-2 infection in children: Transmission dynamics and clinical characteristics. *Journal of the Formosan Medical Association*, 119(3), 670–673. https://doi.org/10.1016/j.jfma.2020.02.009.

[8] Yonker, L. M., Neilan, A. M., Bartsch, Y., Patel, A. B., Regan, J., Arya, P., Gootkind, E., Park, G., Hardcastle, M., St. John, A., Appleman, L., Chiu, M. L., Fialkowski, A., De la Flor, D., Lima, R., Bordt, E. A., Yockey, L. J., D'Avino, P., Fischinger, S. & Fasano, A. (2020). Pediatric SARS-CoV-2: Clinical Presentation, Infectivity, and Immune Responses. *The Journal of Pediatrics*. https://doi.org/10.1016/j.jpeds.2020.08.037.

[9] Dong, L., Tian, J., He, S., Zhu, C., Wang, J., Liu, C. & Yang, J. (2020). Possible Vertical Transmission of SARS-CoV-2 from an Infected Mother to Her Newborn. *JAMA - Journal of the American Medical Association*, 323(18), 1846–1848. https://doi.org/10.1001/ jama.2020.4621.

[10] Dong, Y., Dong, Y., Mo, X., Hu, Y., Qi, X., Jiang, F., Jiang, Z., Jiang, Z., Tong, S., Tong, S. & Tong, S. (2020). Epidemiology of COVID-19 among children in China. *Pediatrics*, 145(6). https://doi.org/10.1542/peds.2020-0702.

[11] Zimmermann, P. & Curtis, N. (2020). Coronavirus infections in children including COVID-19: An overview of the epidemiology, clinical features, diagnosis, treatment and prevention options in children. *Pediatric Infectious Disease Journal*, 39(5), 355–368. https://doi.org/10.1097/INF.0000000000002660.

[12] Brodin, P. (2020). Why is COVID-19 so mild in children? *Acta Paediatrica, International Journal of Paediatrics*, 109(6), 1082–1083. https://doi.org/10.1111/apa.15271.

[13] Foust, A. M., McAdam, A. J., Chu, W. C., Garcia-Peña, P., Phillips, G. S., Plut, D. & Lee, E. Y. (2020). Practical guide for pediatric pulmonologists on imaging management of pediatric patients with COVID-19. In *Pediatric Pulmonology*, (Vol. 55, Issue 9). https://doi.org/10.1002/ppul.24870.

[14] Xia, W., Shao, J., Guo, Y., Peng, X., Li, Z. & Hu, D. (2020). Clinical and CT features in pediatric patients with COVID-19 infection: Different points from adults. *Pediatric Pulmonology*, 55(5), 1169–1174. https://doi.org/10.1002/ppul.24718.

[15] Shema Hameed, Heba Elbaaly, Catriona E. L. Reid, Rui M. F. Santos, Vinay Shivamurthy. & James Wong, K. H. J. (2015). *in Pr E E. ii.*

[16] Mina, A., Besien, K. Van. & Platanias, L. C. (2020). Hematological manifestations of COVID-19. *Leukemia and Lymphoma*, 1–9. https://doi.org/10.1080/10428194.2020.1788017.

[17] Chen, N., Zhou, M., Dong, X., Qu, J., Gong, F., Han, Y., Qiu, Y., Wang, J., Liu, Y., Wei, Y., Xia, J., Yu, T., Zhang, X. & Zhang, L. (2020). Epidemiological and clinical characteristics of 99 cases of 2019 novel coronavirus pneumonia in Wuhan, China: a descriptive study. *The Lancet*, 395(10223), 507–513. https://doi.org/10.1016/ S0140-6736(20)30211-7.

[18] Li, Y. Y., Wang, W. N., Lei, Y., Zhang, B., Yang, J., Hu, J. W., Ren, Y. L. & Lu, Q. F. (2020). [Comparison of the clinical characteristics between RNA positive and negative patients clinically diagnosed with 2019 novel coronavirus pneumonia]. *Zhonghua Jie He He Hu Xi Za Zhi = Zhonghua Jiehe He Huxi Zazhi = Chinese Journal of Tuberculosis and Respiratory Diseases*, 43(0), E023. https://doi.org/10.3760/cma.j.cn112147-20200214-00095.

[19] Wu, C., Chen, X., Cai, Y., Xia, J., Zhou, X., Xu, S., Huang, H., Zhang, L., Zhou, X., Du, C., Zhang, Y., Song, J., Wang, S., Chao, Y., Yang, Z., Xu, J., Zhou, X., Chen, D., Xiong, W. & Song, Y. (2020). Risk Factors Associated with Acute Respiratory Distress Syndrome and Death in Patients with Coronavirus Disease 2019 Pneumonia in Wuhan, China. *JAMA Internal Medicine*, 180(7), 934–943. https://doi.org/10.1001/jamainternmed.2020.0994.

[20] Wang, D., Hu, B., Hu, C., Zhu, F., Liu, X., Zhang, J., Wang, B., Xiang, H., Cheng, Z., Xiong, Y., Zhao, Y., Li, Y., Wang, X. & Peng, Z. (2020). Clinical Characteristics of 138 Hospitalized Patients with 2019 Novel Coronavirus-Infected Pneumonia in Wuhan, China. *JAMA - Journal of the American Medical Association*, 323(11), 1061–1069. https://doi.org/10.1001/jama.2020.1585.

[21] Tan, L., Wang, Q., Zhang, D., Ding, J., Huang, Q., Tang, Y. Q., Wang, Q. & Miao, H. (2020). Lymphopenia predicts disease severity of COVID-19: a descriptive and predictive study. *Signal Transduction and Targeted Therapy*, 5(1), 16–18. https://doi.org/10.1038/s41392-020-0148-4.

[22] Li, T., Lu, H. & Zhang, W. (2020). Clinical observation and management of COVID-19 patients. *Emerging Microbes and Infections*, 9(1), 687–690. https://doi.org/10.1080/22221751.2020.1741327.

[23] Fischer, K., Hoffmann, P., Voelkl, S., Meidenbauer, N., Ammer, J., Edinger, M., Gottfried, E., Schwarz, S., Rothe, G., Hoves, S., Renner, K., Timischl, B., Mackensen, A., Kunz-schughart, L., Andreesen, R., Krause, S. W. & Kreutz, M. (2007). *Inhibitory effect of tumor cell – derived lactic acid on human T cells*. 109(9), 3812–3819. https://doi.org/10.1182/blood-2006-07-035972.

[24] Qu, R., Ling, Y., Zhang, Y. hui zhi, Wei, L. ya, Chen, X., Li, X. mian, Liu, X. yong, Liu, H. mian, Guo, Z., Ren, H. & Wang, Q. (2020). Platelet-to-lymphocyte

ratio is associated with prognosis in patients with coronavirus disease-19. *Journal of Medical Virology*, 92(9), 1533–1541. https://doi.org/10.1002/jmv.25767.

[25] Liu, Y., Sun, W., Guo, Y., Chen, L., Zhang, L., Zhao, S., Long, D. & Yu, L. (2020). Association between platelet parameters and mortality in coronavirus disease 2019: Retrospective cohort study. *Platelets*, 31(4), 490–496. https://doi.org/10.1080/09537104.2020.1754383.

[26] Xu, P., Zhou, Q. & Xu, J. (2020). Mechanism of thrombocytopenia in COVID-19 patients. *Annals of Hematology*, 99(6), 1205–1208. https://doi.org/10.1007/s00277-020-04019-0.

[27] Varga, Z., Flammer, A. J., Steiger, P., Haberecker, M., Andermatt, R., Zinkernagel, A. S., Mehra, M. R., Schuepbach, R. A., Ruschitzka, F. & Moch, H. (2020). Endothelial cell infection and endotheliitis in COVID-19. *The Lancet*, *395*(10234), 1417–1418. https://doi.org/ 10.1016/S0140-6736(20)30937-5.

[28] Loi, M., Branchford, B., Kim, J., Self, C. & Nuss, R. (2020). COVID-19 anticoagulation recommendations in children. *Pediatric Blood and Cancer*, 67(9), 15–17. https://doi.org/10.1002/pbc.28485.

[29] Fan, B. E. (2020). Hematologic parameters in patients with COVID-19 infection: a reply. *American Journal of Hematology*, 95(8), E215. https://doi.org/10.1002/ajh.25847.

[30] Stefely, J. A., Christensen, B. B., Gogakos, T., Cone Sullivan, J. K., Montgomery, G. G., Barranco, J. P. & Van Cott, E. M. (2020). Marked factor V activity elevation in severe COVID-19 is associated with venous thromboembolism. *American Journal of Hematology*. https://doi.org/10.1002/ajh.25979.

[31] Panzeri Carlotti, A. P. de C., de Carvalho, W. B., Johnston, C., Rodriguez, I. S. & Delgado, A. F. (2020). Covid-19 diagnostic and management protocol for pediatric patients. *Clinics*, 75, 1–5. https://doi.org/10.6061/CLINICS/2020/E1894.

[32] [32] Chiotos, K., Hayes, M., Kimberlin, D. W., Jones, S. B., James, S. H., Pinninti, S. G., Yarbrough, A., Abzug, M. J., MacBrayne, C. E., Soma, V. L., Dulek, D. E., Vora, S. B., Waghmare, A., Wolf, J., Olivero, R., Grapentine, S., Wattier, R. L., Bio, L., Cross, S. J. & Nakamura, M. M. (2020). Multicenter initial guidance on use of antivirals for children with COVID-19/SARS-CoV-2. *Journal of the Pediatric Infectious Diseases Society*, *Xx*, 1–15. https://doi.org/10.1093/jpids/piaa045.

[33] Tezer, H. & Bedir Demirdağ, T. (2020). Novel coronavirus disease (Covid-19) in children. *Turkish Journal of Medical Sciences*, 50(SI-1), 592–603. https://doi.org/10.3906/SAG-2004-174.

[34] Al-Bari, A. A. (2014). Chloroquine analogues in drug discovery: New directions of uses, mechanisms of actions and toxic manifestations from malaria to multifarious diseases. *Journal of Antimicrobial Chemotherapy*, 70(6), 1608–1621. https://doi.org/10.1093/jac/dkv018.

[35] Gautret, P., Lagier, J., Parola, P., Doudier, B., Courjon, J., Scola, B. La, Rolain, J., Brouqui, P., Raoult, D., Mailhe, M., Doudier, B. & Courjon, J. (2020). *I fec U1065, Centre Méditerranéen de Médecine Moléculaire, C3M, Virulence Microbienne et [I fec U1065, Mediterranean Center for Molecular Medicine, C3M, Microbial Virulence and] Department of Virology, Biological and Pathological Center, Centre Hospitalier.*

[36] Chen, Z. M., Fu, J. F., Shu, Q., Chen, Y. H., Hua, C. Z., Li, F. B., Lin, R., Tang, L. F., Wang, T. L., Wang, W., Wang, Y. S., Xu, W. Z., Yang, Z. H., Ye, S., Yuan, T. M., Zhang, C. M. & Zhang, Y. Y. (2020). Diagnosis and treatment recommendations for pediatric respiratory infection caused by the 2019 novel coronavirus. *World Journal of Pediatrics*, 16(3), 240–246. https://doi.org/10.1007/s12519-020-00345-5.

[37] Zhu, N., Zhang, D., Wang, W., Li, X., Yang, B., Song, J., Zhao, X., Huang, B., Shi, W., Lu, R., Niu, P., Zhan, F., Ma, X., Wang, D., Xu, W., Wu, G., Gao, G. F. & Tan, W. (2020). A novel coronavirus from patients with pneumonia in China, 2019. *New England Journal of Medicine*, 382(8), 727–733. https://doi.org/10.1056/NEJMoa2001017.

[38] Dulek, D. E., Fuhlbrigge, R. C., Tribble, A. C., Connelly, J. A., Loi, M. M., El Chebib, H., Chandrakasan, S., Otto, W. R., Diorio, C., Keim, G., Walkovich, K., Jaggi, P., Girotto, J. E., Yarbrough, A., Behrens, E. M., Cron, R. Q. & Bassiri, H. (2020). Multidisciplinary Guidance Regarding the Use of Immunomodulatory Therapies for Acute Coronavirus Disease 2019 in Pediatric Patients. *Journal of the Pediatric Infectious Diseases Society*, 2019, (Xx Xxxx), 1–22. https://doi.org/10.1093/jpids/piaa098.

[39] Wang, H., Wang, S. & Yu, K. (2020). COVID-19 infection epidemic: The medical management strategies in Heilongjiang Province, China. *Critical Care*, 24(1), 10–13. https://doi.org/10.1186/s13054-020-2832-8.

[40] Panzeri Carlotti, A. P. de C., de Carvalho, W. B., Johnston, C., Rodriguez, I. S. & Delgado, A. F. (2020). Covid-19 diagnostic and management protocol for pediatric patients. *Clinics*, 75, 1–5. https://doi.org/10.6061/CLINICS/2020/E1894.

[41] Keech C, Albert G, Cho I, Robertson A, Reed P Phase 1-2 Trial of a SARS-COV-2 Rekombinant Spike Protein Nanoparticle Vaccine *N. Engl. J. Med*, September 2, 2020, doi: 1.1056/NEJMoa2026920

[42] Ozdemir, C., Kucuksezer, U. C. & Tamay, Z. U. (2020). Is BCG vaccination affecting the spread and severity of COVID-19? *Allergy: European Journal of Allergy and Clinical Immunology*, 75(7), 1824–1827. https://doi.org/10.1111/all.14344.

In: Coronavirus Disease
Editor: Yildiz Dincer

ISBN: 978-1-53619-296-4

Chapter 11

COVID-19 AND OPHTHALMOLOGY

Ceyhun Arici[1,*], MD and Burak Mergen[2], MD
[1]Istanbul University-Cerrahpasa, Cerrahpasa Medical Faculty, Department of Ophthalmology, Istanbul, Turkey
[2]University of Health Sciences, Basaksehir Cam ve Sakura City Hospital, Department of Ophthalmology Istanbul, Turkey

ABSTRACT

The emergence of coronavirus disease 2019 (COVID-19) pandemic due to severe acute respiratory syndrome coronavirus-2 (SARS-CoV-2) led to a global health crisis. After the report of the first case in Wuhan, China, in December 2019, millions of people were infected with the virus in only a few months. Apart from many systemic findings such as fever, fatigue, dry cough, the disease can also involve the eyes mainly in form of conjunctivitis. Therefore, all patients with red eyes became suspicious of COVID-19 conjunctivitis. Ophthalmologists are at increased risks for COVID-19 because of their close physical proximity to the patients during the eye examination. Thus, eye care providers should use proper ways of protection including wearing an N95 mask, gloves, and protective goggles. The outpatient clinics should be disinfected regularly and social distancing should be provided for all areas. Regular visits without any emergency should be postponed or those patients should be managed via telemedicine. Urgent or visually important cases should be triaged for COVID-19 risk before the ophthalmological examination. International guidelines should be followed for determining the effective and safe treatment protocols for the patients during the pandemic.

Keywords: Ophthalmology, COVID-19, social distancing, severe acute respiratory syndrome

---

* Corresponding Author's Email: ceyhundr@gmail.com.

INTRODUCTION

The severe acute respiratory syndrome coronavirus 2 (SARS-CoV-2) is a highly contagious RNA virus, causes Coronavirus disease 2019 (COVID-19) emerged on the last days of December 2019 in Wuhan city, Hubei province, China. COVID-19 is the third and largest coronavirus outbreak in the 21st century after the severe acute respiratory syndrome (SARS) in 2002 and the Middle East respiratory syndrome (MERS) in 2012. Over 80 million people have been infected and the COVID-19 has caused more than one million deaths.

There are seven types of coronaviruses known to infect humans: 229E (alphacoronavirus), NL63 (alphacoronavirus), OC43 (betacoronavirus), HKU1 (betacoronavirus), MERS-CoV (betacoronavirus), SARS-CoV (betacoronavirus), and the most recent SARS-CoV-2 [1]. Although not proven, the source of the disease has been speculated to be from bats [2].

COVID-19 can potentially be fatal and affects mainly the lungs and airways leading to the most frequent symptoms of the disease including fever (87.9%), dry cough (67.7%), and fatigue (38.1%) [3]. However, apart from the respiratory tract, it can also affect other regions including the gastrointestinal tract and ocular tissues [4, 5]. So, the manifestations of COVID-19 in other organ systems should not be ignored as they can represent an alternative mode of transmission.

From genomic and structural analyses, it has been reported that the SARS-CoV-2 has a similar receptor-binding motif as SARS-CoV, which allows it to infect host cells via the angiotensin-converting-enzyme-2 (ACE2) [6]. ACE2 has been found in the aqueous humor [7], conjunctiva, and corneal epithelium [8].

Conjunctival congestion or conjunctivitis can be an early clinical manifestation of COVID-19. In a study with a large case series, 0.8% prevalence was seen in China [9]. Previous studies reported that SARS-CoV-2 was found in tear samples of patients with COVID-19 [10]. Apart from conjunctivitis, hyperreflective lesions were observed on the papillomacular bundle and between the retinal ganglion cell layer and inner plexiform layer without causing any visual disturbance in optical coherence tomography [11]. Ophthalmoplegia cases related to COVID-19 have also been reported [12, 13].

Ophthalmologists are at increased risks for COVID-19 because of their close physical proximity to the patients during eye examination (less than 30 cm during the slit-lamp examination, and less than 5 cm at direct ophthalmoscopy examination). Also, manipulation of eyelids in some patients required during the slit lamp examination, which increases the risk of contact with tears or other ocular discharge. Ophthalmologists should routinely wear respiratory masks and gloves if contact is required.

Dr. Li Wenliang, who alerted Chinese government officials of an incipient viral syndrome (COVID-19), was a young ophthalmologist. By his account, he believed he contracted the infection from a glaucoma patient he was evaluating for conjunctivitis; a month after exposure, he passed away due to respiratory failure. With the outbreak of COVID-19, ophthalmologists may be the first to identify patients with COVID-19 seeking treatment for acute conjunctivitis before the manifestation of respiratory symptoms. They have an important role in guiding infection control measures to prevent unnecessary exposures to other patients and medical staff.

Old age is a known risk factor for more severe clinical manifestation of COVID-19 with probable additional systemic diseases (e.g., diabetes mellitus, hypertension, etc.). Cataract, glaucoma, and macular degeneration, common ophthalmic conditions, are associated with aging. Thus, additional increased risk portended to ophthalmic practice relates to the increased age of patients in ophthalmology clinics or undergoing ophthalmic procedures.

The above-mentioned factors make the role of ophthalmologists during the pandemic very crucial.

SARS-CoV-2 in Tears and Ocular Findings of COVID-19

From the experience on SARS-CoV, it was known that coronaviruses can be found in tears [4]. However, at the beginning of the pandemic, the ocular involvement of the COVID-19 was unknown. After the report of transmission of the disease in a patient (Guangfa Wang, a member of the national expert panel) who did not wear protective goggles but wore an N95 mask, the possibility of disease transmission via the eyes started to be questioned. Then a report showed that COVID-19 can be transmitted through the mucous membranes including the conjunctiva [14]. Ophthalmologists have also been shown to be infected in several case reports.

Polymerase chain reaction (PCR) analysis of the tear films of the patients with COVID-19 with or without conjunctivitis showed that the virus can be isolated from the patients with COVID-19. The patients with positive PCR in the tear film can be in the early stage of the disease without any systemic symptoms. Therefore, protection of the eyes with goggles is very important to prevent the disease spread during the examination of the patients, and tears of the COVID-19 patients are also potential sources of disease transmission. PCR positivity of the tear of a patient with COVID-19 despite no systemic symptoms 3 weeks after the disease onset should be another warning for the clinicians to be careful with handling ocular tissues or secretions even after the disappearance of the symptoms and negative nasopharyngeal swab [15].

The studies on tear samples of patients with COVID-19 are summarized in Table 1. Ocular findings of the disease were as high as 31.6% and the PCR positivity of the tear samples was as high as 24%. However, a recent meta-analysis showed that the overall prevalence of the ocular involvement in patients with COVID-19 was 5% and 28% of ocular samples showed SARS-CoV-2 PCR positivity [16]. A study on pediatric patients with SARS-CoV-2 positivity showed that asymptomatic COVID-19 pediatric patients could also have positive tear samples [17].

Table 1. List of the studies investigating the PCR positivity in tear samples of patients with COVID-19

Study	Sample size	Patients	Ocular findings	SARS-CoV-2 in Tear Samples
Wu et al., [18]	38	Clinical confirmation	31.6%	5%
Xia et al., [19]	30	Laboratory confirmation	3.3%	3%
Seah et al., [20]	17	Laboratory confirmation	5%	0%
Sun et al., [21]	72	Laboratory confirmation	2.7%	1.3%
Deng et al., [22]	114	Clinical confirmation	0%	0%
Zhou et al., [23]	67	Confirmed/suspects	1.4%	4.4%
Karimi et al., [10]	43	Clinical confirmation	2.3%	7%
Arora et al., [24]	78	Laboratory confirmation	0%	24%

SARS-CoV-2: Severe acute respiratory syndrome coronavirus-2.

Several possible reasons for tear sample positivity for SARS-CoV-2 have been speculated including direct inoculation of the virus, its migration from the respiratory tract through the nasolacrimal duct, or shedding of the virus from an infected lacrimal gland [25]. The last possible transmission way might be the affinity of SARS-CoV-2 to angiotensin-converting-enzyme-2 in the ocular tissues [8].

COVID-19 can lead to some ocular findings including mostly conjunctivitis with complaints of itching and red-eye. Conjunctival congestion was reported in 0.8% (9/1099) of the patients with laboratory-confirmed disease in China [9]. A recent meta-analysis on ocular findings of COVID-19 showed that ocular findings of the disease can be the first presenting sign of the disease [26] and the overall prevalence of the ocular involvement in patients with COVID-19 was 5% [16]. Furthermore, the ocular involvement of the disease has been reported to be as high as 31.6% [18].

The ocular manifestation was earlier than the systemic manifestation in around a quarter of COVID-19 patients with ocular manifestation regardless of the severity [16]. However, the association of the presence of ocular manifestation with disease severity is yet to be determined due to controversial results from different studies. Furthermore, the same meta-analysis showed that one-third of ocular samples (28%) showed SARS-CoV-2 PCR positivity [16]. Therefore, since coronaviruses could be transmitted to the nasopharynx via nasolacrimal duct and tear positivity can be observed in asymptomatic patients, eyes could potentially be the windows to the COVID-19 transmission.

Being healthcare workers, elderly patients (> 60 years), frequent touching of the eyes with hands, lacrimal duct abnormalities, immunosuppression, and swimming are among the reported possible predisposing factors for ocular manifestation of COVID-19 [16].

The ocular manifestation of the disease can be observed together with, before, or after the systemic manifestations. Ocular manifestation in form of conjunctivitis can be the only presenting symptom of the disease [26]. Therefore, all patients who were admitted to the emergency or ophthalmology departments should be investigated for COVID-19 related findings.

The ocular manifestation of the disease improved in all patients reported in the previous studies and did not get worse in time. Therefore, although red eyes in COVID-19 patients should be accepted as ocular involvement of the disease as conjunctivitis until proven otherwise, emergent referral or consultation of the patients to an ophthalmologist may not be needed.

After an autopsy study reporting SARS-CoV-2 positivity in retinal biopsy specimens of three specimens out of 14 COVID-19 patients [27], retinal involvement of the disease started to be questioned. An optic coherence tomography study showed hyper-reflective lesions at the level of ganglion cell and inner plexiform layers [11]. However, this finding became controversial due to many consequent correspondences about this study. Rare neuro-ophthalmic presentations such as cranial nerve palsies, ophthalmoplegia, diplopia, and nystagmus have also been reported in patients with COVID-19 [12, 13].

Control Measures for the Ophthalmological Examination and Surgeries

Since the risk of human-to-human transmission increases closer than 1.5 m distance, the waiting area for the patients should be designed to ensure social distancing between patients by blocking alternating seats (Figure 1).

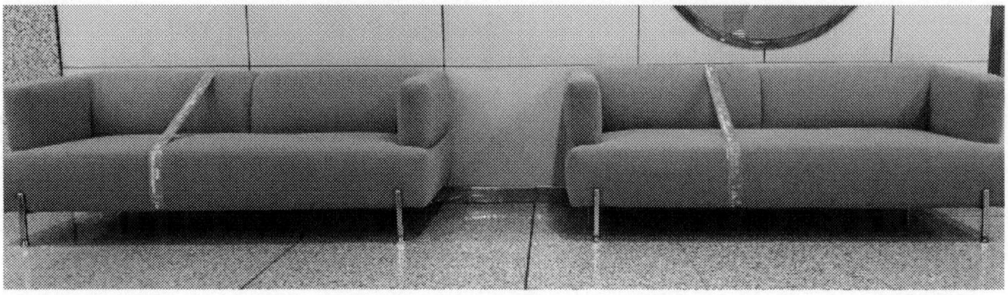

Figure 1. Blocked seats to provide social distancing in the waiting area for the patients.

Because SARS-CoV-2 can live on the inanimate surfaces up to 9 days [28], efficient cleaning of all areas with possible contamination should be disinfected regularly with appropriate disinfectants. Povidone-iodine, a combination of chlorhexidine with ethanol and cetrimide, most alcohol-based solutions such as ethanol or isopropanol significantly reduces the viral titers and is recommended [29,30]. The Centers for Disease Control and Prevention (CDC) specifically recommended the use of alcohol solutions with at least 70% alcohol and diluted household bleach (five tablespoons of bleach per gallon of water) [31]. Some antiseptics-disinfectants formulated with only phenolic or quaternary ammonium compounds, or a combination of chlorhexidine with cetrimide may be ineffective against SARS-CoV-2, therefore should not be preferred for disinfection [32].

Ophthalmic lenses contacting eyes should be disinfected with 1:100 sodium hypochlorite or 3% hydrogen peroxide for 5 minutes followed by washing with water before the next use [33].

Due to the high frequency of fever in COVID-19 patients, all patients admitted to the ophthalmology department should be checked for their body temperature. Patients with an ocular emergency with fever should be examined in an isolated room, but those without any ocular emergency should be referred for COVID-19 exclusion to the relevant department and their ophthalmological examination should be postponed. Patients without fever should also be questioned about COVID-19 related symptoms or risk factors including the history of traveling abroad within the past 2 weeks or any suspicious contact with a COVID-19 patient.

The current recommendation from WHO for general ophthalmology patients would be wearing personal protective equipment according to standard precautions, which is wearing surgical masks in all areas. A complete ophthalmological examination usually takes around 30 minutes. Thus, longer exposure of the ophthalmologists to patients leads to another risk factor for the disease transmission. The distance during the slit lamp examination between patient and examiner varies between 20 and 40 cm. Therefore, a large protective transparent plastic shield should be installed on the biomicroscopes to provide another control measure during slit-lamp examination (Figure 2).

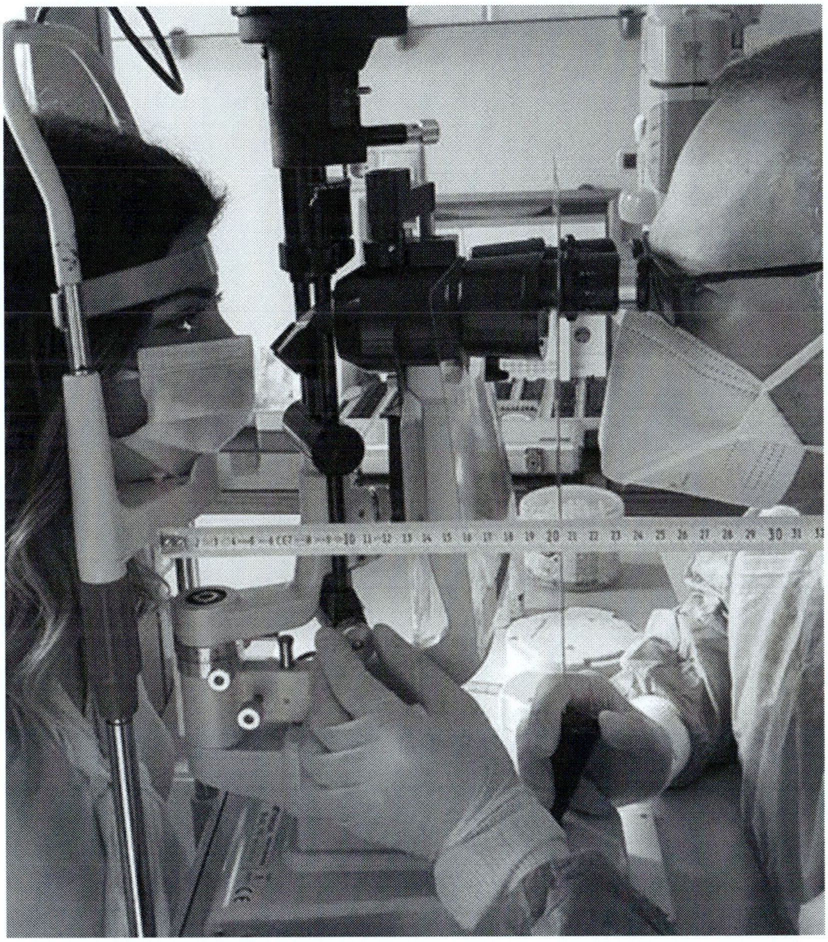

Figure 2. The close proximity of an ophthalmologist to a patient during slit-lamp examination with appropriate personal protective equipment.

Since the tear can be SARS-CoV-2 positive even without any ocular or systemic finding of the COVID-19 and asymptomatic COVID-19 patients were reported to be 15.6% among all patients [34], ophthalmologists should accept all patients as possible infection sources. Therefore, ophthalmologists should wear protective goggles, N95 masks, and gloves during the examination of all patients to prevent disease transmission. While the American Academy of Ophthalmology recommended ophthalmologists to wear masks and eye protection when caring for patients with potential COVID-19 positivity [35], a report from Hong Kong during the SARS-CoV outbreak recommended the use of personal protective equipment (PPE) including the gloves for all patients regardless of SARS status [36]. The patients can be requested to speak less frequently during the examination.

Studies have shown that healthy individuals touch their eyes 10 times per hour [37]. The use of glasses may be protective against this frequent touching. Interestingly, extended daily use of glasses for more than 8 hours per day was shown to be associated with less susceptibility to COVID-19 emphasizing the importance of wearing protective goggles or glasses [38].

Ophthalmologists preferring not to wear gloves should wash his/her hands with disinfectants after each patient and the ones who prefer to wear gloves should change the gloves after each patient. Ophthalmologists should wear isolation gowns while examining the COVID-19 positive or suspicious patients in an isolated room.

The working shifts of all medical staff can be designed to work as small groups to prevent cross-infection between different staff members. To prevent disease spread among medical staff, all meetings should be made as online meetings. The personnel should also be careful about social distancing. Gathering in large groups of more than 10 people should be stopped.

Outpatient and inpatient ophthalmology care should be separated to curtail the risk of cross-infection. Inpatients should be examined at the bedside with portable devices or in an examination room designed only for inpatient use [39].

Recommendations for each subspecialty clinics in ophthalmology are given below under separate subtitles.

Retina

Retina clinics are usually very crowded, and the patient population usually consist of elderly patients. Therefore, some control measures should be administered to decrease the number of unnecessary visits. The physicians should check the patient records to postpone some of the appointments and the patients should be informed via text messages, phone calls, or emails. Implementation of telemedicine applications could also be helpful for virtual visits to determine the emergency status of the condition. During the fundus examination of the patients, indirect ophthalmoscopes can be preferred instead of slit lamp fundus examination.

Patients necessitating intravitreal injections are a major concern for retina specialists. One approach could be increasing the time interval between the injections. Another approach could be the decision of injection only according to the OCT imaging results. The last approach could be postponing any visits or injections until the patient complains about any significant visual loss.

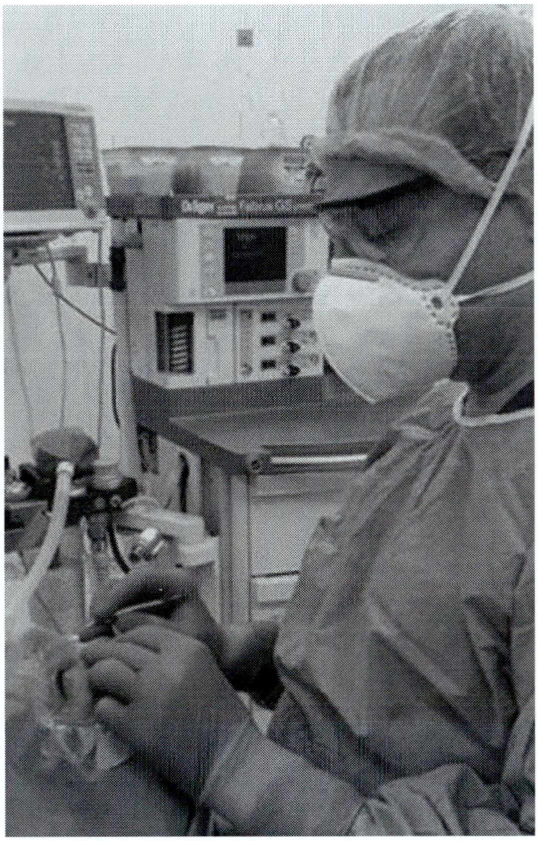

Figure 3. Oculoplasty surgery with appropriate personal protective equipment.

Oculoplasty

Oculoplasty is a subspecialty of ophthalmology with particularly higher-risk for transmission of COVID-19 compared to the other ophthalmologists and other physicians due to the higher viral load in the nasal cavity than in the throat. Oculoplastic surgeons operate on the nasolacrimal area (lacrimal drainage system and sinuses) as well as the orbit and sinuses, they are at risk for aerosolization of viral particles from nasal mucosa and/or other mucosal surfaces [40, 41]. Therefore, protective face shields or goggles should be used during the oculoplastic surgeries (Figure 3).

Contact Lens

During the contact lens clinics' daily routine, ophthalmologists prescribing the contact lenses and contact lens nurses advising the contact lens use are in close contact with the patients. Therefore, special precautions must be taken to prevent any contamination of the equipment and working environment. Application of the contact lens should be accepted as an elective procedure and patient triaging including the COVID-19 risk assessment and the determination of the emergency status of the contact lens users must be done before accepting the patient appointment.

For former contact lens users, any newly developed complaint should be evaluated via telemedicine or clinic visits and control visits should be postponed. British Contact Lens Association recommended postponing the new contact lens examinations.

Since a study showed that extended daily use of glasses more than 8 hours per day was associated with less susceptibility to COVID-19 [38], contact lens users should be recommended the use of glasses during the pandemic for better protection against COVID-19.

Uveitis

Some uveitis patients are under immunomodulatory treatment possibly making them more susceptible to COVID-19. However, the uveitis patients should not be advised to stop their treatment since the treatment discontinuation may lead to more dangerous conditions. Telemedicine, especially evaluation with fundus photography, can be used for the diagnosis of uveitis. However, all active uveitis conditions should be examined by the physician, but the follow-up interval can be longer than usual.

The current recommendation for immunosuppressive treatment includes the continuation of the treatment apart from the patients with high COVID-19 risk and avoiding the use of high-dose steroid treatment. Because steroid use of more than 10 mg/day was shown to be associated with a higher hospitalization risk for COVID-19 patients. Interferon and tocilizumab are highly recommended to be continued in the treatment of uveitis patients due to their possible positive effect on COVID-19 treatment. However, the use of anti-tumor necrosis factor treatment in uveitis patients is controversial [42–44].

Cataract

Cataracts are the second most common cause of treatable visual impairment globally. Since cataract surgeries are among the elective surgeries except for some relatively urgent conditions (phacolytic glaucoma, phacomorphic glaucoma, etc.), almost all cataract surgeries were canceled or postponed due to the COVID-19 pandemic. However, the increased cataract patient volume will be a big concern for the future practice of the ophthalmologists.

Some countries recommended the ophthalmologists to start some elective surgeries including cataract surgery. However, precautions should be taken to prevent cross-infection by wearing appropriate PPE including an N95 mask and protective goggles during the surgery (Figure 4).

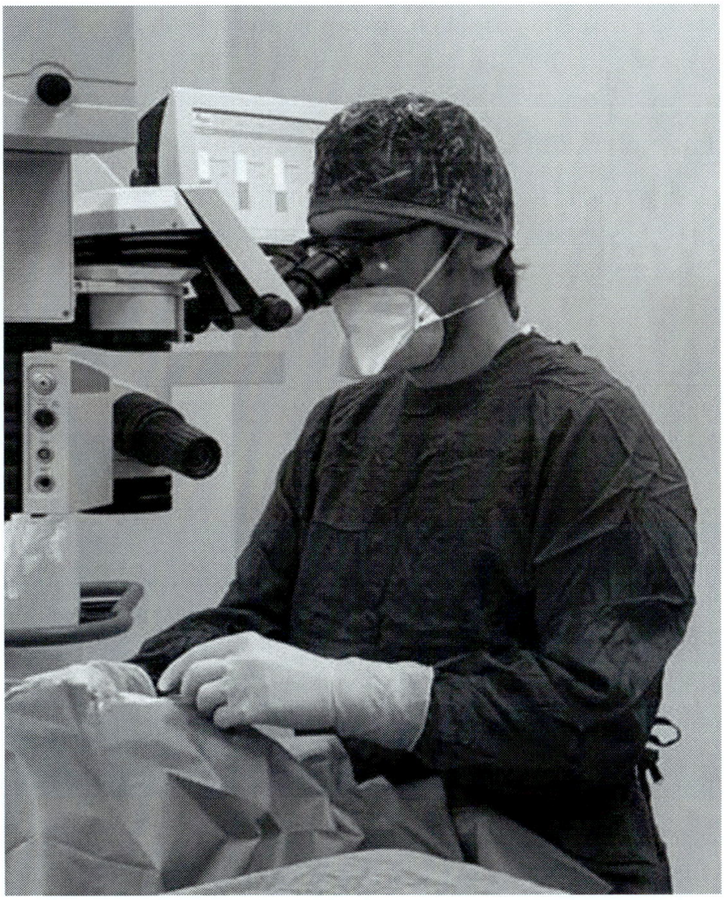

Figure 4. Cataract surgery with appropriate personal protective equipment including an N95 mask, gloves, and protective goggles.

Cataract surgery training for ophthalmology residents was also impaired. Wet labs can be a useful tool for the training of the residents during the pandemic.

Cataract surgery may have the potential of aerosol formation. A recent study showed that aerosol formation can be reduced with hydroxypropyl methylcellulose (HPMC) coating of the cornea every 1 minute or when 2.2 mm phaco tip was used instead of 2.75 mm [45]. On the other hand, povidone-iodine is used for surgical antisepsis before the cataract surgery and is virucidal to SARS-CoV-2 [46]. Furthermore, phacoemulsification cataract surgery occurs in a closed system preventing the intraocular fluid to contact with the outer environment [45]. However, the safety of the cataract surgery with phacoemulsification regarding the COVID-19 transmission is still unknown.

Cornea

Foreign bodies that necessitate removal, active keratitis, corneal ulcers, corneal perforation, or melt, corneal graft rejection are among the corneal pathologies requiring a visit to the ophthalmology clinic. Elective surgeries including keratoplasties should be postponed. However, therapeutic tectonic keratoplasty can be performed in urgent conditions. The donors should also be checked for COVID-19 before the harvesting process. Theoretically, due to the presence of ACE2 in cornea epithelium, the viruses can be transmitted via corneal transplantation. However, further postmortem studies on corneal tissues should be conducted to better understanding the possibility of transmission via transplantation.

The use of cauterization during ocular surface-related surgeries possess a risk for aerosol formation. Therefore, irrigation will be important during cauterization and the use of cautery should be minimized in terms of power and duration. The smoke should also be evacuated effectively during cauterization.

Glaucoma

Glaucoma is an incipient disease causing painless peripheral vision loss due to progressive optic nerve damage. The well-known risk factor for the disease is increased intraocular pressure. Non-contact tonometer sprays a gas for measuring the intraocular pressure and possibly creates aerosol around that local area for a long time (3-8 hours) thereby creating a possible environment for the disease transmission [47]. Therefore, for safer intraocular pressure measurement, an applanation tonometer with efficient cleaning or iCare tonometer should be used instead of a non-contact tonometer.

Glaucoma patients can be followed only with OCT-RNFL imaging or visual field test to postpone clinical visits. Home-based IOP monitoring with contact lenses can be used for investigating the diurnal variation.

Pediatric Ophthalmology

Sight threatening conditions such as retinopathy of prematurity, congenital cataract, congenital glaucoma, or severe amblyopia can be followed and managed without postponing any visit to prevent any permanent visual loss. Telemedicine can be used for the follow up with more benign conditions such as strabismus.

Surgery

Hospitalization should be approved only for the SARS-CoV-2 negative cases. However, in conditions requiring urgent intervention such as corneal rupture, the operation can be done without waiting for the PCR test result.

PCR tests should be implemented in all patients before their surgery. For the procedures possibly not causing any aerosol formation, wearing only a surgical mask for the patient can be enough. However, we recommend the use of N95 masks for all ophthalmological interventions.

COVID-19 positive patients should be operated in operating rooms with negative pressure, if possible. Hospitals should provide operating rooms with negative pressure given the possible long duration of the pandemic. The frequency of air change should be high in standard operating rooms. All patients should wear surgical masks.

COVID-19 and Telemedicine in Ophthalmology

Telemedicine is a way of transmitting any information to support healthcare by using communication technologies. Video examination visits can be used during the pandemic to postpone any elective case or to determine the emergency status of the patient. However, the limitations and medicolegal concerns of virtual visits should be understood by the eye care provider and explained in detail to the patients.

Conclusion

In conclusion, ophthalmologists are at increased risks for COVID-19 because of their close physical proximity to the patients during the eye examination. All eye care providers should take precautions against COVID-19 by wearing appropriate PPE including protective goggles, gloves, and N95 masks. Social distancing in outpatient clinics should be warranted for preventing cross-infection. Elective surgeries should be postponed, and only relatively urgent cases should be seen in the clinics. Telemedicine applications should be implemented for patient triaging or virtual visits. Conjunctivitis can be the presenting sign of COVID-19 as well as it can be observed concurrently with the other symptoms. Therefore, all patients with red eyes can be accepted as COVID-19 conjunctivitis until proven otherwise during the pandemic.

References

[1] Corman, V. M., Muth, D., Niemeyer, D., and Drosten, C. (2018) Hosts and Sources of Endemic Human Coronaviruses. *Advances in Virus Research*. 100: 163–188.

[2] Shereen, M. A., Khan, S., Kazmi, A., Bashir, N., and Siddique, R. (2020) COVID-19 infection: Origin, transmission, and characteristics of human coronaviruses. *Journal of Advanced Research*. 24: 91–98.

[3] (2020) *Report of the WHO-China Joint Mission on Coronavirus Disease 2019 (COVID-19).* 2019 (February), 16–24. Available at: https://www.who.int/docs/default-source/coronaviruse/who-china-joint-mission-on-covid-19-final-report.pdf. Date of citation: Sep 28, 2020.

[4] Loon, S. C., Teoh, S. C. B., Oon, L. L. E., Se-Thoe, S. Y., Ling, A. E., Leo, Y. S., et al., (2004) The severe acute respiratory syndrome coronavirus in tears. *British Journal of Ophthalmology*. 88 (7): 861–863.

[5] Yeo, C., Kaushal, S., and Yeo, D. (2020) Enteric involvement of coronaviruses: is faecal–oral transmission of SARS-CoV-2 possible? *The Lancet Gastroenterology and Hepatology*. 5 (4): 335–337.

[6] Wan, Y., Shang, J., Graham, R., Baric, R. S., and Li, F. (2020) Receptor Recognition by the Novel Coronavirus from Wuhan: an Analysis Based on Decade-Long Structural Studies of SARS Coronavirus. *Journal of Virology*. 94 (7).

[7] Holappa, M., Vapaatalo, H., and Vaajanen, A. (2017) Many Faces of Renin-angiotensin System - Focus on Eye. *The Open Ophthalmology Journal*. 11 (1): 122–142.

[8] Zhou, L., Xu, Z., Castiglione, G. M., Soiberman, U.S., Eberhart, C. G., and Duh, E. J. (2020) ACE2 and TMPRSS2 are expressed on the human ocular surface, suggesting susceptibility to SARS-CoV-2 infection. *Ocular Surface*. 18 (4): 537–544.

[9] Guan, W., Ni, Z., Hu, Y., Liang, W., Ou, C., He, J., et al., (2020) Clinical characteristics of coronavirus disease 2019 in China. *New England Journal of Medicine*. 382 (18): 1708–1720.

[10] Karimi, S., Arabi, A., Shahraki, T., and Safi, S. (2020) Detection of severe acute respiratory syndrome Coronavirus-2 in the tears of patients with Coronavirus disease 2019. *Eye (Basingstoke)*. 34 (7): 1220–1223.

[11] Marinho, P. M., Marcos, A. A. A., Romano, A. C., Nascimento, H., and Belfort, R. (2020) Retinal findings in patients with COVID-19. *The Lancet*. 395 (10237): 1610.

[12] Dinkin, M., Gao, V., Kahan, J., Bobker, S., Simonetto, M., Wechsler, P., et al., (2020) COVID-19 presenting with ophthalmoparesis from cranial nerve palsy. *Neurology*. 95 (5): 221–223.

[13] Lantos, J. E., Strauss, S. B., and Lin, E. (2020) COVID-19-Associated miller fisher syndrome: MRI findings. *American Journal of Neuroradiology*. 41 (7): 1184–1186.

[14] Dockery, D. M., Rowe, S. G., Murphy, M. A., and Krzystolik, M. G. (2020) The Ocular Manifestations and Transmission of COVID-19: Recommendations for Prevention. *Journal of Emergency Medicine*. 59 (1): 137–140.

[15] Colavita, F., Lapa, D., Carletti, F., Lalle, E., Bordi, L., Marsella, P., et al., (2020) SARS-CoV-2 Isolation From Ocular Secretions of a Patient With COVID-19 in Italy With Prolonged Viral RNA Detection. *Annals of Internal Medicine*. 173 (3): 242–243.

[16] La Distia Nora, R., Putera, I., Khalisha, D. F., Septiana, I., Ridwan, A.S., and Sitompul, R. (2020) Are eyes the windows to COVID-19? Systematic review and meta-analysis. *BMJ Open Ophthalmology*. 5 (1): e000563.

[17] Valente, P., Iarossi, G., Federici, M., Petroni, S., Palma, P., Cotugno, N., et al., (2020) Ocular manifestations and viral shedding in tears of pediatric patients with coronavirus disease 2019: a preliminary report. *Journal of AAPOS*. S1091-8531(20)30115-4.

[18] Wu, P., Duan, F., Luo, C., Liu, Q., Qu, X., Liang, L., et al., (2020) Characteristics of Ocular Findings of Patients with Coronavirus Disease 2019 (COVID-19) in Hubei Province, China. *JAMA Ophthalmology*. 138 (5): 575–578.

[19] Xia, J., Tong, J., Liu, M., Shen, Y., and Guo, D. (2020) Evaluation of coronavirus in tears and conjunctival secretions of patients with SARS-CoV-2 infection. *Journal of Medical Virology*. 92 (6): 589–594.

[20] Seah, I. Y. J., Anderson, D. E., Kang, A. E. Z., Wang, L., Rao, P., Young, B. E., et al., (2020) Assessing Viral Shedding and Infectivity of Tears in Coronavirus Disease 2019 (COVID-19) Patients. *Ophthalmology*. 127 (7): 977–979.

[21] Sun, C., Wang, Y., Liu, G., and Liu, Z. (2020) Role of the Eye in Transmitting Human Coronavirus: What We Know and What We Do Not Know. *Frontiers in Public Health*. 8: 155.

[22] Deng, C., Yang, Y., Chen, H., Chen, W., Chen, Z., Ma, K., et al., (2020) Ocular Dectection of SARS-CoV-2 in 114 Cases of COVID-19 Pneumonia in Wuhan, China: An Observational Study. *SSRN Electronic Journal*.

[23] Zhou, Y., Zeng, Y., Tong, Y., and Chen, C. (2020) Ophthalmologic evidence against the interpersonal transmission of 2019 novel coronavirus through conjunctiva. *MedRxiv*. 2020.02.11.20021956.

[24] Arora, R., Goel, R., Kumar, S., Chhabra, M., Saxena, S., Manchanda, V., et al., (2020) Evaluation of SARS-CoV-2 in tears of moderate to severe COVID-19 patients. *Ophthalmology*. S0161-6420(20): 30847-2.

[25] Seah, I. and Agrawal, R. (2020) Can the Coronavirus Disease 2019 (COVID-19) Affect the Eyes? A Review of Coronaviruses and Ocular Implications in Humans and Animals. *Ocular Immunology and Inflammation*. 28 (3): 391–395.

[26] Scalinci, S. Z. and Trovato Battagliola, E. (2020) Conjunctivitis can be the only presenting sign and symptom of COVID-19. *IDCases*. 20: e00774

[27] Casagrande, M., Fitzek, A., Püschel, K., Aleshcheva, G., Schultheiss, H.-P., Berneking, L., et al., (2020) Detection of SARS-CoV-2 in Human Retinal Biopsies of Deceased COVID-19 Patients. *Ocular Immunology and Inflammation*. 28 (5): 721–725.

[28] Kampf, G., Todt, D., Pfaender, S., and Steinmann, E. (2020) Persistence of coronaviruses on inanimate surfaces and their inactivation with biocidal agents. *Journal of Hospital Infection*. 104 (3): 246–251.

[29] Geller, C., Varbanov, M., and Duval, R. (2012) Human Coronaviruses: Insights into Environmental Resistance and Its Influence on the Development of New Antiseptic Strategies. *Viruses*. 4 (11): 3044–3068.

[30] Rabenau, H. F., Cinatl, J., Morgenstern, B., Bauer, G., Preiser, W., and Doerr, H. W. (2005) Stability and inactivation of SARS coronavirus. *Medical Microbiology and Immunology*. 194 (1–2): 1–6.

[31] *Cleaning and Disinfection for Households* | CDC. (2019) Available at: https://www.cdc.gov/coronavirus/2019-ncov/prevent-getting-sick/cleaning-disinfection.html?CDC_AA_refVal=https%3A%2F% 2Fwww.cdc.gov%2Fcoronavirus%2F2019-ncov%2Fprepare%2Fcleaning-disinfection.html. Date of citation: Sep 28, 2020.

[32] Sattar, S. A., Springthorpe, V. S., Karim, Y., and Loro, P. (1989) Chemical disinfection of non-porous inanimate surfaces experimentally contaminated with four human pathogenic viruses. *Epidemiology and Infection*. 102 (3): 493–505.

[33] Amesty, M. A., Alió del Barrio, J. L., and Alió, J. L. (2020) COVID-19 Disease and Ophthalmology: An Update. *Ophthalmology and Therapy*. 9 (3): 1.

[34] He, J., Guo, Y., Mao, R., and Zhang, J. (2020) Proportion of asymptomatic coronavirus disease 2019: A systematic review and meta-analysis. *Journal of Medical Virology*. jmv.26326.

[35] (2020) *Important coronavirus updates for ophthalmologists* - American Academy of Ophthalmology. Available at: https://www.aao.org/headline/alert-important-coronavirus-context. Date of citation: Sep 28, 2020.

[36] Chan, W. M., Liu, D. T. L., Chan, P. K. S., Chong, K. K. L., Yuen, K. S. C., Chiu, T. Y. H., et al., (2006) Precautions in ophthalmic practice in a hospital with a major acute SARS outbreak: An experience from Hong Kong. *Eye*. 20 (3): 283–289.

[37] Kwok, Y. L. A., Gralton, J., and McLaws, M. L. (2015) Face touching: A frequent habit that has implications for hand hygiene. *American Journal of Infection Control*. 43 (2): 112–114.

[38] Zeng, W., Wang, X., Li, J., Yang, Y., Qiu, X., Song, P., et al., (2020) Association of Daily Wear of Eyeglasses With Susceptibility to Coronavirus Disease 2019 Infection. *JAMA Ophthalmology*. doi: 10.1001/jamaophthalmol.2020.3906.

[39] Lim, L. W., Yip, L. W., Tay, H. W., Ang, X. L., Lee, L. K., Chin, C.F., et al., (2020) Sustainable practice of ophthalmology during COVID-19: challenges and

solutions. *Graefe's Archive for Clinical and Experimental Ophthalmology*. 258 (7): 1427–1436.

[40] Vukkadala, N., Qian, Z. J., Holsinger, F. C., Patel, Z. M., and Rosenthal, E. (2020) COVID-19 and the Otolaryngologist: Preliminary Evidence-Based Review. *Laryngoscope*. doi: 10.1002/ lary.28672.

[41] *Modes of transmission of virus causing COVID-19: implications for IPC precaution recommendations.* Available at: https://www.who.int/news-room/ commentaries/detail/modes-of-transmission-of-virus-causing-covid-19-implications-for-ipc-precaution-recommendations. Date of citation: Sep 28, 2020.

[42] Hsieh, J., Honda, A. F., Suárez-Fariñas, M., Samson, C. M., Kedhar, S., Mauro, J., et al., (2013) Fundus image diagnostic agreement in uveitis utilizing free and open source software. *Canadian Journal of Ophthalmology*. 48 (4): 227–234.

[43] Thng, Z. X., De Smet, M. D., Lee, C. S., Gupta, V., Smith, J. R., McCluskey, P. J., et al., (2020) COVID-19 and immunosuppression: A review of current clinical experiences and implications for ophthalmology patients taking immunosuppressive drugs. *British Journal of Ophthalmology*. doi: 10.1136/bjophthalmol-2020-316586.

[44] Gianfrancesco, M., Hyrich, K. L., Hyrich, K. L., Al-Adely, S., Al-Adely, S., Carmona, L., et al., (2020) Characteristics associated with hospitalisation for COVID-19 in people with rheumatic disease: Data from the COVID-19 Global Rheumatology Alliance physician-reported registry. *Annals of the Rheumatic Diseases*. 79 (7): 859–866.

[45] Darcy, K., Elhaddad, O., Achiron, A., Keller, J., Leadbetter, D., Tole, D., et al., (2020) Reducing visible aerosol generation during phacoemulsification in the era of Covid-19. *Eye (Basingstoke)*. https://doi.org/10.1038/s41433-020-1053-3.

[46] Kariwa, H., Fujii, N., and Takashima, I. (2006) Inactivation of SARS coronavirus by means of povidone-iodine, physical conditions and chemical reagents. *Dermatology*. 212 Suppl 1(Suppl 1): 119-23.

[47] Britt, J. M., Clifton, B. C., Barnebey, H. S., and Mills, R. P. (1991) Microaerosol Formation in Noncontact 'Air-Puff' Tonometry. *Archives of Ophthalmology*. 109 (2): 225–228.

In: Coronavirus Disease
Editor: Yildiz Dincer
ISBN: 978-1-53619-296-4

Chapter 12

The Impact of the COVID-19 Pandemic on Patients with Diabetes

Zeynep Mine Coskun*[1]*, PhD and Sema Bolkent*[2,*]*, PhD
[1]Demiroglu Bilim University, Faculty of Arts and Sciences, Department of Molecular Biology and Genetics, Istanbul Turkey
[2]Istanbul University-Cerrahpasa, Cerrahpasa Medical Faculty, Department of Medical Biology, Istanbul Turkey

Abstract

The purpose of the present chapter is to explain the impact of coronavirus disease 2019 (COVID-19) on diabetes and implications for treatment. The SARS-CoV-2 outbreak affected millions all around the world and the number of infected cases is still increasing. The available scientific data from clinical studies of COVID-19 show that is worse with comorbidities such as diabetes. According to statistical data, the mortality rate in diabetic patients is higher than non-diabetics. SARS-CoV-2 can cause acute diabetes using angiotensin-converting enzyme-2 (ACE-2), which is abundant in Langerhans islets. Anti-diabetic drugs during COVID-19 may be a novel strategy to reduce virus entry and replication in individuals with or without type II diabetes. Studies to date have shown that some drugs tried in the treatment of COVID-19 improve glucose profile but the others cause impairment of glucose metabolism and β-cell function. Dipeptidyl peptidase 4 (DPP-4) inhibitors may prevent the progression of the hyperinflammatory state associated with COVID-19. Therefore, since it is important to maintain glucose homeostasis in COVID-19 treatment, more studies are needed on the hyperglycemia or hypoglycemia molecular mechanisms of anti-diabetic drugs. Telemedicine or digital medicine plays a crucial role in monitoring glycemic control in diabetic patients with COVID-19.

Keywords: COVID-19, diabetes, hyperglycemia, ketoacidosis, anti-diabetic therapeutics

---

* Corresponding Author's Email: bolkent@istanbul.edu.tr.

INTRODUCTION: SARS-COV-2 AND DIABETES

Diabetes, a metabolic disease, characterized by inappropriately raised blood glucose concentrations. Diabetes can be categorized as type I diabetes, type II diabetes, gestational diabetes, and specific types of diabetes due to other causes. The two major types of diabetes are type I diabetes and type II diabetes, which are caused by absolute insulin deficiency (type I diabetes) and/or insulin resistance (type II diabetes). Type I diabetes is caused by the destruction of the pancreatic β-cells and is found in children and adolescents, while type II diabetes results from an imbalance between insulin sensitivity and insulin levels and commonly present in older adults. Type II diabetes also called "adult-onset diabetes", accounts for approximately 90-95% of all diabetic individuals. A combination of genetic and lifestyle is involved in the development of type II diabetes. For example, middle-aged and older adults can have prolonged hyperglycemia due to poor lifestyle and an unhealthy diet [1].

According to the International Diabetes Federation (IDF), 1 in 11 people aged 20-79 years worldwide has diabetes in the global population. It has been estimated that the prevalence of diabetes will increase from 463 to 578 million by 2030. Unfortunately, the number will jump to 700 million by 2045. Furthermore, diabetes is among the top 10 causes of death [2]. Thus, the disease is a serious growing problem for global health.

Currently, a new coronavirus, rapidly spreading, remains a threat to most of the human population worldwide. The new virus, SARS-CoV-2, which induce the COVID-19 disease in humans, first appeared in China. One of the coronaviruses (CoVs), SARS-CoV-2, belongs to the large *Coronaviridae* family. It is known that these CoVs, a large family, are enveloped viruses with a single-strand, positive-sense RNA genome. Despite a long history of coronavirus research starting in the 1930s, with the first appearance of SARS-CoV in 2002, many scientists have realized the potential for this virus group to cause fatal infections in humans [3]. It is reported that seven types of CoVs can infect humans [4]. Human coronaviruses (HCoVs), respiratory pathogens, cause respiratory infections such as severe acute respiratory syndrome-CoV (SARS-CoV), and the Middle East respiratory syndrome-CoV (MERS-CoV) [5].

According to the latest data, the COVID-19 outbreak has caused over 1.839.660 deaths and 83.910.386 infected cases and these numbers are increasing [6]. Li et al., [7] reported that angiotensin-converting enzyme-2 (ACE-2) is a functional receptor for SARS-CoV and it infects humans through this receptor. After ACE-2, dipeptidyl peptidase 4 (DPP4) has been identified as a receptor for coronaviruses. One of the highly pathogenic CoV, MERS-CoV uses DPP4 as a cellular receptor [8]. To infect humans, SARS-CoV-2 is also used the ACE-2 cell receptor [9].

Recent evidence has presented that patients with underlying metabolic conditions of diabetes show higher morbidity and mortality than individuals without diabetes [10]. It has been reported that blocking the renin-angiotensin system (RAS) with ACE inhibitors or angiotensin II receptor blockers reduced the development of diabetes in adults [11]. On the other hand, these therapeutics upregulate the ACE-2 receptor on the surface of the host cell and so, the SARS-CoV-2 virus can enter the host cells [12]. This suggests that individuals with diabetes are more likely to be infected with SARS-CoV-2 compared to healthy humans. On the contrary, diabetes disease does not cause an increase in the risk of SARS-CoV-2 infection but may contribute to worsening the outcome of COVID-19 disease [13]. Another thought is that the anti-viral drugs used cause deficiency in glucose metabolism and other endocrine disorders, and even cause ketoacidosis [14, 15].

Hyperglycemia Is a Risk in COVID-19

There is an association between hyperglycemia and elevated risk of mortality in stroke, pneumonia, acute myocardial infarction, trauma, and surgery [16]. Hyperglycemia was shown as a risk factor of morbidity and mortality in SARS and MERS [17, 18].

The fact that type II diabetes is the second most common comorbidity of COVID-19 is evidence that these two outbreaks are related. According to the study on adult patients with COVID-19, patients with diabetes disease have a higher probability of in-hospital death compared with non-diabetics [19]. In a study of 7337 COVID-19 patients, 952 of whom had diabetes, it was reported that type II diabetes significantly increases the risk of medical interventions and mortality. However, among the individuals with type II diabetes, patients with well-controlled blood glucose regulation (3.9 to 10.0 mmol/L) were found to perform better compared with patients with poorly controlled blood glucose (> 10.0 mmol/L) [20]. Deng et al., [14] suggested that the prevention of diabetes can contribute to reducing COVID-19 mortality. It is reported that high glucose not only damages cells and tissues but also activates interferon regulatory factor 5 (IRF5), thereby promoting cytokine storm (CS) caused by a virus [14, 21]. Furthermore, it is predicted that SARS-CoV-2 infection induces the CS as a systemic immune response. The CS can cause the progression of the disease and lead to multiple organ failure or even death [22]. Due to the CS caused by high blood glucose and SARS-CoV-2, it is estimated that patients with diabetes have a higher mortality rate.

COVID-19 on the Regulation of Blood Glucose

Some non-diabetes-related diseases, such as systemic inflammation response syndrome, traumatic brain injury, and severe sepsis tend to have high blood glucose levels [23]. This condition is defined as stress hyperglycemia (glucose value > 7.8 mmol/L or 140 mg/dl). Stress hyperglycemia was frequently found in patients not diagnosed with diabetes [24]. Stress hyperglycemia may be occurred as a result of insulin deficiency, worsening of insulin resistance, and increased hepatic glucose production [25]. Similarly, it is thought that COVID-19 patients may also have stress hyperglycemia. The importance of well-controlled blood glucose in COVID-19 patients was reported in recent studies. Wang et al., [16] emphasized that fasting blood glucose at admission is a significant factor for the prognosis of COVID-19. They suggested that the rise of fasting blood glucose elevates the incidence of in-hospital complications. Therefore, since most COVID-19 patients tend to glucose metabolic disorders, glycemic control is significant for all COVID-19 patients, even without pre-existing diabetes. According to another study, in 29 of 184 patients, SARS-CoV-2 infection caused new and permanent hyperglycemia. Thus, the dysregulation of glucose metabolism in patients may be induced by the SARS-Co-2 infection and, this increases the development of severe COVID-19 in patients [26]. On the contrary, Liu et al., [27] specified that a high level in admission fasting blood glucose was not a dependent risk factor for developing critical diseases of COVID-19 patients. They suggested that fasting blood glucose may be associated with systemic inflammatory reactions and immune status. Continuous glucose monitoring may prevent infections and complications, thereby contributing to the recovery of the patient with COVID-19. According to Li et al., [28], under the persistent hypoxia state hyperglycemia can develop in the COVID-19 patients. They also recommended that to prevent the progressive COVID-19 from getting worse, adequate oxygen intake for patients are monitored, as well as blood glucose levels.

Pancreas Failure

The pancreas is an important gland in diabetic patients as well as in patients with COVID-19. Recent studies have reported that patients with COVID-19 show not only fever and respiratory disease but also an increasing number of patients with gastrointestinal symptoms such as nausea, vomiting, and abdominal pain [29]. Hadi et al., [30] reported that acute pancreatitis is a complication related to COVID-19. The researchers emphasized that if patients with COVID-19 suffer from abdominal pain, lipase and amylase should be measured. In a study on 52 patients with Covid-19, 17% of COVID-19 cases showed pancreas injury that was defined as increased lipase [31]. Ding et al., [32] reported that SARS-CoV was found not only in the lung, liver, intestine, and kidney tissues but also in the pancreas. Thus, the pancreas may be a potential target of SARS-CoV infection. Consistent with the report of Ding et al., [32], the high damage level of SARS-CoV in the pancreas is correlated with ACE-2 expression in the pancreas. Moreover, ACE-2 expression is localized especially in the endocrine part of the pancreas. SARS-CoV may enter Langerhans islets using ACE-2, the receptor of SARS-CoV, and it may cause acute diabetes after damaging the islets [33]. According to Wang et al., [31], the pancreatic damage in COVID-19 may be induced directly by the cytopathic effect mediated by SARS-CoV-2 replication. Indirectly, the damage in the pancreas may be originated from immune-mediated and systemic inflammatory cellular responses induced by SARS-CoV-2 infection. Researchers found that the expression of ACE-2 in the pancreas of healthy individuals is slightly higher than in the lungs. Similar to SARS-CoV, SARS-CoV-2 may also bind to ACE-2 in the pancreas and enter into the tissue. Therefore, SARS-CoV-2 causes damage to the pancreas. Moreover, the expression of ACE-2 has been shown in both the exocrine and endocrine regions of the pancreas [34]. In the same study on 121 cases with COVID-19, the authors found an increase in amylase and lipase levels depending on the severity of the disease. It was emphasized that more attention should be paid to the pancreas in patients with SARS-CoV-2 infection, particularly, in severe cases. Otherwise, it has been suggested that there may be pancreatic injuries associated with the use of antipyretic drugs [31].

Diabetic Ketoacidosis

Diabetic ketoacidosis (DKA), one of the most serious complications of diabetes, is characterized by the triad of hyperglycemia (blood glucose level > 13.9 mmol/L), acidosis (arterial pH less than 7.3 and serum bicarbonate level less than 18 mEq/L) and ketosis (ketonemia or ketonuria) [35].

DKA has been noticed in COVID-19 as well as in other serious infections [36]. DKA can be triggered by SARS-CoV-2 in poorly controlled diabetic patients [10]. In a case study, researchers reported that COVID-19 could cause DKA and multiorgan failure even without lung involvement in patients with diabetes [37]. Similarly, Chee et al., [38] found that DKA may be occurred by SARS-CoV-2 in a 37-years-old male diabetic patient. In the period from January 1 to March 3, 2020, a Chinese cohort study on 658 patients was reported that COVID-19 infection may cause ketosis and ketoacidosis in non-diabetic individuals, and can induce DKA in diabetic patients [39]. According to another case study, in a 54-years-old male patient with newly diagnosed diabetes, COVID-19 infection may cause an increase in DKA [40]. When SARS-CoV-2 enters pancreatic islet cells, it damages β-cells, which may induce precipitated DKA in patients.

Anti-Diabetic Therapeutics

According to the last International Diabetes Federation (IDF) atlas, the control of blood glucose is usually initiated with metformin as a first-line drug. In cases where treatment with a single anti-diabetic drug is not sufficient, there are combination treatment options such as sulfonylureas, DPP4 inhibitors, glucagon-like peptide 1 (GLP-1) analogs. Insulin injections may be needed if oral anti-diabetic drugs are unable to control hyperglycemia [2].

Studies have shown that some of the drugs tried in the treatment of COVID-19 improve glucose profile, but some drugs cause impaired glucose metabolism [41]. On the other hand, although ACE-2 and DPP4, two coronavirus receptor proteins, are known to be important in the regulation of glucose homeostasis and inflammation, there is insufficient clinical evidence that drugs targeting these receptors benefit human coronavirus infections [42]. One study suggested that ACE inhibitor (ACEI) and angiotensin receptor antagonist (ARB) use should be considered in diabetic patients during the COVID-19 outbreak, while another study reported that the use of ACEI and ARB in diabetic patients may increase the morbidity and mortality of COVID-19 [43, 44].

The potential benefits of anti-diabetic drugs during COVID-19 are as follows.

METFORMIN

Metformin, which has been used for decades, is the most preferred drug worldwide for every diabetic patient. Jean Sterne introduced this drug as 'Glucophage', which means 'glucose eater', in 1957 [45]. Interestingly, Sharma et al., [46] suggested that when there is no specific agent against COVID-19, metformin should be among the drugs used to fight the virus. Rena et al., [47] have mentioned that metformin affects the improvement of glucose metabolism through the AMP-activated protein kinase (AMPK) dependent mechanism. Metformin is thought to provide conformational and functional changes to the ACE-2 receptor through AMPK activation that causes phosphorylation of ACE-2. As a result, binding of SARS-CoV-2 to the receptor-binding site can be prevented, so that the virus is not able to enter the cell [46]. By contrast with Sharma et al., [46], the researchers have suggested that metformin may promote SARS-CoV2 infection by increasing the presence of ACE-2 in the respiratory system. On the other hand, researchers still not sure whether metformin is friendly or not [48]. According to a retrospective study on 283 patients by Luo et al., [49], the fasting blood glucose level in diabetic patients infected with COVID-19 using anti-diabetic drugs other than metformin was lower than in those using metformin. However, other laboratory parameters were similar in patients taking metformin and other anti-diabetic drugs. This study also suggested that the mortality of metformin users was lower than that of non-users in diabetic patients infected with COVID-19.

Dipeptidyl Peptidase 4 (DPP4) Inhibitors

DPP4 inhibitors are commonly used to control glucose in patients with diabetes [42]. To facilitate virus entry, SARS-CoV-2 uses co-receptors as ACE-2 partners. DPP4, a membrane protein, has also been reported among these co-receptors [50]. It has been reported that DDP4 inhibitor anti-diabetic drugs such as gliptins (sitagliptin, vildagliptin, or linagliptin) can prevent coronavirus / DPP4 interaction and thus protect the cell from virus entry [51]. Consistent with this study, Solerte et al., [52] suggested that the inhibition of DPP4 may be a new strategy to strengthen COVID-19 therapy in diabetic patients or not. Besides, DPP4 inhibitors may also be used to prevent the progression of the hyperinflammatory condition associated with COVID-19, thanks to its inflammatory healing properties [53]. In a review article by Bassendine et al., [54], it was emphasized that DPP4 activity is higher in elderly individuals and the increase of DPP4 in plasma is an indicator of the onset of metabolic syndrome. Thus, gliptins used in DPP4 inhibition may be a treatment strategy to reduce the severity of COVID-19 disease.

Glucagon-Like Peptide 1 (GLP-1) Receptor Agonists

GLP-1 receptor agonists, which are more widely used in the treatment of diabetes in recent years, reduce cardiovascular risk [55]. Beyond their anti-diabetic effects, GLP-1 receptor agonists have anti-inflammatory effects [56]. Thus, Ceriello et al., [57] suggested that GLP-1 receptor agonists might be useful in COVID-19 patients due to their anti-inflammatory effects. Similarly, Longo et al., [58] also reported that GLP-1 receptor agonists could be used in diabetic patients with COVID-19 due to their glucose-lowering and anti-inflammatory effects. However, they suggested that data on the use of GLP-1 receptor agonists in these patients were insufficient.

Sulfonylureas and Thiazolidinediones

Sulfonylureas and thiazolidinediones provide excellent improvements in glycemic control in different mechanisms. Sulfonylureas stimulate insulin secretion and act immediately on HbA1c, whereas thiazolidinediones sensitize insulin and take longer to express their effect [59]. According to Derosa and Maffioli [60], thiazolidinediones may provide a more adequate control in diabetic patients compared to sulfonylureas due to their cardiovascular risk lowering effect. Sulfonylureas have been reported to show no interaction with ACE-2 and its use can be safely continued [61].

It has been reported that sulfonylurea treatment affects the risk of hypoglycemia in diabetic patients with COVID-19 [62]. Thiazolidinediones treatment may reduce the development of pulmonary fibrosis (PF) in patients with COVID-19 and thus be a valuable approach to alleviating the course of the disease, especially in diabetic patients. However, due to insulin sensitivity, it is recommended that diabetic patients be followed carefully for any signs of hypoglycemia [63]. Other than these features, thiazolidinediones have anti-inflammatory properties through PPAR-γ activation and affect severe viral pneumonia [64].

INSULIN

To control glucose in hospitalized diabetic patients, insulin treatment has been used extensively for decades. Some case studies have shown that intravenous insulin administration accompanies anti-viral agents and empirical antibiotics for the treatment of both COVID-19 and DKA [10,37]. According to Nakhleh and Shehadeh [65], there is a relationship between SARS-CoV-2-induced lung injury and hyperglycemia. Researchers defend that insulin can be promising in the treatment of COVID-19 patients, thanks to its immunomodulatory effect, its ability to prevent the spread of cytokine storm and lung damage by regulating ACE-2 expression and angiotensin II levels, and its ability to reduce the risk of developing DKA or hyperglycemic hyperosmolar states. Similarly, in a study conducted on 59 patients with COVID-19, it was stated that insulin therapy could be an effective method to control glycemic targets and reduce mortality [66].

SODIUM GLUCOSE TRANSPORTER-2 (SGLT-2) INHIBITORS

Current guidelines for the management of type II diabetes recommend SGLT-2 inhibitors can use in patients with type II diabetes and heart failure to reduce heart failure, major adverse cardiovascular events, and cardiovascular disease death [67]. However, according to the study by Hamblin et al., [68], the use of SGLT-2 inhibitors has been associated with an increase in DKA. In the study, it was observed that SGLT-2 inhibitor users were more likely to develop DKA than non-SGLT-2 inhibitor users. In the same way, Orioli et al., [69] also recommend discontinuation of SGLT-2 inhibitors in patients with serious forms of COVID-19 because of the risks of ketoacidosis and lactic acidosis. On the other hand, it is predicted that the careful use of dapagliflozin, an SGLT-2 inhibitor, and insulin together avoiding dehydration in COVID-19 may be beneficial in the treatment of diabetes [70].

CONCLUSION

Diabetes plays a significant role in further deterioration of the clinical severity of COVID-19. It is a fact that blood glucose levels should be monitored regularly in COVID-19 patients. Unfortunately, the impact of anti-diabetic drugs on COVID-19 outcomes remains unclear. It is important to investigate how SARS-CoV-2 interacts with glucose metabolism to understand disease pathogenesis and improve treatments.

REFERENCES

[1] American Diabetes Association. 2020. "2. Classification and diagnosis of diabetes: standards of medical care in diabetes-2020." *Diabetes Care*. 43(1):S14-S31.

[2] International Diabetes Federation. "*IDF Diabetes Atlas 9th edition 2019*." Available 25 July, 2020. http://www. diabetesatlas.org/en.

[3] Weiss, S-R. 2020. "Forty years with coronaviruses." *J. Exp. Med*. 217(5): e20200537.

[4] Centers for Disease Control and Prevention. *"Human Coronavirus Types."* Available 15 July, 2020. https://www.cdc.gov/coronavirus/ types.html.

[5] Lim, Y-X., Ng, Y-L., Tam, J-P., Liu, D-X. 2016. "Human coronaviruses: a review of virus-host interactions." *Diseases*. 4(3):26.

[6] World Health Organization. "*WHO Coronavirus Disease (COVID-19) Dashboard*." Available 4 January, 2021. https://covid 19.who.int.

[7] Li, W., Moore, M-J., Vasilieva, N., Sui, J., Wong, S-K., Berne, M-A., Somasundaran, M., et al. 2003. "Angiotensin-converting enzyme 2 is a functional receptor for the SARS coronavirus." *Nature*. 426:450-4.

[8] Lu, G., Hu, Y., Wang, Q., Qi, J., Gao, F., Li, Y., Zhang, Y., et al. 2013. "Molecular basis of binding between novel human coronavirus MERS-CoV and its receptor CD26." *Nature*. 500(7461):227-31.

[9] Yan, R., Zhang, Y., Li, Y., Xia, L., Guo, Y., Zhou, Q. 2020. "Structural basis for the recognition of SARS-CoV-2 by full-length human ACE2." *Science*. 367(6485):1444-8.

[10] Kim, N-Y., Ha, E., Moon, J-S., Lee, Y-H., Choi, E-Y. 2020. "Acute hyperglycemic crises with coronavirus disease-19: Case Reports." *Diabetes Metab. J*. 44(2):349-53.

[11] Gillespie, E-L., White, C-M., Kardas, M., Lindberg, M., Coleman, C-I. 2005. "The impact of ACE inhibitors or angiotensin II type 1 receptor blockers on the development of new-onset type 2 diabetes." *Diabetes Care*. 28(9):2261-6.

[12] Mahmoud, I-S., Jarrar, Y-B., Alshaer, W., Ismail, S. 2020. "SARS-CoV-2 entry in host cells-multiple targets for treatment and prevention." *Biochimie*. 175:93-8.

[13] Fadini, G-P., Morieri, M-L., Longato, E., Avogaro, A. 2020. "Prevalence and impact of diabetes among people infected with SARS-CoV-2." *J. Endocrinol. Invest*. 43(6):867-9.

[14] Deng, M., Jiang, L., Ren, Y., Liao, J. 2020. "Can we reduce mortality of COVID-19 if we do better in glucose control?" *Med. Drug. Discov*. 7:100048.

[15] Zhang, W., Zhao, Y., Zhang, F., Wang, Q., Li, T., Liu, Z., Wang, J., et al. 2020. "The use of anti-inflammatory drugs in the treatment of people with severe coronavirus disease 2019 (COVID-19): The perspectives of clinical immunologists from China." *Clin. Immunol.* 214:108393.

[16] Wang, S., Ma, P., Zhang, S., Song, S., Wang, Z., Ma, Y., Xu, J., et al. 2020. "Fasting blood glucose at admission is an independent predictor for 28-day mortality in patients with COVID-19 without previous diagnosis of diabetes: a multi-centre retrospective study." *Diabetologia*. 63(10):2102-11.

[17] Alanazi, K-H., Abedi, G-R., Midgley, C-M., Alkhamis, A., Alsager, T., Almoaddi, A., Algwizani, A., et al. 2020. "Diabetes mellitus, hypertension, and death among 32 patients with MERS- CoV infection." *Saudi Arabia. Emerg. Infect. Dis.* 26(1):166-8.

[18] Yang, J-K., Feng, Y., Yuan, M-Y., Yuan, S-Y., Fu, H-J., Wu, B-Y., Sun, G-Z., et al. 2006. "Plasma glucose levels and diabetes are independent predictors for mortality and morbidity in patients with SARS." *Diabet. Med.* 23(6):623-8.

[19] Zhou, F., Yu, T., Du, R., Fan, G., Liu, Y., Liu, Z., Xiang, J., et al. 2020. "Clinical course and risk factors for mortality of adult inpatients with COVID-19 in Wuhan, China: a retrospective cohort study." *Lancet*. 395(10229):1054-62.

[20] Zhu, L., She, Z-G., Cheng, X., Qin, J-J., Zhang, X-J., Cai, J., Lei, F., et al. 2020. "Association of blood glucose control and outcomes in patients with COVID-19 and pre-existing type 2 diabetes." *Cell Metab.* 31(6):1068-77.

[21] Wang, Q., Fang, P., He, R., Li, M., Yu, H., Zhou, L., Yi, Y., et al. 2020. "*O*-GlcNAc transferase promotes influenza A virus-induced cytokine storm by targeting interferon regulatory factor-5." *Sci. Adv*. 6(16): eaaz7086.

[22] Song, P., Li, W., Xie, J., Hou, Y., You, C. 2020. "Cytokine storm induced by SARS-CoV-2." *Clin. Chim. Acta*. 509:280-7.

[23] Bar-Or, D., Rael, L-T., Madayag, R-M., Banton, K-L., Tanner II, A., Acuna, D-L., Lieser, M-J., et al. 2019. "Stress hyperglycemia in critically Ill patients: insight into possible molecular pathways." *Front. Med. (Lausanne)*. 6:54.

[24] Goyal, N., Kaur, R., Sud, A., Ghorpade, N., Gupta, M. 2014. "Non diabetic and stress induced hyperglycemia [SIH] in orthopedic practice what do we know so far?" *J. Clin. Diagn. Res*. 8(10): LH01-LH3.

[25] Mifsud, S., Schembri, E-L., Gruppetta, M. 2018. "Stress-induced hyperglycaemia." *Br. J. Hosp. Med. (Lond)*. 79(11):634-9.

[26] Smith, S-M., Boppana, A., Traupman, J-A., Unson, E., Maddock, D-A., Chao, K., Dobesh, D-P., et al. 2020. "Impaired glucose metabolism in patients with diabetes, prediabetes, and obesity is associated with severe COVID-19." *J. Med. Virol.* doi: 10.1002/jmv.26227.

[27] Liu, Q., Chen, H., Li, J., Huang, X., Lai, L., Li, S., Zeng, Q. 2020. "Fasting blood glucose predicts the occurrence of critical illness in COVID-19 patients: a multicenter retrospective cohort study." *J. Infect.* S0163-4453(20):30464-3.

[28] Li, Z., Liu, G., Wang, L., Liang, Y., Zhou, Q., Wu, F., Yao, J., et al. 2020. "From the insight of glucose metabolism disorder: Oxygen therapy and blood glucose monitoring are crucial for quarantined COVID-19 patients." *Ecotoxicol. Environ. Saf.* 197:110614.

[29] Patel, K-P., Patel, P-A., Vunnam, R-R., Hewlett, A-T., Jain, R., Jing, R., Vunnam, S-R. 2020. "Gastrointestinal, hepatobiliary, and pancreatic manifestations of COVID-19." *J. Clin. Virol.* 128:104386.

[30] Hadi, A., Werge, M., Kristiansen, K-T., Pedersen, U-G., Karstensen, J-G., Novovic, S., Gluud, L-L. 2020. "Coronavirus disease-19 (COVID-19) associated with severe acute pancreatitis: Case report on three family members." *Pancreatology*. 20(4):665-7.

[31] Wang, F., Wang, H., Fan, J., Zhang, Y., Wang, H., Zhao, Q. 2020. "Pancreatic injury patterns in patients with coronavirus disease 19 pneumonia." *Gastroenterology*. S0016-5085(20)30409-1.

[32] Ding, Y., He, L., Zhang, Q., Huang, Z., Che, X., Hou, J., Wang, H., et al. 2004. "Organ distribution of severe acute respiratory syndrome (SARS) associated coronavirus (SARS-CoV) in SARS patients: implications for pathogenesis and virus transmission pathways." *J. Pathol.* 203(2):622-30.

[33] Yang, J-K., Lin, S-S., Ji, X-J., Guo, L-M. 2010. "Binding of SARS coronavirus to its receptor damages islets and causes acute diabetes." *Acta Diabetol.* 47(3):193-9.

[34] Liu, F., Long, X., Zhang, B., Zhang, W., Chen, X., Zhang, Z. 2020. "ACE2 expression in pancreas may cause pancreatic damage after SARS-CoV-2 infection." *Clin. Gastroenterol. Hepatol.* 18(9):2128-30.

[35] Misra, S., Oliver, N-S. 2015. "Diabetic ketoacidosis in adults." *BMJ*. 351:h5660.

[36] Palermo, N-E., Sadhu, A-R., McDonnell, M-E. 2020. "Diabetic ketoacidosis in COVID-19: unique concerns and considerations." *J. Clin. Endocrinol. Metab.* 105(8): dgaa360.

[37] Kabashneh, S., Ali, H., Alkassis, S. 2020. "Multi-organ failure in a patient with diabetes due to COVID-19 with clear lungs." *Cureus*. 12(5):e8147.

[38] Chee, Y-J., Ng, S-J-H., Yeoh, E. 2020. "Diabetic ketoacidosis precipitated by COVID-19 in a patient with newly diagnosed diabetes mellitus." *Diabetes Res. Clin. Pract.* 164:108166.

[39] Li, J., Wang, X., Chen, J., Zuo, X., Zhang, H., Deng, A. 2020. "COVID-19 infection may cause ketosis and ketoacidosis." *Diabetes Obes. Metab.* doi: 10. 1111/dom.14057.

[40] Heaney, A-I., Griffin, G-D., Simon, E-L. 2020. "Newly diagnosed diabetes and diabetic ketoacidosis precipitated by COVID-19 infection." *Am. J. Emerg. Med.* S0735-6757(20)30488-5.

[41] Wang, Y., Zhang, D., Du, G., Du, R., Zhao, J., Jin, Y., Fu, S., et al. 2020. "Remdesivir in adults with severe COVID-19: a randomised, double-blind, placebo-controlled, multicentre trial." *Lancet.* 395 (10236):1569-78.

[42] Drucker, D-J. 2020. "Coronavirus infections and type 2 diabetes-shared pathways with therapeutic implications." *Endocr. Rev.* 41(3): bnaa011.

[43] Pal, R., Bhansali, A. 2020. "COVID-19, diabetes mellitus and ACE2: The conundrum." *Diabetes Res. Clin. Pract.* 162:108132.

[44] Cure, E., Cure, M-C. 2020. "Angiotensin-converting enzyme inhibitors and angiotensin receptor blockers may be harmful in patients with diabetes during COVID-19 pandemic." *Diabetes Metab. Syndr.* 14(4):349-50.

[45] Patede, G-R., Marita, A-R. 2014. "Metformin: A journey from countryside to the bedside." *J. Obes. Metab. Res.* 1(2):127-30.

[46] Sharma, S., Ray, A., Sadasivam, B. 2020. "Metformin in COVID-19: A possible role beyond diabetes." *Diabetes Res. Clin. Pract.* 164:108183.

[47] Rena, G., Hardie, D-G., Pearson, E-R. 2017. "The mechanisms of action of metformin." *Diabetologia.* 60(9):1577-85.

[48] Ursini, F., Ciaffi, J., Landini, M-P., Meliconi, R. 2020. "COVID-19 and diabetes: Is metformin a friend or foe?" *Diabetes Res. Clin. Pract.* 164:108167.

[49] Luo, P., Qiu, L., Liu, Y., Liu, X-l., Zheng, J-I., Xue, H-Y., Liu, W-H., et al. 2020. "Metformin treatment was associated with decreased mortality in COVID-19 patients with diabetes in a retrospective analysis." *Am. J. Trop. Med. Hyg.* 103(1):69-72.

[50] Qi, F., Qian, S., Zhang, S., Zhang, Z. 2020. "Single cell RNA sequencing of 13 human tissues identify cell types and receptors of human coronaviruses." *Biochem. Biophys. Res. Commun.* 526(1): 135-40.

[51] Mirabelli, M., Chiefari, E., Puccio, L., Foti, D-P., Brunetti, A. 2020. "Potential benefits and harms of novel antidiabetic drugs during COVID-19 crisis." *Int. J. Environ. Res. Public. Health.* 17(10):3664.

[52] Solerte, S-B., Di Sabatino, A., Galli, M., Fiorina, P. 2020. "Dipeptidyl peptidase-4 (DPP4) inhibition in COVID-19." *Acta Diabetol.* 57(7):779-83.

[53] Strollo, R., Pozzilli, P. 2020. "DPP4 inhibition: Preventing SARS-CoV-2 infection and/or progression of COVID-19?" *Diabetes Metab. Res. Rev.* e3330.

[54] Bassendine, M-F., Bridge, S-H., McCaughan, G-W., Gorrell, M-D. 2020. "COVID-19 and comorbidities: A role for dipeptidyl peptidase 4 (DPP4) in disease severity?" *J. Diabetes.* 12(9):649-58.

[55] Rizzo, M., Nikolic, D., Patti, A-M., Mannina, C., Montalto, G., McAdams, B-S., Rizvi, A-A., et al. 2018. "GLP-1 receptor agonists and reduction of cardiometabolic risk: Potential underlying mechanisms." *Biochim. Biophys. Acta Mol. Basis Dis.* 1864(9 Pt B):2814-21.

[56] Lee, Y-S., Jun, H-S. 2016. "Anti-inflammatory effects of GLP-1-based therapies beyond glucose control." *Mediators Inflamm.* 2016:3094642.

[57] Ceriello, A., Standl, E., Catrinoiu, D., Itzhak, B., Lalic, L-M., Rahelic, D., Schnell, O., et al. 2020. "Issues of cardiovascular risk management in people with diabetes in the COVID-19 era." *Diabetes Care.* 43(7):1427-32.

[58] Longo, M., Caruso, P., Maiorino, M-I., Bellastella, G., Giugliano, D., Esposito, K. 2020. "Treating type 2 diabetes in COVID-19 patients: the potential benefits of injective therapies." *Cardiovasc. Diabetol.* 19(1):115.

[59] Hanefeld, M. 2007. "Pioglitazone and sulfonylureas: effectively treating type 2 diabetes." *Int. J. Clin. Pract. Suppl.* 61(153):20-27.

[60] Derosa, G., Maffioli, P. 2010. "Effects of thiazolidinediones and sulfonylureas in patients with diabetes." *Diabetes Technol. Ther.* 12(6):491-501.

[61] Pal, R., Bhadada, S-K. 2020. "Should anti-diabetic medications be reconsidered amid COVID-19 pandemic?" *Diabetes Res. Clin. Pract.* 163:108146.

[62] Shah, K., Tiwaskar, M., Chawla, P., Kale, M., Deshmane, R., Sowani, A. 2020. "Hypoglycemia at the time of Covid-19 pandemic." *Diabetes Metab. Syndr.* 14(5):1143-6.

[63] Kruglikov, I-L., Scherer, P-E. 2020. "The role of adipocytes and adipocyte-like cells in the severity of COVID-19 infections." *Obesity (Silver Spring).* 28(7):1187-90.

[64] Ciavarella, C., Motta, I., Valente, S., Pasquinelli, G. 2020. "Pharmacological (or synthetic) and nutritional agonists of PPAR-γ as candidates for cytokine storm modulation in COVID-19 disease." *Molecules.* 25(9):2076.

[65] Nakhleh, A., Shehadeh, N. 2020. "Interactions between antihyperglycemic drugs and the renin-angiotensin system: Putative roles in COVID-19. A mini-review." *Diabetes Metab. Syndr.* 14(4):509-12.

[66] Sardu, C., D'Onofrio, N., Balestrieri, M-L., Barbieri, M., Rizzo, M-R., Messina., V., Maggi, P., et al. 2020. "Outcomes in patients with hyperglycemia affected by COVID-19: Can we do more on glycemic control?" *Diabetes Care.* 43(7):1408-15.

[67] Buse, J-B., Wexler, D-J., Tsapas, A., Rossing, P., Mingrone, G., Mathieu, C., D'Alessio, D-A., et al. 2020. "2019 update to: management of hyperglycaemia in

type 2 diabetes, 2018. A consensus report by the American Diabetes Association (ADA) and the European Association for the Study of Diabetes (EASD)." *Diabetologia*. 63(2):221-8.

[68] Hamblin, P-S., Wong, R., Ekinci, E-I, Fourlanos, S., Shah, S., Jones, A-R., Hare, M-J-L., et al. 2019. "SGLT2 inhibitors increase the risk of diabetic ketoacidosis developing in the community and during hospital admission." *J. Clin. Endocrinol. Metab.* 104(8):3077-87.

[69] Orioli, L., Hermans, M-P., Thissen, J-P., Maiter, D., Vandeleene, B., Yombi, J-C. 2020. "COVID-19 in diabetic patients: Related risks and specifics of management." *Ann. Endocrinol. (Paris)*. 81(2-3):101-9.

[70] Cure, E., Cure, M-C. 2020. "Can dapagliflozin have a protective effect against COVID-19 infection? A hypothesis." *Diabetes Metab. Syndr*. 14(4):405-6.

In: Coronavirus Disease
Editor: Yildiz Dincer
ISBN: 978-1-53619-296-4

Chapter 13

THE IMPACT OF COVID-19 PANDEMIC ON THE PATIENTS WITH CHRONIC RESPIRATORY DISEASES

Buket Caliskaner Ozturk*, MD
Istanbul University-Cerrahpasa, Cerrahpasa Medical Faculty, Department of Pulmonology, Istanbul Turkey

ABSTRACT

The process beginning with some cases of pneumonia of unknown etiology in the city of Wuhan in China at the end of 2019 has continued with the agent being defined as a new virus and announced as a pandemic by World Health Organization (WHO). It has been seen to spread by droplet route and direct contact and usually locate to and cause disease condition in the respiratory tract. It may present asymptomatically or cause a clinical presentation ranging from mild upper respiratory tract infection to adult respiratory distress syndrome due to viral pneumonia. The clinical condition it causes has been named *coronavirus disease* 2019 (COVID-19).

The first impressions on the disease have shown that the disease caused by this new type of virus presents with higher rates of mortality and morbidity in the elderly patients with several co-morbidities including cardiovascular conditions, immune suppressive diseases, metabolic, and chronic respiratory tract diseases. In the initial phase of the pandemic, it has been predicted that the presence of an underlying chronic respiratory tract disease may cause serious co-morbidity because the disease involves the respiratory tract particularly. In the forthcoming period, it has been found that cardiovascular and metabolic diseases might cause more severe co-morbidity compared to respiratory tract diseases.

---

* Corresponding Author's Email: drbuketozturk@gmail.com.

Chronic respiratory tract diseases that may lead to serious co-morbidity during the pandemic include chronic obstructive and restrictive respiratory tract diseases, and respiratory sleep disorders.

The first and most important recommendation for patients with chronic respiratory tract diseases should be protection and the precautions. Concern on this point is whether the inhaler and systemic steroids used in the treatment of chronic obstructive pulmonary disease (COPD) and asthma are an extra risk factor. While research on this topic continues, it has been recommended that the patients should continue their treatment as always because no data exists suggesting that they increase the risk. Thus, it has been aimed to maintain stabilization of the disease, decrease hospital exposure, and reduce the risk of COVID-19 contamination. Pulmonary rehabilitation should be recommended to these patients in this process.

The similarity between the radiological findings of COVID-19 and interstitial pulmonary diseases is of importance in the differential diagnosis. Additionally, the patients with COVID-19 are a candidate to be a patient with interstitial pulmonary disease because fibrosis may occur in the recovery process of the disease.

Patients with obstructive sleep apnea syndrome (OSAS) also have several cardiovascular and metabolic disorders. Thus, OSAS is an extra high-risk factor for COVID-19. Furthermore, positive airway pressure (PAP) devices used in its treatment are additional important threats because they spread aerosols.

Keywords: COVID-19, chronic respiratory diseases, pandemic

INTRODUCTION

A virus that emerged in Wuhan city of China in December 2019 and was found to be originating from the livestock market has spread among the humans and caused a pandemic. The virus named Severe Acute Respiratory Syndrome-Coronavirus-2 (SARS-CoV-2) spreads by route of the droplet or direct contact.

With the emergence of the first cases, it was observed that SARS- CoV-2 was characterized by the upper and lower respiratory tract infection in particular and presented with more severe clinical courses especially in the elderly, immune-suppressive, and with co-morbid patients. It utilizes the receptors of angiotensin-converting enzyme-2 (ACE-2) for entering the cells. ACE-2 receptor is a protein present on the cell surface. It is most abundantly present in the lungs, heart, blood vessels, kidneys, liver, and gastrointestinal tract [1]. The virus binds to the ACE-2 receptor via the spike protein on its surface. The nasal mucosa, bronchi, and lung parenchyma all of which have a high degree of expression of ACE-2 receptors are more sensitive to the SARS-CoV-2 virus. Thus, the respiratory tract is frequently involved by the disease.

The primary viral replication is considered to occur primarily and frequently in the mucosal epithelium of the upper respiratory tract including the nasopharynx and then to continue in the lower respiratory tract. It may be asymptomatic or show clinical presentation ranging from mild upper respiratory tract infection to acute respiratory distress syndrome (ARDS) due to viral pneumonia. Although it primarily causes clinical disease of the respiratory tract, it may also involve other systems.

Advanced age and presence of co-morbid conditions are predisposing factors for both infection with SARS-CoV-2 and increased severity of the infection. Especially the conditions such as hypertension, ischemic heart diseases, diabetes mellitus, chronic obstructive lung disease have been reported as the most important risk factors for the severe course of the disease [2–8].

It has been thought that the presence of chronic respiratory tract diseases might be a cause of serious co-morbidity because the virus involves the respiratory tract after it begins to spread. For a virus that may involve the respiratory tract, the presence of underlying pathology of the respiratory tract will facilitate contamination of the infection as well as it will lead to a worse clinical course. Thus, a high rate of mortality and morbidity is expected in the cases of COVID-19 with chronic lung diseases. Additionally, considering that these patients are elderly, the risk is much higher. Based on the first impressions and data, however, lung diseases have been observed to cause lower risk for COVID-19 compared to other chronic diseases. In a meta-analysis on 1.576 patients with COVID-19, the frequency of hypertension was reported as 21.1%, diabetes mellitus as 9.7%, and cardiovascular diseases as 8.4% whereas the frequency of the lung diseases was reported as 1.5% [8]. Studies are still going on because of the short time from the emergence of the disease.

COVID-19 Pandemic and the Patients with Asthma

Asthma is a heterogeneous disease related to hypersensitivity of the airway to the direct or indirect stimulants and is characterized by chronic airway inflammation [9]. Genetic factors usually play role in the development of asthma. Its exacerbations, however, are usually due to environmental factors. The infections and exposure to allergens are leading causes of asthma attacks. The most common infectious causes are viral respiratory tract infections. Virus-related attacks may present with poorer clinical findings, especially in uncontrolled asthma.

During the initial phase of the pandemic, asthma was considered to be an important risk factor for COVID-19 because of its chronic nature as well as its risk of exacerbation. It was also predicted that the inhaler and systemic steroids used in the treatment of asthma might trigger this risk by predisposing to the infections. But surprisingly, the first analyses on COVID-19 revealed that the patients with asthma showed a similar presentation to the general population, and studies were published supporting that asthma was not a risk factor for being contaminated with COVID-19 and for mortality [10–13]. Consequently, a few opinions were suggested for a lower prevalence of asthma than expected in patients with COVID-19.

The first of these opinions was that patients with asthma were protected from the disease because they used medication regularly and because of their conscious behaviors. Although it was expected that long- acting inhaler steroids used in the treatment of asthma might increase this risk, it is also possible that they might decrease the risk because they suppress replication of the coronavirus and the production of cytokines [14]. The studies on budesonide and cyclosonide suggested that these agents had effects of inhibiting HCoV-229E replication and cytokine production in the human nasal and tracheal epithelial cells, that cyclosonide blocked in vitro COVID-19 RNA replication and prevented cytopathic activity of the virus [15, 16]. Data on this topic, however, are limited, and comprehensive and new studies are needed.

The second opinion is that the most common symptoms in COVID-19 are dyspnea and cough, and there was a possibility of missing out on the presence of COVID-19 in the patients with asthma because of the similarity of symptoms. Accuracy of this possibility, however, was weakened after the first impressions on the pandemic. COVID-19 shows different presentations from asthma exacerbations radiologically as well as in terms of laboratory findings. While cough and dyspnea occur in both of them, a sudden increase in dyspnea and wheezing are in the foreground in the asthma exacerbations and sore throat, high fever, anosmia and ageusia, and diarrhea are predominant findings in COVID-19. On the laboratory findings high level of D-dimer and ferritin, presence of lymphopenia, and radiological view of dispersed viral pneumonia are supportive findings for COVID-19. However, the theory may be validated by confirmation by the studies on the patients with COVID-19 and asthma together.

Another point on the lower prevalence of COVID-19 than expected in asthma may be that prevalence of smoking is lower in patients with asthma compared to the general population. Studies have shown that smoking is an important risk factor for contamination with and poorer clinical course of COVID-19. This may be associated with a lower risk for patients with asthma than that predicted for COVID-19 [17].

Another opinion was that presence of chronic respiratory tract disease might have protected from COVID-19 through a different mechanism. It has been demonstrated that the virus utilizes the ACE-2 for entering the cells. ACE-2 expression is known to be lower or less active in asthma [18], which means protection for patients with asthma from COVID-19.

Even though it has been understood that asthma isn't a risk at the predicted level in patients with COVID-19, SARS-Cov-2 is an important risk factor for exacerbations of asthma similar to other viruses. It may cause severe clinical course in patients with asthma. Thus, the approach that patients with asthma will follow during the pandemic process is of importance. National Institute for Health and Care Excellence (NICE) and Global Initiative for Asthma (GINA) published interim reports to give recommendations on the management of asthma during the pandemic [19, 20]. The main items suggested are as follows:

- To prevent contamination risk of the infection, the patients should be educated on social isolation, keeping the distance, not contacting, hand hygiene, and using the masks correctly.
- Patients with asthma are recommended to continue their current medications during the pandemic; the dose of the inhaler steroids may be increased, if necessary, and lowering the line of medication is not recommended even though asthma is controlled during the pandemic. Discontinuing the disease-modifying drugs or lowering their dose may jeopardize controlling asthma, increase the risk of exacerbation, and consequently may cause the risk of contamination of the virus by leading to presentation to the hospital.
- During the attacks, using short-acting systemic steroids shouldn't be avoided.
- During the attacks, using nebulizers should be avoided because they may spread aerosols; metered-dose inhalers should be preferred and the spacer may be used when necessary.
- Allergic rhinitis is one of the diseases accompanying asthma and its treatment is important in controlling asthma. It is recommended that patients with asthma using nasal steroids for allergic rhinitis should continue their treatment during the pandemic in order not to impair asthma control.
- The pandemic process during which social isolation and time at home are increased has been a disadvantage for the patients with allergy, especially to house dust mites. In contrast, increasing time at home has been an advantage for the patients with allergy to the pollens. Controlling the signs of coughing and sneezing by giving the right patient symptomatic treatment at the right time is of great importance in decreasing the attacks as well as the spread of the aerosols.
- Routine examination of the patients with asthma should be delayed to protect them from exposure to the hospital environment and the virus. Interviews may be done and required recommendations may be given via telephone, internet, e-mail, etc.
- Spirometric tests should be avoided as much as possible. If they should be performed absolutely, all individual protective equipment should be worn by the technician because of asymptomatic and unknown COVID-19. The room should be well ventilated, and it should be carried out in a negative-pressure room, if possible.

Treatment with anti-IgE, anti-interleukin (IL)-5/IL-5 alpha, IL-4-alpha receptor antagonists used to control patients with severe asthma have been reported not to increase the risk for COVID-19. Although it has been recommended that the patients using biological agents should continue their treatment, it is also recommended that these patients should extend the interval between the treatments to decrease hospital exposure [21].

In conclusion, based on the information collected so far asthma is not considered as a factor increasing the risk for COVID-19 although more comprehensive studies are needed to confirm the validity of and discuss reasons for this. COVID-19, however, may be a poor prognostic and exacerbation factor for asthma. Thus, taking measures for protection from the infection as well as giving optimal treatments to control asthma during the pandemic process is considered as the most important factor in patients with asthma.

COVID-19 Pandemic and the Patients with Chronic Obstructive Pulmonary Disease

COPD is a disease characterized by irreversible and progressive airway obstruction. This condition develops as a consequence of the inflammatory process to the harmful gases and particles. Being a preventable and treatable disease, COPD presents with exacerbations of which severity and frequency increases in time. It is an important cause of morbidity and mortality in the world. The most common cause of COPD exacerbations is tracheobronchial infections. It is known that these infections are mostly viral.

COPD is considered as a co-morbidity factor for COVID-19. Its prevalence ranges between 1.1% and 2.9% [2, 8, 11]. COPD is a chronic respiratory disease condition although it has a lower prevalence for COVID-19 compared to other co-morbid diseases. Thus, question marks and research are still going on. COPD has been reported to have 5 folds higher risk for severe COVID-19 infection [22]. It may be suggested that this is due to advanced age, inhaler steroid use, structural damage, suppressed immunity, and exacerbations in the patients with COPD. Difficulties in adapting the protective measure due to advanced age in the patients with COPD is another factor increasing the risk of contamination of the infection. A short time from the beginning of the pandemic and the limited number of studies conducted on this topic so far leave controversial areas behind.

The main harmful particle leading to the development of COPD is tobacco. Nicotine, which is present in tobacco causes increased expression of the ACE-2 receptors. This is considered to facilitate entry of the virus to the cell and development of the disease for COPD patients [23, 24].

Differential diagnosis between exacerbations of COPD and COVID-19 may be difficult due to the similarity of the symptoms at the time of presentation. High fever, cough, and dyspnea are present in both of them. In the laboratory findings, a high level of D-dimer and fibrinogen is supportive of COVID-19 although they may be elevated in the patients with COPD due to several confounding factors such as co-morbidity and advanced age and these may not be helpful in the differential diagnosis. Imaging studies may be helpful in the differential diagnosis. Even though findings supportive of COVID-

19 may facilitate diagnosis, alterations that may be present in the background of the lung in the COPD such as emphysema, bronchiectasis, peribronchial thickening may overlap with findings of COVID-19 and cause difficulties in diagnosis. At this point, comparative evaluations with the previous radiological examinations may be utilized.

The rate of development of severe disease with oxygen desaturation and rates of admission in the intensive care unit, intubation, and mortality in COVID-19 has been reported to be higher in the patients with COPD. This may be suggested to be related to structural parenchymal disorders of the lung and reduced respiratory function.

The measures that should be taken for patients with COPD are as follows:

- In addition to the rules of social distance and routine hygiene for being protected from the pandemic, extra measures should be taken for the patients with COPD not to encounter the virus. First of these should be delaying routine controls of the patients.
- Several studies exist indicating that the use of inhaler corticosteroids might cause an increased risk of pneumonia in COPD [25]. At the beginning of the pandemic, this was predicted to be an extra risk for COVID-19, and the opinion that using inhaler and steroid treatments will not be appropriate during the pandemic was proposed. However, the Global Initiative of COPD (GOLD) noted that the opinion that use of the inhaler and systemic steroids will not be appropriate during the pandemic of COVID-19 didn't have a scientific basis by publishing an interim report in 2020. It was reported that destabilizing COPD as a consequence of interrupting the treatment would be a higher risk for the patients. The recommendation of the patient with COPD during the pandemic would be continuing the current treatment exactly as usual. Even previously planned interruptions have been recommended to be delayed [26]. It has been recommended to wait until the efficacy of the pandemic will cease to switch the treatment. The main objective during the pandemic is to decrease hospital exposure of the patients by avoiding the exacerbations without destabilizing COPD.
- In the context of pulmonary rehabilitation with a multidisciplinary approach, the patients receive education on nutrition, psychosocial support, regulation of the daily life activities, and exercise. It is appropriate to incorporate a pulmonary rehabilitation support program to the medical treatment in the patients not receiving such supportive treatments because pulmonary rehabilitation will contribute positively to the respiratory reserve and thus, it will provide an advantage in the case of encountering COVID-19.
- Spirometric tests should be avoided in the patients presenting admitted to the hospital in the presence of attacks or symptoms. Assisting devices such as nebulizers, high-flow oxygen, and non-invasive mechanic ventilators cause the

spread of the aerosols and carry a high risk for contamination; their use should be limited as much as possible. In the case of using them for mandatory reasons, negative-pressure rooms should be preferred [27]. NICE guideline for the nebulizers states that the use of the nebulizer by the patients will not be an additional risk factor for contamination because the aerosol comes from the reservoir of the nebulizer and doesn't carry viral particles from the patient [26]. Nonetheless, it would be useful to limit their use as much as possible. Metered-dose inhalers should be preferred instead of nebulizer; spacer may be used. In the case of using nebulizer in the patients not being able to use metered-dose inhalers, the patient should be alone in the room and the room should be ventilated well after their use.

- If it is mandatory to provide non-invasive mechanical ventilator (NIMV) support in the case of problems of limited sources of intensive care bed and available invasive mechanical ventilator, it should be given with a full-face mask with Helmet mask to minimize the risk.
- The procedures should be avoided such as sputum induction and nasotracheal aspiration creating a high risk for contamination of COVID-19 because of the risk of development of aerosols in patients with COPD.

In conclusion, COPD is a risk factor for COVID-19. Risk in COPD, however, is lower compared to other chronic diseases related to other systems (i.e., diabetes mellitus, hypertension) although it is a chronic lung disease. The diagnostic process of the patients is of importance because of the similar clinical presentation of both conditions. As in other chronic diseases, the main objective in patients with COPD should be to protect the patient from the virus. For this purpose, the current treatment should be continued in the usual manner and the dose of the inhaler steroid shouldn't be reduced in order not to destabilize the treatment. Use of the nebulizers, high-flow oxygen, and NIMV should be avoided as much as possible.

COVID-19 Pandemic and the Patients with Interstitial Lung Disease

Interstitial lung diseases is a common name of diseases presenting with varying degrees of fibrosis, inflammation, and structural alterations in the lung parenchyma and affecting the lungs diffusely. The fact that immune- suppressive agents are usually used for their treatment is a facilitating factor for being contaminated with SARS-CoV-2. Additionally, destruction in the lung parenchyma and reduced respiratory reserve may also cause severe clinical presentation of COVID-19.

Both interstitial lung diseases and COVID-19 have similar clinical and radiological features. Clinically dyspnea, the non-productive cough may be present in both; the presence of fever, sore throat, anosmia and ageusia, muscle pain, and diarrhea should suggest a diagnosis of COVID-19. Radiologically, lesions of ground-glass density may be seen in both diseases. Comparing with the previous images is of importance in distinguishing the new appearing ground-glass lesions.

In COVID-19, apoptosis of the epithelial and endothelial cells occurs in the early periods along with rapid viral replication and increased pro- inflammatory/chemokine responses [28–30], followed by vascular leakage, edema, and uncontrolled inflammatory response [31–34]. In the later periods, these are followed by widespread lung damage, fibrosis in the interstitium and alveolar space, hyperplasia of the pneumocytes, and uncontrolled cellular proliferation. These alterations are accompanied by the abnormal immune response to the viral invasion and consequent imbalance in the increased production of cytokines. During this process, pulmonary epithelial cells and alveolar microvascular endothelial cells become the target organs attacked by the inflammatory mediators and lead to characteristic damage of ARDS.

Tissue injury on one hand and impaired remodeling on the other hand increase mortality. In the patients surviving ARDS develop pulmonary fibrosis. On the other hand, there is a possibility that pulmonary involvement of COVID-19 may heal with fibrotic scar tissue in the patients not developing ARDS. Thus, all patients with COVID-19 are a candidate for interstitial lung disease independent of the development of ARDS. Thus, preventing and treating pulmonary fibrosis may be one of the targets in treating COVID-19. Several options exist to resolve the cytokine storm and inflammatory factors including cytokine inhibiting agents, plasma replacement therapy, and blood/plasma filtration. The long-time effects of these medicines are not known yet.

Recommendations for patients with interstitial lung diseases are as follows [35]:

- First of all, the patients should take measures of using a mask, hygiene, and social distance for protection from the disease.
- Routine controls should be delayed during the pandemic and they should be instructed on that they shouldn't apply to the hospital if they don't have symptoms.
- Respiratory function tests should be avoided even though they are presented to the hospital with new symptoms.
- In addition to the medical treatment, the patients should be recommended pulmonary rehabilitation.
- Idiopathic pulmonary fibrosis (IPF) is an important group of interstitial lung diseases. Anti-fibrotic agents are used for theirtreatment. Using anti-fibrotic agents for IPF isn't an additional risk for COVID-19. Continuing to use the drugs should be recommended during the pandemic.

- In the case of making a diagnosis of COVID-19 in the patients with IPF using anti-fibrotic agents, the drugs may be discontinued for 4 to 8 weeks; in the case of discontinuation, however, the risk of exacerbation of IPF should be kept in mind and the decision should be tailored on an individual basis.
- Discontinuing medication in patients using immune suppressive therapy may exacerbate the findings of the present disease. There is no consensus on this topic.
- If a patient with interstitial lung disease is diagnosed as having COVID-19, immune suppressive therapy is discontinued during the active infection and then for 2 weeks following the recovery of the disease (or for a longer period if the patient can tolerate). Discontinuing the immune-suppressive treatment should be considered if COVID-19 is detected in patients with interstitial lung disease.

COVID-19 Pandemic and the Patients with Obstructive Sleep Apnea Syndrome

OSAS is a condition characterized by a complete or partial obstruction of the upper airway during sleep. It manifests with apnea or hypopnea episodes followed by desaturation and subsequent arousals [36].

OSAS is usually accompanied by cardiovascular and metabolic conditions. Several factors including advanced age, male gender, obesity, hypertension, cardiovascular diseases, and diabetes mellitus make the high risk for both OSAS and COVID-19, increasing the frequency of development of COVID-19 in the patients with OSAS. COVID-19 presents mortality for the group of elderly patients with serious co-morbidities [37].

OSAS is one of the most common chronic respiratory diseases. The presence of quality sleep is of great importance to boosting immunity and for a healthy life. Treatment of patients with sleep apnea is much more important during the pandemic process because they have poor sleep unless they are treated. Thus, measures for the patients with OSAS gain extra importance during the pandemic.

OSAS and obesity have been suggested to worsen clinical course in the patients with coronavirus infection by increasing hypoxemia and cytokine storm.

The most effective therapeutic option for OSAS is PAP. Regularly and appropriately using the treatment during the pandemic is of great importance for quality sleep [38].

In contrast, another opinion exists advocating to discontinue PAP treatment during the pandemic. It suggests that treating the asymptomatic virus-carrying patients with OSAS with PAP at home may contaminate the virus to the household [39]. In this case, considering the risk-benefit ratio, it would be more appropriate to recommend the patients without diagnosis of COVID-19 to continue the treatment during the indeterminate pandemic period. If the patient having a diagnosis of COVID-19 is being followed at home, treatment may be interrupted for 2 weeks to protect the household again considering the risk-benefit ratio.

If the patient with a diagnosis of COVID-19 has been admitted to the hospital:

- It is recommended to discontinue the treatment until the attendant physician allows using PAP [38].
- If a PAP device will be used, it should be used in negative- pressure rooms, or if unavailable in the single rooms in which the health providers use full individual protective equipment [27].
- In the hospital, if the one-circuit device of the patients own will be used and the mask has an expiration valve, changing it with a mask without a valve and mounting a viral/bacterial filter will substantially reduce the risk of droplet contamination [40].

REFERENCES

[1] Zhou, P., Yang, X. L., Wang, X. G., Hu, B., Zhang, L., Zhang, W., Si, H. R., Zhu, Y., Li, B., Huang, C. L., Chen, H. D., Chen, J., Luo, Y., Guo, H., Jiang, R. D., Liu, M. Q., Chen, Y., Shen, X. R., Wang, X., Zheng X. S., Zhao, K., Chen, Q. J., Deng, F., Liu, L. L., Yan, B., Zhan, F. X., Wang, Y. Y., Xiao, G. F., Shi, Z. L. 2020. "A Pneumonia Outbreak Associated with a New Coronavirus of Probable Bat Origin." *Nature.* 579; 270–273.

[2] Guan, W. J., Ni, ZY., Hu, Y., Liang, W. H., Ou,C. Q., He, J. X., Liu, L., Shan, H., Lei, C. L., Hui, D. S. C,, Du, B., Li, L. J., Zeng, G., Yuen, K. Y., Chen, R. C., Tang, C. L., Wang, T., Chen, P. Y., Xiang, J., Li, S. Y., Wang, J. L., Liang, Z. J., Peng, Y. X., Wei, L., Liu, Y., Hu, Y. H., Peng, P., Wang, J. M., Liu, J. Y., Chen, Z., Li, G., Zheng, Z. J., Qiu, S. Q., Luo, J., Ye, C. J., Zhu, S. Y., Zhong, N. S. 2020. "Clinical Characteristics of Coronavirus Disease 2019 in China." *New England Journal of Medicine*. 30; 382(18):1708-1720.

[3] Zhu, N., Zhang, D., Wang, W., Li, X., Yang, B., Song, J., Zhao, X., Huang, B., Shi, W., Lu, R., Niu, P., Zhan, F., Ma, X., Wang, D., Xu, W., Wu, G., Gao, G. F., Tan, W. 2020. "A Novel Coronavirus from Patients with Pneumonia in China, 2019." *New England Journal of Medicine*. 382(8):727-733.

[4] Lauer, S. A., Grantz, K. H., Bi, Q., Jones, F. K., Zheng, Q., Meredith, H. R., Azman, A. S., Reich, N. G., Lessler, J. "The Incubation Period of Coronavirus Disease 2019 (CoVID-19) from Publicly Reported Confirmed Cases: Estimation and Application." *Annals of Internal Medicine.* 172(9):577-582.

[5] Kenneth, M., Hirsch, M. S., Bloom, A. 2020. "Coronavirus Disease 2019 (COVID-19)." UpToDate Hirsch MS B2 020. "Coronavirus Disease 2019 (COVID-19)." *UpToDate* Hirsch MS Bloom 5.

[6] Zhou, F., Yu, T., Du, R., Fan, G., Liu, Y., Liu, Z., Xiang, J., Wang, Y., Song, B., Gu, X., Guan, X., Wei, Y., Li, H., Wu, X., Xu, J., Tu, S., Zhang, Y., Chen, H., Cao, B. 2020. "Clinical Course and Risk Factors for Mortality of Adult Inpatients with COVID-19 in Wuhan, China: A Retrospective Cohort Study." *The Lancet.* 395(10229): 1054-1062.

[7] Team, Eurosurveillance Editorial. 2020. "Updated Rapid Risk Assessment from ECDC on the Outbreak of COVID-19: Increased Transmission Globally." *Eurosurveillance* 25, no. 9.

[8] Wang, D., Hu B., Hu C., Zhu, F., Liu, X., Zhang, J., Wang, B., Xiang, H., Cheng, Z., Xiong, Y., Zhao,Y., Li, Y., Wang, X., Peng, Z. 2020. "Clinical Characteristics of 138 Hospitalized Patients with 2019 Novel Coronavirus-Infected Pneumonia in Wuhan, China." *JAMA - Journal of the American Medical Association.* 323(11):1061-1069.

[9] Global Initiative for Asthma: Global Strategy for Asthma Management and Prevention (Updated 2020). 2020." *Revue Francaise d'Allergologie et d'Immunologie Clinique*.

[10] Zhang, J. J., Dong, X., Cao, Y. Y., Yuan, Y. D., Yang, Y. B., Yan, Y. Q., Akdis, C. A., Gao, Y. D. 2020. "Clinical Characteristics of 140 Patients Infected with SARS-CoV-2 in Wuhan, China." *Allergy: European Journal of Allergy and Clinical Immunology.* 75(7):1730- 1741.

[11] Dong, X., Cao, Y. Y., Lu X. X., Zhang, J. J., Du, H., Yan, Y. Q., Akdis, C. A., Gao, Y. D. 2020. "Eleven Faces of Coronavirus Disease 2019." *Allergy: European Journal of Allergy and Clinical Immunology.* 75(7):1699-1709.

[12] Zhang, J. J., Cao, Y. Y., Dong, X., Wang, B. C., Liao, M. Y., Lin, J., Yan, Y. Q., Akdis, C. A., Gao, Y. D. 2020. "Distinct Characteristics of COVID-19 Patients with Initial RRT-PCR-Positive and RRT- PCR-Negative Results for SARS-CoV-2." *Allergy: European Journal of Allergy and Clinical Immunology.* 75(7):1809-1812.

[13] Garg, S., Kim, L., Whitaker, M., O'Halloran, A., Cummings, C., Holstein, R., Prill, M., Chai, S. J., Kirley, P. D., Alden, N. B., Kawasaki, B., Yousey-Hindes, K., Niccolai, L., Anderson, E. J., Openo, K. P., Weigel, A., Monroe, M. L., Ryan, P., Henderson, J., Kim, S., Como-Sabetti, K., Lynfield, R., Sosin, D., Torres, S., Muse, A., Bennett, N. M., Billing, L., Sutton, M., West, N., Schaffner, W., Talbot, H. K., Aquino, C., George, A., Budd, A., Brammer, L., Langley, G., Hall, A. J., Fry A. 2020. "Hospitalization Rates and Characteristics of Patients Hospitalized with Laboratory-Confirmed Coronavirus Disease 2019 — COVID-NET, 14 States,

March 1–30, 2020." *MMWR. Morbidity and Mortality Weekly Report.* 17; 69(15):458-464.

[14] Halpin, D. M. G., Singh, D., Hadfield, R. M. 2020. "Inhaled Corticosteroids and COVID-19: A Systematic Review and Clinical Perspective." *Eur Respiratory Soc.* 7;55(5):2001009.

[15] Yamaya, M., Nishimura, H., Deng, X., Sugawara, M., Watanabe, O., Nomura, K., Shimotai, Y., Momma, H., Ichinose, M., Kawase, T. 2020. "Inhibitory Effects of Glycopyrronium, Formoterol, and Budesonide on Coronavirus HCoV-229E Replication and Cytokine Production by Primary Cultures of Human Nasal and Tracheal Epithelial Cells." *Respiratory Investigation.* 58(3):155-168.

[16] Matsuyama, S., Kawase, M., Nao, N., Shirato, K., Ujike, M., Shimojima, M., Fukushi, S. 2020. "The Inhaled Steroid Ciclesonide Blocks SARS-CoV-2 RNA Replication by Targeting Viral Replication-Transcription Complex in Culture Cells 2 3." *Journal of Virology.* 14; JVI.01648-20.

[17] Zhao, Q., Meng M., Kumar, R., Wu, Y., Huang, J., Lian, N., Deng, Y., Lin, S. 2020. "The Impact of COPD and Smoking History on the Severity of COVID-19: A Systemic Review and Meta-Analysis." *Journal of Medical Virology.* 15; 10.1002/jmv.25889.

[18] Jin, Y., Yang, H., Ji, W., Wu, W., Chen, S., Zhang, W., Duan G. 2020. "Virology, Epidemiology, Pathogenesis, and Control of COVID- 19." *Viruses.* 27;12(4):372.

[19] NICE. "*COVID-19 Rapid Guideline: Severe Asthma*," no. April (2020): 11.

[20] Global Initiative for Asthma. "*COVID-19 : GINA Answers to Frequently Asked Questions on Asthma Management*," 2020.

[21] Shaker, M. S., Oppenheimer, J., Grayson, M., Stukus, D., Hartog, N., Hsieh, E. W. Y., Rider, N., Dutmer, C. M., Leek, T. K. V., Kim, H., Chan, E. S., Mack, D., Ellis, A. K., Lang, D., Lieberman, J, Fleischer, D., Golden, D. B. K., Wallace, D., Portnoy, J. Mosnaim, G., Greenhawt M. 2020. "COVID-19: Pandemic Contingency Planning for the Allergy and Immunology Clinic." *Journal of Allergy and Clinical Immunology: In Practice.* 8(5):1477-1488.

[22] Lippi, G., Henry B. M. 2020. "Chronic Obstructive Pulmonary Disease Is Associated with Severe Coronavirus Disease 2019 (COVID-19): COPD and COVID-19." *Respiratory Medicine.* 167: 105941.

[23] Oakes, JM., Fuchs, R. M., Gardner, J. D, Lazartigues, E., Yue, X. 2018. |"Nicotine and the renin-angiotensin system." *The American Journal of Physiology-Regulatory, Integrative and Comparative.* 1;315(5):R895-R906.

[24] Brake, S. J., Barnsley, K., Lu, W., McAlinden, K. D., Eapen, M. S., Sohal, S. S. 2020. "Smoking Upregulates Angiotensin-Converting Enzyme-2 Receptor: A Potential Adhesion Site for Novel Coronavirus SARS-CoV-2 (COVID-19)." *Journal of Clinical Medicine.* 20;9(3):841.

[25] Wedzicha, J. A., Banerji, D., Chapman, K. R., Vestbo, J., Roche, N., Ayers, R. T., Thach, C., Fogel, R., Patalano, F., Vogelmeier, C. F. 2016. "Indacaterol-Glycopyrronium versus Salmeterol-Fluticasone for COPD." *New England Journal of Medicine*. 9; 374(23):2222-34.

[26] Jamil, S., Mark, N., Carlos, G., Cruz, J. S. D., Gross, J. E., Pasnick, 2020. "Diagnosis and Management of COVID-19 Disease." *American Journal of Respiratory and Critical Care Medicine*. 201(10): P19–22.

[27] Kryger, M. H., Thomas, R. 2020. "Home PAP Devices in COVID-19 Infected Patients." *Journal of Clinical Sleep Medicine*. 15; 16(7):1217-1219.

[28] Susanne, H., Steinmueller, M., Wulffen, W. V., Cakarova, L., Pinto, R., Pleschka, S., Mack, M., Kuziel, W. A., Corazza, N., Brunner, T., Seeger, W., Lohmeyer, J. 2008. "Lung Epithelial Apoptosis in Influenza Virus Pneumonia: The Role of Macrophage-Expressed TNF-Related Apoptosis-Inducing Ligand." *Journal of Experimental Medicine*. 205(13):3065-77.

[29] Högner, K., Wolff, T., Pleschka, S., Plog, S., Gruber, A. D., Kalinke, U., Walmrath, H. D., Bodner, J., Gattenlöhner, S., Lewe-Schlosser, P., Matrosovich, M., Seeger, W., Lohmeyer, J., Herold, S. 2013. "Macrophage-Expressed IFN-β Contributes to Apoptotic Alveolar Epithelial Cell Injury in Severe Influenza Virus Pneumonia." *PLoS Pathogens*. 9(2):e1003188.

[30] Rodrigue-Gervais, I. G., Labbé, K., Dagenais, M., Dupaul-Chicoine, J., Champagne, C., Morizot, A., Skeldon, A. Brincks, E. L., Vidal, M., Griffith, T. S., Saleh, M. 2014. "Cellular Inhibitor of Apoptosis Protein CIAP2 Protects against Pulmonary Tissue Necrosis during Influenza Virus Infection to Promote Host Survival." *Cell Host and Microbe*. 15(1):23-35.

[31] Jincun, Z., Zhao, J., Perlman, S. 2010. "T Cell Responses Are Required for Protection from Clinical Disease and for Virus Clearance in Severe Acute Respiratory Syndrome Coronavirus- Infected Mice." *Journal of Virology*. 84(18):9318-25.

[32] Kim, K. D., Zhao, J., Auh, S., Yang, X., Du, P., Tang, H., Fu Y. X. 2007. "Adaptive Immune Cells Temper Initial Innate Responses." *Nature Medicine*. 13(10):1248-52.

[33] Palm, N. W., Medzhitov R. 2007. "Not so Fast: Adaptive Suppression of Innate Immunity." *Nature Medicine*. 13(10):1142-4.

[34] Jincun, Z., Zhao, J., Legge, K., Perlman, S. 2011. "Age-Related Increases in PGD 2 Expression Impair Respiratory DC Migration, Resulting in Diminished T Cell Responses upon Respiratory Virus Infection in Mice." *Journal of Clinical Investigation*. 121(12):4921- 30.

[35] Disease, Interstitial Lung, Most Ild, New Ild, Social Shielding, British Lung Foundation, I L D Outpatient, U K I L D Opd, and I L D Opd. 2020. *"British*

Thoracic Society Advice for Managing Interstitial Lung Disease Patients during COVID-19 Pandemic." no. Ild : 1–6.

[36] Azagra-Calero, E., Espinar-Escalona, E., Barrera-Mora, J. M., Llamas-Carreras, J. M., Solano-Reina, E. 2012. "Obstructive Sleep Apnea Syndrome (OSAS). Review of the Literature." *Medicina Oral, Patologia Oral y Cirugia Bucal*. 1;17(6):e925-9.

[37] McSharry, D., Malhotra, A. 2020. "Potential Influences of Obstructive Sleep Apnea and Obesity on COVID-19 Severity." *Journal of Clinical Sleep Medicine : JCSM : Official Publication of the American Academy of Sleep Medicine*. 15;16(9):1645.

[38] Craig, S., West, S. 2020. "Guidance Regarding Coronavirus (COVID-19) and Obstructive Sleep Apnoea (OSA): For People Who Routinely Use Continuous Positive Airway Pressure (CPAP), *Their Families and Health Care Workers,* 20 March 2020."

[39] Barker, J., Oyefeso, O., Koeckerling, D., Mudalige, N. L., Pan D. 2020. "COVID-19: Community CPAP and NIV Should Be Stopped Unless Medically Necessary to Support Life." *Thorax*. 75(5):367.

[40] Simonds, A. K., Hanak, A., M. Chatwin, M., Morrell, M., Hall, A., Parker, K. H., Siggers, J. H., Dickinson, R. J. 2010. "Evaluation of Droplet Dispersion during Non-Invasive Ventilation, Oxygen Therapy, Nebuliser Treatment and Chest Physiotherapy in Clinical Practice: Implications for Management of Pandemic Influenza and Other Airborne Infections." *Health Technology Assessment.* 14(46):131-172.

In: Coronavirus Disease
Editor: Yildiz Dincer
ISBN: 978-1-53619-296-4

Chapter 14

THE IMPACT OF THE COVID-19 PANDEMIC ON PATIENTS WITH CARDIOVASCULAR DISEASES

Serap Yavuzer[1,*], MD and Veysel Suzan[2], MD
[1]Biruni University, Faculty of Medicine,
Department of Internal Medicine, Istanbul, Turkey
[2]Istanbul University - Cerrahpasa, Cerrahpasa Medical Faculty, Department of Internal Medicine, Division of Geriatrics,
Istanbul, Turkey

ABSTRACT

Cardiovascular diseases are the leading cause of morbidity and mortality in the world, but with the Corona Virus Disease-2019 (COVID-19) pandemic emerging at the end of 2019, this issue has gained different importance. The presence of cardiovascular diseases leads to more severe COVID-19 infection and an increased mortality rate. On the other hand, COVID-19 itself causes myocardial damage and this contributes to morbidity and mortality. At the beginning of the pandemic, there was a concern that angiotensin converting enzyme (ACE) inhibitors or angiotensin receptor blockers (ARB) would up-regulate the ACE2 receptor at the tissue level, increasing viral binding and facilitating the infection. With the current studies, this opinion has lost the influence and it was decided not to change the treatment of patients using ACE inhibitors or ARBs. Another important point is that patients with cardiovascular diseases are now far from the healthcare they could receive before as both pre-hospital and hospital health care is directed towards the COVID-19 pandemic. Considering that the epidemic will not disappear rapidly, a different arrangement may be planned in healthcare services.

Keywords: Cardiovascular Disease, COVID-19, Coronavirus

---

* Corresponding Author's Email: drserapsahin@gmail.com.

INTRODUCTION

The disease caused by "Severe Acute Respiratory Syndrome-Coronavirus-2" (SARS-CoV-2), which is accepted as a global pandemic by the World Health Organisation (WHO), has been named Corona Virus Disease-2019 (COVID-19) [1, 2]. By September 2020, COVID-19 infection affected more than thirty million people and caused nearly one million deaths. SARS-CoV-2 is a highly contagious virus and spreads mainly through droplets and direct contact. The average incubation period is 5.5 days but extension up to 14 days is known [3]. In symptomatic cases, the most common symptoms are fever, fatigue, muscle pain, sore throat, and dry cough, less frequently nausea-vomiting, and diarrhea [4]. It is important not to forget the atypical presentations including delirium, hypothermia, and abdominal pain, especially in elderly patients [5].

SARS-CoV-2 is genetically 79% similar to the SARS-CoV that caused the SARS epidemic between 2002 - 2003 and 96% similar to coronaviruses in bats. The main feature of SARS-CoV-2, thought to be formed as a result of a new mutation, is that the virus causes infection by binding to the human angiotensin converting enzyme 2 (ACE2) receptor, after activation of its spike (S) protein by the transmembrane protease serine 2 enzyme [6]. ACE2 is expressed in the lung, particularly in type 2 alveolar cells, and it appears to be the main gateway for the virus [7]. By this way, it causes lung damage. In addition to the lungs, ACE2 is also expressed in the myocardium, oesophagus and intestinal epithelium, vascular endothelium, bladder urothelial cells, and kidney proximal tubule. So, this is already shown as the reason for the course of Covid-19 infection towards multiorgan failure [8].

COVID-19 infection is much more aggressive and fatal in patients with comorbidities and the geriatric population. Studies show that advanced age is the most important determinant for mortality [9]. Epidemiological data reveal that the risk of death is significantly increased in people over 80 years of age compared to young people [10, 11]. At the same time, the frequency of cardiovascular disease (CVD) is also high in people who die due to COVID-19. In an epidemiological study involving 72.314 patients in China, 22.7% of fatal cases had a history of CVD [12]. In a study including seven hospitals in Spain and comparing 1139 COVID-19 positive patients with 11.390 healthy people, it was found that the CVD (odds ratio, OR, 1.98) and CVD risk factors (OR, 1.46) and comorbid diseases such as hypertension (HT) (OR, 1.27), chronic obstructive pulmonary disease (COPD) (OR, 1.35), diabetes mellitus (DM) (OR, 1.5) and heart failure (HF) (OR, 2.18) are more common in COVID-19 positive patients than in healthy control group [13]. Similarly, with the information we have obtained from "Severe Acute Respiratory Syndrome" (SARS) and "Middle East Respiratory Syndrome" (MERS) infections, the mortality rate is higher in patients with cardiovascular diseases. The prevalence of DM and CVD in SARS was determined to be 11% and 8% respectively, and the presence of these two comorbidities has been shown to increase the risk of death

12 times [14, 15]. In MERS, DM and HT were seen in approximately 50% of the cases, and CVD were seen in approximately 30% of the cases [5]. As a result, the most affected group and the group with the highest mortality rate are the elderly with cardiovascular diseases.

As the symptoms and signs of the disease were recognized, the importance of cardiovascular damage was understood and it attracted more attention [16]. COVID-19 affects the cardiovascular system in many ways. It increases morbidity and aggravates myocardial damage and dysfunction in patients with accompanying cardiovascular diseases. The virus can affect the cardiovascular system and heart direct and/or indirect ways. Hemodynamic compromise, hypoxemia, inflammatory myocarditis, stress cardiomyopathy, microvascular dysfunction, or thrombosis due to hypercoagulability and systemic inflammation may impair the stabilization of coronary artery plaques [17]. In severe COVID-19 infection, the risk of type 2 myocardial infarction (MI) may increase by the need for increased cardiac output with hypoxia due to lung disease. Although the data on Covid-19 are still insufficient, studies are showing that pneumonia and influenza infection increase acute MI 6 times [18, 19].

HYPERTENSION

Considering that there are approximately 1.5 billion hypertensive patients in the world, it is not surprising that HT was the first co-morbid disease to be noted in articles on COVID-19 infection [17]. In a study conducted in the United States of America (USA), while 89.3% of 1482 patients hospitalized due to COVID-19 had at least one chronic disease, HT was the most common one with a frequency of 49.7% [20]. In the meta-analysis of four case-control studies including 1352 patients, HT was found to be the most common comorbidity and it was reported that the risk of the need for intensive care unit (OR, 2.54) increased in cases accompanied by HT [21]. In a retrospective cohort study in which acute respiratory distress syndrome (ARDS) and risk of death were analyzed in 201 COVID-19 positive patients, HT was found in 27.4% of patients who developed ARDS, while this rate was found as 13.7% in those who did not develop ARDS; however, a statistically significant difference could not be demonstrated [22]. In a multi-center study examining the impact of chronic diseases in 1590 COVID-19 positive patients in China, mortality was found higher in patients with HT (10.4%) compared to those without HT (1.7%) [23]. It has been demonstrated in many observational studies originating from China that mortality and morbidity increase in COVID-19 positive patients with HT [24, 25]. In the data from China and Italy, it has been shown that hypertensive patients constitute approximately 70% of the population, and progression to ARDS is significantly higher in patients with HT [26].

These have led to the discussions that the antihypertensive drugs that are effective through ACE, the cell entry protein of the virus, and increasing ACE2 [angiotensin 1 receptor blockade (ARB) and ACE inhibitors] may play a role in the pathogenesis of COVID-19 infection. However, these studies did not investigate the relationship between HT and mortality-morbidity in age-adjusted regression models. In addition, in these studies, HT is highly variable and mostly defined as being on antihypertensive treatment. Drug compliance and blood pressure control parameters were not mentioned.

The SARS-CoV-2 spike (S) protein uses the ACE2 receptor to enter the host cell, as in SARS and MERS [6]. The S protein binds to the catalytic domain of ACE2 with high affinity. The binding of the S protein to ACE2 triggers a conformational change in the S protein of the coronavirus and in this way, viral RNA enters the cell and infects the cell [27]. The concern that the treatment with ACE inhibitors or ARBs will increase viral binding and infection by causing tissue-level up-regulation of the ACE2 receptor in HT patients is the basis of the controversy [28]. Studies are showing increased ACE2 mRNA expression in the left ventricle of normotensive Lewis rats and enalapril in rat heart tissue after treatment with Lisinopril and Losartan [29, 30]. Ishiyama et al. reported the increase of ACE2 mRNA levels in the coronary endothelium after the treatment with ARBs in their study with coronary artery ligation [31]. On the other hand, there are also experimental studies that have not shown a similar effect. In a study, after coronary artery ligation and treatment with ramipril, no increase in ACE2 mRNA compared to control was shown [32].

Also, Burchill et al. observed no increase in ACE2 protein in rat coronary endothelium after coronary artery ligation and treatment with valsartan, ramipril, or both [33]. The human studies showing ACE2 up-regulation with the renin-angiotensin aldosterone system (RAAS) are highly contradictory. In the study of Walters et al., no association was found in plasma ACE2 levels with the use of ACE inhibitors or ARBs [34]. Furuhashi et al. showed increased urinary ACE2 levels in patients with HT after using Olmesartan [35].

As can be seen from the current literature, the ACE2 receptor up-regulation hypothesis with RAAS blockers is based only on limited in-vitro and in-vivo animal experiments, and the studies in which this hypothesis cannot be demonstrated in humans and animals are also available in the literature.

In none of the accessible studies, there is no data on ACE2 up-regulation in respiratory epithelium and type 2 pneumocytes, the entrance gate used by SARS-CoV2 to infect the body. On the other hand, it has been shown in animal experiments that ACE2 transforms angiotensin 2 to angiotensin 1 - 7, and this vasodilatory effect occurring in this way can reduce lung damage in viral pneumonia [24]. Similarly, it has been suggested that ACE2, which is down-regulated by the SARS-CoV-2 surface spike protein, can be increased by RAAS blockade, thus antagonizing the effects of SARS-CoV-2 [36]. The guideline published by the American Heart Association and the

American College of Cardiology (AHA/ACC) recommends the continuation of RAAS antagonists, which have proven useful in diseases such as heart failure, ischaemic heart disease, and HT, in COVID-19 patients [37]. In a study including seven hospitals in Spain, it was shown that there was no increase in the risk of hospitalization due to COVID-19 in patients using RAAS inhibitors, and there was no significant difference between long and short-term drugs use. One of the important findings of this study is that DM patients using RAAS inhibitors have a lower risk of hospitalization due to COVID-19 (OR 0.53, $p = 0.004$) [13].

Roffi et al. suggested that ARBs may be protective for COVID-19 depending on their mechanism of action [38]. However, since there is not enough evidence to support these hypotheses, it is not appropriate to use ACE inhibitors and ARBs as a potential treatment for COVID-19. As a result, if there is no contraindication such as hypotension or acute kidney damage, patients using ACE inhibitors or ARBs should continue their medication during COVID-19 infection.

Coronary Artery Disease

It is known that the prevalence of coronary artery disease (CAD) among cardiovascular diseases varies depending on the society. For this reason, there are significant differences in the frequency of CAD among patients diagnosed with COVID-19. The studies about COVID-19 have also reported a wide range from 4.2 to 25% for CAD [39, 40]. These numbers are much higher when considering patients treated in intensive care units [40]. In a large series of 72,314 people in China, the death rate was 2.3%, while the mortality rate over 80 years old was 14.8%. While 4.2% of all patients had a history of CAD, 22.7% of those who died had CAD [41].

ACE2, the cell-entry receptor of SARS-CoV-2, is also found in endothelial cells. Whether the vascular irregularities in COVID-19 infection are caused by the endothelial cell involvement of the virus or not is currently unclear but SARS-CoV-2 has been shown to infect human blood vessel organoids in-vitro [42]. Varga et al. demonstrated viral inclusion patterns in endothelial cells in an autopsy analysis of a 71-year-old male patient who died of COVID-19 and had CAD, HT, and kidney transplant, the recipient. This way, they found evidence of direct virus infection and widespread endothelial inflammation in the endothelial cell [43]. The vascular endothelium is an active paracrine, endocrine, and autocrine organ indispensable for regulating vascular tone and maintaining vascular homeostasis. Endothelial dysfunction is the main determinant of microvascular dysfunction by shifting the vascular balance to more vasoconstriction with organ ischemia, inflammation, and a pro-clotting state [44]. Thus, interest in treatments for stabilizing the endothelium has increased. Statins commonly used in the treatment of CAD are inhibitors of the inflammatory pathway MYD88 and have been shown to stabilize MYD88 at in-vitro and animal studies [43]. The instability of MYD88 has been associated with negative consequences in SARS-COV and MERS-COV infections, but this relationship has not been identified with SAR-COV-2. Statins may be useful in treating COVID-19 infection, but further studies are needed for a recommendation. It is also important for the patient to use statin therapy regularly, as COVID-19 is also a risk factor for acute cardiac damage.

Continuation of the drugs used in the routine treatment of CAD has been recommended as it is recommended in hypertensive patients. None of the medications we use in treatment such as acetylsalicylic acid, beta-blockers, statins, and nitrate have been associated with poor results in the management of COVID-19 infection.

Pulmonary involvement of COVID-19 infection can cause arterial hypoxia and acidosis, and this can result in myocardial dysfunction. Although there are no cardiac complaints due to myocardial damage and microvascular deterioration, an increase in cardiac biomarkers (troponin and natriuretic peptide) and nonspecific ECG changes can be observed [43]. Studies showing the SARS-CoV2 primarily attacking pericytes in the heart may explain the capillary endothelial cell dysfunction and an increase in cardiac damage markers [45]. COVID-19 infection may also be present with type 1 and type 2 myocardial infarction (MI) as a result of respiratory failure and exposure to hypoxia, especially in elderly patients, or COVID-19 may be tested positive in the course of MI.

It should be kept in mind that the patient considered to have the acute coronary syndrome in clinical and laboratory terms, should be questioned in terms of COVID-19 and tested for SARS-CoV2. When the intervention is to be performed, the patients are accepted as positive only if there is a suspicious contact history. Percutaneous coronary intervention may be preferred instead of coronary artery bypass graft surgery in suitable patients for revascularisation to reduce exposure. In addition, in low-risk ST-segment elevation myocardial infarction (STEMI), thrombolytic therapy can be considered instead of the invasive procedure [45]. A separate catheter laboratory for COVID-19 patients can also be beneficial for both the patient and the healthcare team.

COVID-19 can cause MI, myocarditis, or arrhythmia directly and indirectly. In addition, hydroxychloroquine and chloroquine used in the treatment of COVID-19 infection may cause prolongation of the QT distance, development of the atrioventricular block, sick sinus syndrome, and bundle branch block by making sodium/potassium/calcium channel blockade. Hydroxychloroquine and chloroquine are widely used in the world due to their antiviral activity as well as their anti-inflammatory activity, but there are some points to be careful about when using these drugs. These agents are relatively well tolerated but may cause rare and serious side effects (<10%) such as heart conduction system, hypoglycemia, neuropsychiatric effects, and retinopathy.

Monitoring the patient by electrocardiography is recommended especially in critically ill patients and in patients receiving concomitant agents that prolong the QT interval (such as macrolides, fluoroquinolones, amiodarone). Efficiency and side effects will be revealed better as the studies continue.

As the health system is overburdened due to the COVID-19 pandemic, neglecting the patients with CAD is a serious problem. In Hong Kong, Tam et al. showed that the rate of care for STEMI cases was seriously affected after COVID-19. In Hong Kong, the time for the ambulance to reach the patient after the call has increased from 80-90 minutes to 318 minutes on average [46].

In a study from Italy, they found that there was a 48.4% total decrease in STEMI and Non-ST segment elevation myocardial infarction (NSTEMI) cases taken to the catheter laboratory during the COVID-19 pandemic, a decrease of 26.5% in STEMIs and a 65% decrease in NSTEMIs compared to the same period of the previous year ($p < 0.001$). The mortality rate of STEMI increased significantly with the pandemic compared to the previous year (risk ratio (RR) = 3.3; $p < 0.001$) and there was a significant increase in complications (RR = 1.8; $p = 0.009$). This situation is a serious alarm finding for public health and should be emphasized [47]. The reasons for this situation can be caused by the patient or the healthcare system.

The most important reasons arising from the patient could be considered as disruptions in drug usage and health control, delaying hospitalization due to the fear of the virus.

Considering the reasons caused by the healthcare system, the home care system is not adequately provided, and a safe intervention system cannot be organized.

HEART FAILURE

Heart failure (HF) can be triggered by COVID-19 infection in patients with previously known or undiagnosed HF. In addition to the infection increases the workload of the heart, acute myocardial damage may develop due to events such as acute MI, stress cardiomyopathy, cytokine storm, and this way, heart failure may develop or the existing disease may be decompensated. It is not clear whether the underlying heart failure is exacerbated or a de novo HF is developing in COVID-19 positive patients [48]. In the study of Zhou et al., they retrospectively evaluated the patients presenting with COVID-19 and found that although HF was observed in 23% of the patients during the follow-up, HF ratio among people lost was 52% [49]. In a study where 799 patients in Wuhan were screened, heart failure was found in 49% of the patients who died and 3% of those who recovered [50].

In patients infected with COVID-19, the clinical picture is usually in the form of acute respiratory failure and may progress to ARDS with a ground-glass opacity in imaging. This clinical presentation is not much different from patients admitted to the hospital with acute HF [51]. Therefore, in patients presenting with acute pulmonary edema, heart-related causes alone, or mixed causes related to COVID-19 infection should also be considered. For differential diagnosis, bilateral multilobar ground-glass opacification with peripheral or posterior distribution mainly in the lower lobes is typical for COVID-19 infection in computed tomography of the chest. Atypical views such as superposed consolidated areas on ground-glass opacity can be seen in the elderly population. Findings starting from a single focus and progressing to bilateral lung involvement are in favor of infection. The use of cardiac biomarkers and, more often, echocardiography are effective in differentiating the clinical picture of infection and heart failure [52].

We do not have any conclusive evidence that will require the cessation of treatments that have proven effects on mortality such as ACE inhibitor, ARB, angiotensin receptor blocker-neprilysin inhibitor (ARNI), and mineralocorticoid receptor antagonist (MRA). In the treatment of HF, drug changes and discontinuation of drugs are not recommended, as in HT and CAD.

Conclusion

As a result, the group most affected by the epidemic and having the highest mortality rate are the elderly with known cardiovascular diseases. In the guideline published by the AHA/ACC, they recommended the continuation of RAAS antagonists proven to be beneficial in diseases such as heart failure, ischaemic heart disease, and hypertension in COVID-19 patients. As the health system is overburdened due to the increase in COVID-19 cases during the pandemic process, it resulted in ignoring the patients with CAD, and thus the death rate of patients with CAD during the pandemic process has increased and this is a serious problem.

References

[1] Zhou, P., Yang, X. L., Wang, X. G., Hu, B., Zhang, L., Zhang, W. et al. A pneumonia outbreak associated with a new coronavirus of probable bat origin. *Nature,* 2020; 579:270 - 3.

[2] *Naming the coronavirus disease* (*COVID-19*) *and the virus that causes it* [Internet]. Available at: https://www.who.int/emergencies/diseases/novel-coronavirus-2019/technicalguidance/naming-the-coronavirus-disease-(covid-2019)-and-the-virus-that-causes-it Accessed September 18, 2020.

[3] Lauer, S. A., Grantz, K. H., Bi, Q., Jones, F. K., Zheng, Q., Meredith, H. R. et al. The Incubation Period of Coronavirus Disease 2019 (COVID-19) From Publicly

Reported Confirmed Cases: Estimation and Application. *Ann. Intern. Med.,* 2020 Mar. 10. [Epub ahead of print].

[4] Guan, W. J., Ni, Z. Y., Hu, Y., Liang, W. H., Ou, C. Q., He, J. X. et al. Clinical Characteristics of Coronavirus Disease 2019 in China. *N Engl. J. Med.,* 2020 Feb. 28. [Epub ahead of print].

[5] Badawi, A., Ryoo, S. G. Prevalence of comorbidities in the Middle East respiratory syndrome coronavirus (MERS-CoV): A systematic review and metaanalysis. *Int. J. Infect. Dis.,* 2016; 49:129 - 133.

[6] Hoffmann, M., Kleine-Weber, H., Schroeder, S., Krüger, N., Herrler, T., Erichsen, S., Schiergens, T. S., Herrler, G., Wu, N. H., Nitsche, A. et al. SARS-CoV-2 cell entry depends on ACE2 and TMPRSS2 and is blocked by a clinically proven protease inhibitor *Cell,* [published online March 5, 2020].

[7] Zhao, Y., Zhao, Z., Wang, Y., Zhou, Y., Ma, Y., Zuo, W. Single-cell RNA expression profiling of ACE2, the putative receptor of Wuhan 2019-nCov. *Biorxiv* [published online January 26, 2020].

[8] Tikellis, C., Thomas, M. C. Angiotensin-converting enzyme 2 (ACE2) is a key modulator of the renin angiotensin system in health and disease. *Int. J. Pept.,* 2012; 2012:256294.

[9] Wang, L., He, W., Yu, X. et al. Coronavirus disease 2019 in elderly patients: characteristics and prognostic factors based on 4-week follow-up. *J. Infect.*, 2020.

[10] Lionakis, N., Mendrinos, D., Sanidas, E. Et al. (2012) Hypertension in the elderly. *World J. Cardiol.,* 4:135 - 147.

[11] Suastika, K., Dwipayana, P., Ratna Saraswati, I. M. Et al. (2011) Relationship between age and metabolic disorders in the population of Bali. *J. Clin. Gerontol.,* 2:47 - 52.

[12] The Novel Coronavirus Pneumonia Emergency Response Epidemiology Team. The epidemiological characteristics of an outbreak of 2019 novel coronavirus diseases (COVID-19): China. *China CDC Weekly,* 2020; 2:113.

[13] de Abajo, F. J., Rodriguez-Martin, S., Lerma, V., Mejia-Abril, G., Aguilar, M., Garcia-Luque, A. et al. Use of renin-angiotensin-aldosterone system inhibitors and risk of COVID-19 requiring admission to hospital: A case-population study. *Lancet,* 2020; 395 (10238):1705 - 14.

[14] Chan, J. W., Ng, C. K., Chan, Y. H., Mok, T. Y., Lee, S., Chu, S. Y., Law, W. L., Lee, M. P., Li, P. C. Short term outcome and risk factors for adverse clinical outcomes in adults with severe acute respiratory syndrome (SARS). *Thorax*, 2003; 58:686 - 689.

[15] Booth, C. M., Matukas, L. M., Tomlinson, G. A., Rachlis, A. R., Rose, D. B., Dwosh, H. A., Walmsley, S. L., Mazzulli, T., Avendano, M., Derkach, P. et al. Clinical features and short-term outcomes of 144 patients with SARS in the greater Toronto area. *JAMA*, 2003; 289:2801 - 2809.

[16] Goetzl, E. J., Huang, M.-C., Kon, J. et al. (2010) Gender specificity of altered human immune cytokine profiles in aging. *FASEB J. Off. Publ. Fed. Am. Soc. Exp. Biol.,* 24:3580 - 3589.

[17] Huang, C., Wang, Y., Li, X., Ren, L., Zhao, J., Hu, Y. et al. Clinical features of patients infected with 2019 novel coronavirus in Wuhan, China. *Lancet,* 2020; 395:497 - 506.

[18] Libby, P., Loscalzo, J., Ridker, P. M. et al. Inflammation, Immunity, and Infection in Atherothrombosis: JACC Review Topic of the Week. *J. Am. Coll. Cardiol.,* 2018; 72:2071.

[19] Kwong, J. C., Schwartz, K. L., Campitelli, M. A. et al. Acute Myocardial Infarction after Laboratory-Confirmed Influenza Infection. *N Engl. J. Med.,* 2018; 378:345.

[20] Garg, S., Kim, L., Whitaker, M. et al. Hospitalization Rates and Characteristics of Patients Hospitalized with Laboratory-Confirmed Coronavirus Disease 2019 - COVID-NET, 14 States, March 1 - 30, 2020. *MMWR Morb. Mortal. Wkly Rep.,* 2020; 69(15):458 - 464.

[21] Roncon, L., Zuin, M., Zuliani, G., Rigatelli, G. Patients with arterial hypertension and COVID-19 are at higher risk of ICU admission. *Br. J. Anaesth.,* 2020.

[22] Wu, C., Chen, X., Cai, Y., Xia, Ja., Zhou, X., Xu, S. et al. Risk factors associated with acute respiratory distress syndrome and death in patients with coronavirus disease 2019 pneumonia in Wuhan, China. *JAMA Internal Medicine,* 2020.

[23] Guan, W. J., Liang, W. H., Zhao, Y., Liang, H. R., Chen, Z. S., Li, Y. M., et al. Comorbidity and its impact on 1590 patients with COVID-19 in China: a nationwide analysis. *Eur. Respir. J.,* 2020; 55(5):2000547.

[24] Patel, A. B., Verma, A. COVID-19 and angiotensin-converting enzyme inhibitors and angiotensin receptor blockers: what is the evidence? *JAMA,* 2020. 20.

[25] Mao, B., Liu, Y., Chai, Y. H., Jin, X. Y., Lu, H. W., Yang, J. W. et al. Assessing risk factors for SARS-CoV-2 infection in patients presenting with symptoms in Shanghai, China: a multicentre, observational cohort study. *The Lancet Digital Health,* 2020.

[26] Wu, C., Chen, X., Cai, Y., Xia, J., Zhou, X., Xu, S. et al. Risk Factors Associated with Acute Respiratory Distress Syndrome and Death in Patients with Coronavirus Disease 2019 Pneumonia in Wuhan, China. *JAMA Intern. Med.,* 2020 Mar. 13.

[27] Hamming, I., Timens, W., Bulthuis, M. L., Lely, A. T., Navis, G., van Goor, H. Tissue distribution of ACE2 protein, the functional receptor for SARS coronavirus. A first step in understanding SARS pathogenesis. *J. Pathol.,* 2004; 203:631 - 7.

[28] Wan, Y., Shang, J., Graham, R., Baric, R. S., Li, F. Receptor recognition by the novel coronavirus from Wuhan: An analysis based on decade-long structural studies of SARS coronavirus. *J. Virol.,* 2020; 94(7):e00127 - 20.

[29] Ferrario, C. M., Jessup, J., Chappell, M. C., Averill, D. B., Brosnihan, K. B., Tallant, E. A. et al. Effect of angiotensin-converting enzyme inhibition and

angiotensin II receptor blockers on cardiac angiotensin-converting enzyme 2. *Circulation,* 2005; 111: 2605 - 10.

[30] Ocaranza, M. P., Godoy, I., Jalil, J. E., Varas, M., Collantes, P., Pinto, M. et al. Enalapril attenuates downregulation of Angiotensin-converting enzyme 2 in the late phase of ventricular dysfunction in myocardial infarcted rat. *Hypertension,* 2006; 48:572 - 8.

[31] Ishiyama, Y., Gallagher, P. E., Averill, D. B., Tallant, E. A., Brosnihan, K. B., Ferrario, C. M. Upregulation of angiotensin-converting enzyme 2 after myocardial infarction by blockade of angiotensin II receptors. *Hypertension,* 2004; 43:970 - 6.

[32] Burrell, L. M., Risvanis, J., Kubota, E., Dean, R. G., MacDonald, P. S., Lu, S. et al. Myocardial infarction increases ACE2 expression in rat and humans. *Eur. Heart J.*, 2005; 26:369 - 75.

[33] Burchill, L. J., Velkoska, E., Dean, R. G., Griggs, K., Patel, S. K., Burrell, L. M. Combination renin-angiotensin system blockade and angiotensin-converting enzyme 2 in experimental myocardial infarction: Implications for future therapeutic directions. *Clin. Sci.,* (Lond) 2012; 123:649 - 58.

[34] Walters, T. E., Kalman, J. M., Patel, S. K., Mearns, M., Velkoska, E., Burrell, L. M. Angiotensin converting enzyme 2 activity and human atrial fibrillation: Increased plasma angiotensin converting enzyme 2 activity is associated with atrial fibrillation and more advanced left atrial structural remodelling. *Europace,* 2017; 19:1280 - 7.

[35] Furuhashi, M., Moniwa, N., Mita, T. et al. Urinary angiotensin-converting enzyme 2 in hypertensive patients may be increased by olmesartan, an angiotensin II receptor blocker. *Am. J. Hypertens*., 2015; 28(1):15 - 21.

[36] Messerli, F. H., Siontis, G. C. M., Rexhaj, E. COVID-19 and renin angiotensin blockers: current evidence and recommendations. *Circulation,* 2020.

[37] *HFSA/ACC/AHA statement addresses concerns re: using RAAS antagonists in COVID-19* [Available from: https://www.acc.org/latest-in-cardiology/articles/2020/03/17/08/59/hfsa-acc-aha-statement-addresses-concerns-re-using-raasantagonists-in-covid-19.

[38] Roffi, M., Guagliumi, G., Ibanez, B. The Obstacle Course of Reperfusion for ST-Segment-Elevation Myocardial Infarction in the COVID-19 Pandemic. *Circulation,* 2020; 141:1951.

[39] Madjid, M., Safavi-Naeini, P., Solomon, S. D., Vardeny, O. Potential Effects of Coronaviruses on the Cardiovascular System: A Review. *JAMA Cardiol.,* 2020.

[40] Chen, T., Wu, D., Chen, H. et al. Clinical characteristics of 113 deceased patients with coronavirus disease 2019: Retrospective study. *BMJ,* 2020; 368:m1091.

[41] Wu, Z., McGoogan, J. M. Characteristics of and Important Lessons From the Coronavirus Disease 2019 (COVID-19) Outbreak in China: Summary of a Report

of 72 314 Cases from the Chinese Center for Disease Control and Prevention. *JAMA*, 2020; 10.1001.

[42] Monteil, V., Kwon, H., Prado, P. et al. Inhibition of SARS-CoV-2 Infections in Engineered Human Tissues Using Clinical-Grade Soluble Human ACE2. *Cell*, 2020; 181(4):905 - 913.e7. doi: 10.1016/ j.cell.2020.04.004.

[43] Varga, Z., Flammer, A. J., Steiger, P. et al. Endothelial cell infection and endotheliitis in COVID-19. *Lancet*, 2020; 395:1417.

[44] Bonetti, P. O., Lerman, L. O., Lerman, A. Endothelial dysfunction: A marker of atherosclerotic risk. *Arterioscler. Thromb Vasc. Biol.*, 2003; 23(2):168 - 175.

[45] Thum, T. SARS-CoV-2 receptor ACE2 expression in the human heart: cause of a post-pandemic wave of heart failure? *Eur. Heart J.*, 2020.

[46] Tam, C. F., Cheung, K. S., Lam, S., Wong, A. et al. (2020). Impact of Coronavirus Disease 2019 (COVID-19) Outbreak on ST-Segment-Elevation Myocardial Infarction Care in Hong Kong, China. *Circ. Cardiovasc. Qual. Outcomes*, Mar. 17: CIRCOUTCOMES120006631.

[47] De Rosa, S., Spaccarotella, C., Basso, C. et al. Reduction of hospitalizations for myocardial infarction in Italy in the COVID-19 era. *Eur. Heart J.*, 2020; 41(22):2083 - 2088.

[48] Rinaldi, L., Milione, S., Fascione, M. C. et al. Relevance of lung ultrasound in the diagnostic algorithm of respiratory diseases in a real-life setting: A multicentre prospective study. *Respirology*, 2019.

[49] Zhou, F., Yu, T., Du, R. et al. Clinical course and risk factors for mortality of adult inpatients with COVID-19 in Wuhan, China: A retrospective cohort study. *Lancet*, 2020 Mar. 28; 395(10229):1038.

[50] Chen, T., Wu, D., Chen, H. et al. Clinical characteristics of 113 deceased patients with coronavirus disease 2019: Retrospective study [published correction appears in *BMJ*, 2020 Mar. 31; 368:m1295]. *BMJ*, 2020; 368:m1091.

[51] Zompatori, M., Ciccarese, F., Fasano, L. Overview of current lung imaging in acute respiratory distress syndrome. *Eur. Respir. Rev.*, 2014; 23:519 - 30.

[52] Komiya, K., Ishii, H., Teramoto, S., Takahashi, O., Eshima, N., Yamaguchi, O. et al. Diagnostic utility of C-reactive protein combined with brain natriuretic peptide in acute pulmonary edema: A cross sectional study. *Respir. Res.*, 2011; 12:83.

In: Coronavirus Disease
Editor: Yildiz Dincer

ISBN: 978-1-53619-296-4

Chapter 15

THE IMPACT OF THE COVID-19 PANDEMIC ON CANCER PATIENTS

Hande Turna**, *MD
Istanbul University- Cerrahpasa, Cerrahpasa Medical Faculty, Department of Medical Oncology, Istanbul Turkey

ABSTRACT

COVID-19 infection in patients with cancer is associated with a significantly increased risk of case fatality. Strategies to reduce the likelihood of infection and improve early identification in this immunocompromised patient population is crucial. Clinicians must balance the risks of delaying cancer treatments versus the risks for SARS-CoV-2 exposure and the potential increased adverse outcomes of COVID-19 infection in cancer patients. Physical distancing rules and contact limitations should be essential components of cancer care delivery. Mortality from COVID-19 in cancer patients appears to be principally driven by age, gender, and comorbidities such as diabetes and obesity. Likelihood of severe illness from COVID-19 is higher among patients with lung cancer and hematologic malignancies. There is no identified evidence that cancer patients on cytotoxic chemotherapy or other anticancer treatment are at an increased risk of mortality from COVID-19 disease compared with those not on active treatment. Anti-CD20 monoclonal antibodies causing B cell depletion and lymphopenia may contribute to the severity of COVID-19 infection. Treatment with immune checkpoint inhibitors may have the potential to alleviate inflammation in COVID-19 infection. In retrospective cohort studies there are conflicting results but there is no clear data for increasing the severity of the infection. The management of COVID-19 infection in cancer patients is generally the same as in the general population. Mild cases and asymptomatic infections can be managed conservatively at home Agents used specifically for COVID-19 are reserved for

* Corresponding Author's Email: hande.turna@gmail com.

patients with severe disease. Clinicians delivering cancer care should have discussions with their patients about goals of care and future care planings.

Keywords: COVID-19, cancer patient, lung cancer, cancer treatment

INTRODUCTION

COVID- 19 pandemic has a tremendous effect on daily life, economic conditions, and the health care system all over the world. This impact of the pandemic on health care of cancer patients is also very challenging because of the competitive risks of death from cancer versus death from infection, and the higher lethality of SARS-CoV-2 infection in immunocompromised hosts.

Cancer patients are more prone to infections because of their immunosuppressive state resulting from their malignancy and anti-cancer treatments. Delaying cancer treatments should be balanced with SARS-Cov-2 exposure and the increased risk of severe infection in an immunocompromised group of patients.

A survey study involving health care representatives from the international oncology community from 18 countries presented by Jerusalem et al. At the European Society for Medical Oncology (ESMO) Congress 2020, highlighted the extent to which COVID-19 has challenged the organization and delivery of cancer care. Overall, 60.9% reported that clinical activity was reduced at the peak of the pandemic, while nearly two-thirds (64.2%) cited undertreatment as a major concern, and 37% expected to see significant reductions in a clinical trial data. Cancer treatments canceled or delayed were surgery (in 44.1% of centers), chemotherapy (25.7%), and radiotherapy (13.7%). Earlier cessation of palliative care was observed in 32.1% of centers. Thirty-four percent of respondents reported that surgery was the treatment modality that was most affected by the pandemic, followed by chemotherapy (22.0%), radiotherapy (13.7%), checkpoint inhibitor therapy (9.1%), monoclonal antibodies (9.0%), and oral targeted therapy (3.7%) Increased use of granulocyte colony-stimulating factor in 34.8% and a decreased corticosteroid use in 21.9% was observed. Telemedicine, or teleconsultations were reportedly performed for 94.5% of follow-up visits. Also, approximately 82% of participants projected that they would continue with the use of telemedicine more frequently in their practices after the pandemic [1].

INCIDENCE OF COVID 19 INFECTION IN CANCER PATIENTS

Though most data suggest a higher incidence of COVID-19 infection in cancer patients when compared to the general population, there are conflicting results. Chinese reports the incidence of COVID infection to be 1% in cancer patients; a higher ratio when compared with 0.29% of infection rate in the general population [2].

A study of 1069 cancer patients in Madrid, Spain the incidence of COVID-19 infection was found to be 4.2% much higher than 0.62% incidence of the city population but an Austrian study found a similar and even lower incidence of SARS-Cov-2 infection in cancer patients compared to the general population [3, 4].

CLINICAL OUTCOMES OF COVID-19 INFECTION IN CANCER PATIENTS

The clinical presentation and outcome of COVID-19 infection in cancer patients can be heterogeneous. Some meta-analysis suggests that severe and lethal COVID-19 infection rate is higher in cancer patients particularly with hematological malignancies, lung cancer, metastatic disease, and in older patients having comorbidities including obesity. [5].

A meta-analysis including 32 international studies from Europe, Asia and the United studies for a total of 46499 patients including 1776 cancer patients showed that cause mortality rates were found to be higher in cancer patients (RR, 1.66; 95% CI, 1.33 to 2.07; $P < .0001$; However, in a prespecified subgroup analysis of patients > 65 years of age, all-cause mortality was comparable between those with versus without cancer (RR, 1.06; 95% CI, 0.79 to 1.41; $P = .71$); and the intensive care unit (ICU) admission was also more likely in patients with cancer (26 studies, 15,375 patients; (RR 1.56, 95% CI 1.31-1.87). The authors concluded that cancer is associated with worse clinical outcomes among patients with COVID-19. However, elderly patients with cancer may not be at increased risk of death when infected with COVID-19 [6].

In Spain, a hospital-based study showed that the fatality rate was 9.8% in Covid-19 infected patients however, the mortality rate in cancer patients was 42.2% ($p = 0.0001$) [7].

In a study conducted in New York City Hospital, a total of 218 COVID-19-positive patients from a malignant diagnosis were identified. A total of 61 (28%) patients with cancer died from COVID-19 with a case fatality rate (CFR) of 37% (20/54) for hematologic malignancies and 25% (41/164) for solid malignancies. Six of 11 (55%) patients with lung cancer died from COVID-19 disease. Increased mortality was significantly associated with older age, multiple comorbidities, need for ICU support, and elevated levels of D-dimer, lactate dehydrogenase, and lactate in multivariate analysis. Age-adjusted CFRs in patients with cancer compared with noncancer patients reported a significant increase in case of fatality for patients with cancer. The authors suggest the need for proactive strategies to reduce the likelihood of infection and improve early identification of Covid-19 infection in vulnerable cancer patient population. It remains uncertain if cancer patients other than those with hematologic malignancies or lung cancer are at increased risk of severe outcomes from COVID-19 when the analysis is controlled for age, the mortality/morbidity associated with their cancer, and other comorbidities [8].

Lung cancer is a leading cause of cancer related mortality but also case fatality rates from COVID-19 infection are high in patients with lung cancer. One of the challenging issues in delivering cancer care for patients with lung cancer is that discrimination of clinical symptoms and radiological findings from COVID-19 infection, lung cancer involvement, and progression or other infective conditions can sometimes be very difficult. This difficulty may render the clinicians from delivering the optimal treatment. The Thoracic Cancers International COVID-19 Collaboration (TERAVOLT) registry is a multi-centre observational study composed of a cross-sectional component and a longitudinal cohort component 200 patients with COVID-19 and thoracic cancers from eight countries were identified and included in the TERAVOLT registry. 152 (76%) patients were hospitalized and 66 (33%) died. 13 (10%) of 134 patients who met the criteria for ICU admission were admitted to ICU; the remaining 121 were hospitalized, but were not admitted to ICU Univariable analyses revealed that being older than 65 years (OR 1·88, 95%1·00–3·62), being a current or former smoker (4·24, 1·70–12·95), receiving treatment with chemotherapy alone (2·54, 1·09–6·11), and the presence of any comorbidities (2·65, 1·09–7·46) were associated with increased risk of death. However, in multivariable analysis, only smoking history (OR 3·18, 95% CI 1·11–9·06) was associated with an increased risk of death [9].

The Effect of Cancer Treatment on Covid-19 Infection

The international COVID-19 and Cancer Consortium registry including 928 cancer patients from the United States, Canada, and Spain with confirmed SARS-CoV-2 infection over one month (The most prevalent malignancies were breast (21%) and prostate cancer (16%) percent); 43 percent had active cancer and 39 percent had received chemotherapy treatment within four weeks of virus diagnosis. The use of any form of anticancer therapy (cytotoxic or noncytotoxic) within four weeks of infection was ***not*** associated with higher 30-day mortality rates. In multivariate analysis, independent factors associated with greater 30-day mortality included older age, male sex, former smoker, two or more comorbidities, Eastern Cooperative Oncology Group (ECOG) performance status of 2 or worse and active cancer (versus those in remission; OR 5.2, 95% CI 2.77-9.77) [10].

Cancer, patients who are receiving systemic anticancer treatments, have been postulated to be at increased risk of mortality from COVID-19 infection. In the UK Coronavirus Cancer Monitoring Project (UKCCMP), a study including 800 cancer patients with COVID- 19 infection, 52 percent of patients had a mild COVID-19 disease course while 28% of patients died. After adjusting for age, gender, and comorbidities, chemotherapy and other forms of cancer treatments such as immunotherapy, hormonal and targeted therapies and radiotherapy in the past 4 weeks had no significant effect on mortality from COVID-19 disease [11].

Immunotherapy in the form of Immune Check Point Inhibitors (ICI) is being used in cancer therapy especially in metastatic lung cancer patients in recent years. The answer to the question of whether programmed death 1 (PD-1) blockade therapy which has an immunostimulating effect can alleviate the severity of disease from COVID-19 in patients with cancer is not clear. A study in New York State Memorial Sloan Kettering Cancer Center; 423 cases of symptomatic COVID-19 were diagnosed (from a total of 2,035 patients with cancer tested). Hospitalization rate was, 40% in the patient group, and 20% developed a severe respiratory illness and 12% died within 30 days. Age older than 65 years and treatment with ICIs were predictors for hospitalization and severe disease, whereas receipt of chemotherapy and major surgery was not [12].

A retrospective study of a single-center 69 patients with lung cancer who were diagnosed with COVID-19 examined the severity of the infection based on no or prior receipt of PD-1 blockade. Overall, the severity of COVID-19 in patients with lung cancer was found to be high, including the need for hospitalization in more than half of patients and death in nearly a quarter. After adjustment for smoking status, PD-1 blockade exposure was not found to be associated with an increased risk of severity of COVID-19 [13].

Testing for Covid 19 in Cancer Patients

Patients with cancer ***with*** symptoms concerning for COVID-19 (e. g., fever, cough, dyspnea, hypoxia), ***or*** those with exposure to someone with COVID-19, should be offered to test. Alternative causes for their symptoms (eg, influenza, bacterial pneumonia, cancer progression, treatment-related side effects) must also be considered. For patients with cancer ***without*** symptoms of COVID-19, guidance regarding SARS-CoV-2 testing is evolving, and the approach among is variable. Given the risk of transmission from asymptomatic carriers, some institutions are routinely testing all cancer patients before immunosuppressive therapies, as long as testing capacity is not limited However, this is not a widespread practice and it is not supported by guidelines from the *American Cancer Society* and *ASCO*. On the other hand, this policy is supported by updated guidelines from the *Infectious Disease Society of America,* which now recommends SARS-CoV-2 RNA testing in asymptomatic individuals before immunosuppressive procedures, regardless of known exposure to COVID-19. According to these guidelines, immunosuppressive procedures are defined as cytotoxic chemotherapy, solid organ or stem cell transplantation, long-acting biologic therapy, cellular immunotherapy, or high-dose corticosteroids [14-15].

Unnecessary testing could lead to a delay in the administration of antineoplastic therapy and additionally could increase the risk of exposure to COVID-19. SARS-CoV-2 RNA can be detected for several weeks after initial infection but does not distinguish between active and resolved infection. In patients with mild to moderate illness, replicating the virus cannot be detected after the first testing for the asymptomatic patient without a history of COVID-19 The task force recommended that only patients with hematologic malignancies should be tested for COVID-19 RNA before the initiation of outpatient antineoplastic [16].

Resuming antineoplastic treatment therapy in a patient who previously tested positive for COVID-19 or who has had presumed recent COVID-19 infection. The task force recommended that in a previously symptomatic patient with COVID-19, resumption of antineoplastic therapy be considered when COVID-related fevers have resolved for at least 7 days without the use of fever-reducing medications, there has been a substantial improvement in respiratory symptoms, and at least 14 days have elapsed since the onset of symptoms and/or initial positive COVID-19 test, whichever came earlier. Repeat COVID-19 RNA testing is not recommended. In a previously asymptomatic patient with COVID-19, resumption of antineoplastic therapy can be considered when at least 14 days have elapsed since the initial positive COVID-19 test and no symptoms have developed during this time. [16].

The task force recognized that certain patients may require additional time to recover before resumption of antineoplastic treatment. These include patients who experienced more severe symptoms due to COVID-19 (i.e., required hospitalization and/or supplemental oxygen), older patients, and patients with certain malignancies, such as lung cancer, hematologic malignancies [16].

COVID-19 testing is not recommended for most asymptomatic cancer outpatients, and antineoplastic treatment can be resumed after the resolution of fever or the passage of time in patients who have tested positive, according to an expert task force. Clinicians must weigh the benefits of initiating or resuming antineoplastic therapy against the risk of worsening outcomes related to COVID-19 [16].

SARS-CoV-2 RNA testing of asymptomatic patients without a history of COVID-19 only for those with hematologic malignancies before the initiation of outpatient antineoplastic therapy. For patients with solid tumors, including lung cancer, routine pretreatment SARS-CoV-2 RNA testing was not recommended, according to the online report in the Journal of the National Cancer Institute [16].

Previously symptomatic patients with COVID-19 can resume antineoplastic therapy when COVID-19-related fevers have resolved for at least 7 days without use of fever-reducing medications, there has been a substantial improvement in respiratory symptoms, and at least 14 days have elapsed since the onset of symptoms and/or initial positive SARS-CoV-2 test, whichever came earlier [16].

In previously asymptomatic patients who tested positive for SARS-CoV-2, resumption of antineoplastic therapy can be considered when at least 14 days have elapsed since the initial positive test if no symptoms have emerged during this time. Patients who experienced more severe symptoms due to COVID-19, older patients, and patients with certain malignancies (lung cancer and hematologic malignancies, for example) might require additional time to recover before resumption of antineoplastic treatment [16].

Other institutions leave the decision to individual clinician's judgment as to the immunosuppressive potential of the specific regimen. At some institutions, testing of asymptomatic outpatients before initiating anticancer treatment is limited to those with hematologic malignancies especially for patients with a B-cell hematologic malignancy who are receiving anti-CD20 monoclonal antibodies, which are associated with B-cell depletion, and severe lymphopenia.At many institutions, testing is offered to lung cancer patients who present for surgery, bronchoscopy, or high-risk outpatient testing (eg, pulmonary function tests), as well as to those who are symptomatic or potentially exposed to a virus carrier, but not to others [16, 17, 18].

TREATMENT OF COVID-19 INFECTION IN CANCER PATIENTS

All patients should be informed regarding the symptoms of COVID-19, trained in proper handwashing and hygiene, and advised to wear facial masks in public and minimize exposure to large crowds [14].

COVID-19 disease management is the same in cancer patients as in the general population. Many mild cases (eg, fever, cough, and/or myalgias without dyspnea or hypoxia) and asymptomatic infections can be managed conservatively at home if individuals can be adequately isolated. However, patients with more severe disease may warrant a higher level of care. Agents used specifically for COVID-19 are reserved for patients with severe disease [19].

One area of the potential impact of specific COVID-19 treatments is in cancer patients who have been receiving anti-CD20 therapies, which induce rapid and prolonged B cell depletion. In a case report of a patient with persistent viremia from SARS-CoV-2 who had received rituximab for lymphoma, convalescent plasma resulted in rapid recovery [20].

Another issue is drug interactions between COVID-19 therapies and anticancer agents. The French Society for Oncology Pharmacy has published detailed information about these potential interactions that may be of value in decision-making around the choice of both anti-COVID and anticancer therapy [21].

ASCO recommends that until more definitive information emerges, decisions about interrupting anticancer treatment in patients with active COVID-19 should be based on a clinical benefit: risk assessment that considers the risk of interrupting cancer treatment versus the still poorly defined risk of adverse COVID-19 outcomes in patients receiving active cancer treatment [14].

Although data are very limited, one small study and at least two case reports have suggested that the use of Bruton tyrosine kinase (BTK) inhibitors for patients with a chronic hematologic malignancy may be associated with less severe infection [22, 23].

Glucocorticoids may be beneficial for patients who are hospitalized with severe SARS-CoV-2 infection In other situations, for patients who are receiving glucocorticoids for management of their cancer or treatment-associated toxicities, the decision as to whether to continue or discontinue in a patient diagnosed with COVID-19 must be individualized, and depends in part on the dose and indication for the glucocorticoid. As an example, decision-making for high-dose glucocorticoids in a patient with brain metastases or epidural spinal cord compression, or a serious immunotherapy-related adverse event, is more difficult and must be addressed on a case-by-case basis [24].

Some oral none immunosuppressive therapies such as hormonal therapies, including androgen deprivation therapy or drugs targeting activating mutations (epidermal growth factor receptor inhibitors or BRAF/MEK inhibitors) may be continued on a case-by-case basis [14].

According to ASCO guidelines, cancer therapy can be reinitiated if at least 24 hours have passed since the resolution of fever without the use of antipyretics, and there is an improvement in symptoms (eg, cough, shortness of breath). For asymptomatic patients, waiting at least 20 days after the initial positive test is recommended. For most patients, obtaining at least one negative SARS-CoV-2 test before reinitiating anticancer therapy is preferred [14].

Cancer patients who have a persistently positive test, despite symptom resolution should avoid treatment in the same infusion room with other uninfected cancer patients receiving chemotherapy until they convert to a negative test. ASCO guidelines suggest that specific areas and dedicated staff be designated for treatment of COVID-19-positive patients physical distancing rules and contact limitations remain essential components of cancer treatments amid the pandemic to protect the patient, the health care workers, and other non-COVID-19 patients being treated in the same center [14].

REFERENCES

[1] Jerusalem G. Expected medium and longterm impact of the COVID-19 outbreak in oncology. Presented at: *European Society for Medical Oncology (ESMO) 2020 Opening Press Conference.* September 10, 2020. Virtual. Abstract LBA76.

[2] Liang W, Guan W, Chen R, Wang W, Li J, Xu K, Li C, Ai Q, Lu W, Liang H, Li S, He J. Cancer patients in SARS-CoV-2 infection: a nationwide analysis in China. *The Lancet Oncology* 2020; 21(3):335.

[3] Rogado J, Obispo B, Pangua C, Serrano-Montero G, Martín Marino A, Pérez-Pérez M, López-Alfonso A, Gullón P, Lara MÁ. Covid-19 transmission, outcome and associated risk factors in cancer patients at the first month of the pandemic in a Spanish hospital in Madrid. *Clin. Transl. Oncol.* 2020: May 25.

[4] Berghoff A S, Gansterer M, Bathke A C, Trutschnig W, Hungerländer P, Berger J M, Kreminger J, Starzer A M, Strassl R, Schmidt R, Willschke H, Lamm W, Raderer M,Gottlieb A D, Mauser N J, Preusser M SARS-CoV-2 Testing in Patients with Cancer Treated at a Tertiary Care Hospital During the COVID-19 Pandemic. *J. Clin. Oncol.* 2020:38:1-10.

[5] V T, Girdhar P, Advani P, Sharma A, Elumalai T, Hsieh C, Elghazawy H I, Verma V, Krishnan S A systematic review and meta-analysis of cancer patients affected by a novel coronavirus. *medRxiv*. 2020; 10.1101/2020.05.27.20115303.

[6] Giannakoulis V G, Papoutsi E, Siempos II Effect of Cancer on Clinical Outcomes of Patients With COVID-19: A Meta-Analysis of Patient Data. *JCO Glob. Oncol.* 2020; 6:799.

[7] Rogado J, Obispo B, Pangua C, Serrano-Montero G, Martín Marino A, Pérez-Pérez M, López-Alfonso A, Gullón P, Lara MÁ Covid-19 transmission, outcome and associated risk factors in cancer patients at the first month of the pandemic in a Spanish hospital in Madrid. *Clin. Transl. Oncol.* 2020.

[8] Mehta V, Goel S, Kabarriti R, Cole D, Goldfinger M, Acuna-Villaorduna A, Pradhan K, Thota R, Reissman S, Sparano J A, Gartrell B A, Smith R V, Ohri N, Garg M, Racine A D, Kalnicki S, Perez-Soler R, Halmos B, Verma A Case Fatality Rate of Cancer Patients with COVID-19 in a New York Hospital System. *Cancer Discov.* 2020;10(7):935.

[9] Marina Chiara Garassino, Jennifer G Whisenant, Li-Ching Huang, Annalisa Trama, Valter Torri, Francesco Agustoni et al., on behalf of the TERAVOLT investigators COVID-19 in patients with thoracic malignancies (TERAVOLT): first results of an international, registry-based, cohort study. *Lancet Oncol.* 2020; 21: 914–22.

[10] Kuderer N M, Choueiri T K, Shah D P, Shyr Y, Rubinstein S M, Rivera D R et.al., on behalf of COVID-19 and Cancer Consortium Clinical impact of COVID-19 on patients with cancer (CCC19): a cohort study. *Lancet.* 2020; 395(10241):1907.

[11] Lee L Y, Cazier J B, Angelis V, Arnold R, Bisht V et.al. UK Coronavirus Monitoring Project Team, Kerr R, Middleton G COVID-19 mortality in patients with cancer on chemotherapy or other anticancer treatments: a prospective cohort study. *Lancet.* 2020; 395(10241):1919.

[12] Robilotti E V, Babady N E, Mead P A, Rolling T, Perez-Johnston R, Bernardes M, et al. Determinants of COVID-19 disease severity in patients with cancer. *Nat. Med.* 2020;26(8):1218.

[13] Luo J, Rizvi H, Egger J V, Preeshagul I R, Wolchok J D, Hellmann M D mpact of PD-1 Blockade on Severity of COVID-19 in Patients with Lung Cancers. *Cancer Discov.* 2020;10(8):1121.

[14] American Society of Clinical Oncology (ASCO) *Guidelines.*

[15] Madariaga A, McMullen M, Sheikh S, Kumar R, Liu F F, Zimmermann C, Husain S, Zadeh G, Oza A M COVID-19 Testing in Patients with Cancer: Does One Size Fit All? *Clin. Cancer Res.* 2020;26(18):4737.

[16] Diane Reidy-Lagunes, MD, MS, Leonard Saltz, MD, Michael Postow, MD, Michael Scordo, MD, Alison Moskowitz, MD, William Tew, MD, Dmitriy Zamarin, MD, PhD, Gil Redelman-Sidi, MD, PhD Recommendations for Testing and Treating Outpatient Cancer Patients in the Era of COVID-19 *JNCI: Journal of the National Cancer Institute*, online August 14 https://doi.org/10.1093/jnci/djaa111.

[17] Passaro A, Peters S, Mok T S K, Attili I, Mitsudomi T, de Marinis F Testing for COVID-19 in lung cancer patients. *Ann. Oncol.* 2020;31(7):832.

[18] CalabròL, Peters S, Soria J C, Di Giacomo A M, Barlesi F, Covre A, Altomonte M, Vegni V, Gridelli C, Reck M, Rizvi N, Maio M Challenges in lung cancer therapy during the COVID-19 pandemic. *Lancet Respir. Med.* 2020;8(6):542.

[19] Rivera D R, Peters S, Panagiotou O A, Shah D P, Kuderer N M, Hsu C Y et.al on behalf of, COVID-19 and Cancer Consortium Utilization of COVID-19 Treatments and Clinical Outcomes among Patients with Cancer: A COVID-19 and Cancer Consortium (CCC19) *Cohort Study Cancer Discov.* 2020.

[20] Clark E, Guilpain P, Filip I L, Pansu N, Le Bihan C, Cartron G, Tchernonog E, Roubille C, Morquin D, Makinson A, Tuaillon E, Le Moing V Convalescent plasma for persisting COVID-19 following therapeutic lymphocyte depletion: a report of rapid recovery. *Br. J. Haematol.* 2020;190(3):154.

[21] Slimano F, Baudouin A, Zerbit J, Toulemonde-Deldicque A, Thomas-Schoemann A, Chevrier R, Daouphars M, Madelaine I, Pourroy B, Tournamille J F, Astier A, Ranchon F, Cazin J L, Bardin C, Rioufol C. Cancer, immune suppression and Coronavirus Disease-19 (COVID-19): Need to manage drug safety (French Society for Oncology Pharmacy [SFPO]guidelines) *Cancer Treat Rev.* 2020; 88:102063.

[22] Treon S P, Castillo J J, Skarbnik A P, Soumerai J D, Ghobrial I M, Guerrera M L, Meid K, Yang G. The BTK inhibitor ibrutinib may protect against pulmonary injury in COVID-19-infected patients. *Blood.* 2020;135(21):1912.

[23] Thibaud S, Tremblay D, Bhalla S, Zimmerman B, Sigel K, Gabrilove J Protective role of Bruton tyrosine kinase inhibitors in patients with chronic lymphocytic leukaemia and COVID-19. *Br J. Haematol.* 2020;190(2): e73.

[24] Lamontagne F, Agoritsas T, Macdonald H, Leo YS, Diaz J, Agarwal A et al. A living WHO guideline on drugs for covid-19 *BMJ.* 2020;370:m3379.

In: Coronavirus Disease
Editor: Yildiz Dincer
ISBN: 978-1-53619-296-4

Chapter 16

COVID-19 FROM GENERAL SURGERY PERSPECTIVE

Selen Soylu[1], MD and Serkan Teksoz[2,*], MD
[1]Basaksehir Cam and Sakura City Hospital, Department of General Surgery, Istanbul, Turkey
[2]Istanbul University, Cerrahpasa, Cerrahpasa Medical Faculty, Department of General Surgery, Istanbul, Turkey

ABSTRACT

With the rapid incline of Coronavirus Disease 2019 (COVID-19) cases, healthcare staff was urged to get organized for this new period. While preserving personal protective equipment, general ward beds, and intensive care unit beds physicians face difficulties. Getting infected for surgical teams mean additional workload for the remaining staff and in some cases, loss of the senior surgeon. Only emergent surgical cases are suggested to be performed to keep the healthcare staff ready and healthy for further months. Surgical staff should be minimized and personal protective equipment should be provided for hospital staff. Basic knowledge of COVID-19, action plans, algorithms for emergency and elective surgeries are necessary for surgical teams.

Keywords: surgery, COVID-19, personal protective equipment

INTRODUCTION

In Wuhan, China, pneumonia cases with unknown cause occurred in December 2019 [1]. Then it was discovered that this pneumonia is caused by severe acute respiratory

* Corresponding Author's Email: serkanteksoz@gmail.com.

syndrome coronavirus 2 (SARS-CoV-2). The disease spread throughout the world and on March 11, 2019.World Health Organisation declared pandemic and the disease was started to be called as Coronavirus Disease 2019 (COVID-19) [2].

Diagnosis

In patients with COVID-19 diagnosis; fever, dyspnea, fatigue, and muscle pain are the most common symptoms encountered [3]. Also nearly half of the infected patients remain asymptomatic. The diagnosis is confirmed by the real-time reverse transcription-polymerase chain reaction of viral nucleic acid [4]. In the laboratory evaluation; elevated D-Dimer, ferritin, alanine aminotransferase, aspartate aminotransferase, creatine kinase, lactate dehydrogenase, leukopenia, and lymphopenia are detected [5]. Radiologically, multiple ground-glass appearance and bilateral opacities, infiltrates are reported in chest X-rays. It should be kept in mind that patients with normal X-rays can also be diagnosed with COVID-19. In patients with suspected clinical, laboratory, and X-ray findings, chest computed tomography (CT) is the next step for diagnosis. Ground glass opacities and parenchymal consolidation are some characteristical findings in chest CT. These findings are usually seen bilaterally, in peripheral zones and lower lobes of lungs [3].

Precautions in the COVID Era

With the rapid incline of COVID-19 cases, healthcare staff was urged to get organized for this new period. To reduce the exposure and keep the healthcare staff safe, it is important to minimize the number of surgical teams and healthcare providers. In high-risk interventions producing aerosols, healthcare providers should use personal protective equipment (PPE) such as disposable head caps, gloves, long sleeve waterproof coats, long shoe covers, FFP2 (filtering facepiece) and FFP3 facial masks [6]. Disease Control Center suggested canceling all the elective procedures to keep healthcare providers safe. So, the healthcare staff have a reduced exposure risk and canprovide longer healthcare service for emergency surgeries [7].

Also, face-to-face outpatient visits of non-emergent patients were postponed in many hospitals. In the pandemic, all of the hospitals in Turkey, reduced the staff in the operating theater, rounds, canceled clinical routine meetings and student lectures were held online.

WHICH CASES AND HOW SHOULD WE OPERATE?

With the high transmission rate of the disease, workload and stress are high among healthcare providers. Getting infected in surgical teams mean additional workload for the remaining staff and at some cases, loss of the senior surgeon [8]. Only emergent surgical cases such as patients with life-threatening situations, active symptoms, and malignancy diagnosis should be performed in order to keep the healthcare staff ready and healthy for further months. Surgical staff should be minimized and personal protective equipment should be provided for hospital staff [6]. Efficiency in resource usage and reduction of the contamination risk may be provided by prioritizing the emergency surgeries and postponing elective surgeries, nonurgent procedures, and outpatient visits. To provide healthcare for nonemergent patients who were diagnosed with a disease; followup and treatment of these patient groups may benefit from remote medical care. Face-to-face visits may be replaced by video conferences [9].

Turkish Surgical Society suggests that in emergency surgery, patients should be tested for COVID-19 and every patient should be treated as positive unless proven otherwise. Personal protective equipment should be used [8]. Also, if the abdominal computed tomography (CT) is performed, thorax CT should be added. In elective surgeries, risk evaluation for COVID-19 should be done and a consent form stating that surgery has a high risk for COVID-19 disease, should be taken from the patient [10]. In the safe surgery algorithm, only emergency upper gastrointestinal endoscopies should be done. The laparoscopic procedure should not be used rather open procedures should be preferred. However, during the COVID-19 period, there is not a consensus on whether to do laparoscopy or laparotomy in emergency surgeries. Morris et al. suggested that laparoscopy can be used safely since no studies show COVID-19 is transmitted through aerosolized laparoscopic gas [11]. Also, with the laparoscopic approach, a hospital stay will be shorter so that more bed capacity could be provided for infected patient care and there will be less infection risk for the operated patient.

In the operating theater, a minimum number of medical staff should be assigned and all of them should wear PPE [6]. Positive pressure ventilation is preferred in the operating theater. All patients should wear a face mask if they are not intubated during the procedure. If a patient is proven to be COVID-19, the surgical procedures should be postponed if possible [10]. If resource usage is not done in a planned fashion, it is possible that soon, there will be a shortage of healthy senior surgeons, experienced medical staff due to infection .

When dealing with COVID-19 surgical patients, it is important to have a preemptive plan to minimize the risk of contamination. There should be separate pathways for suspected patients for operating theater transit. So that medical staff shortage is prevented due to unexpected viral spread [12]. A dedicated operation room is needed for COVID-19 patients and this room should be the nearest to the theater block entrance. Transfer routes should be short and transfer through these paths should be as quick as possible with a trained medical staff who wear PPE [12]. In the operating theater for COVID-19 surgical patients, a minimal number of medical staff should work and minimal material and if possible disposable material should be used. The operating theaters usually have positive pressure air exchange [13]. Negative pressure operating rooms with a high air exchange of $\geq$ 25 cycles/hour is suggested to minimize the infection risk [14]. Surgical theater should be sanitized after each procedure [12].

Alcoholic solutions are suggested to be used for hand sanitation. Also, PPE should be worn during the whole procedure. Goggles is crucial for preventing conjunctiva from viral transmission [15]. There is no research on whether there is a viral load in tissue samples or body fluid of the infected patient. But still, precautions with PPE should be taken before entering the surgery. Disposable materials are preferred to be used but if reusable materials are utilized they should be sterilized carefully. Also, ventilators should be disinfected with chloroderivate solution in a concentration $\geq$ 0.1% or 1000 parts per million [16].

Each hospital should have a detailed internal protocol for emergencies with COVID-19 patients so that a safe surgical procedure may be planned for all medical staff [12].

Oncological Operations During the Pandemic

In this public health emergency period, other than emergency surgeries, how to handle oncological surgeries is crucial. Postponing elective surgeries in order to maintain capacity in the healthcare system reduces the risk of additional exposure to infection [10]. There is an erratic dilemma in dealing with cancer patients. On one hand, there is a concern of tumor progression, a decline in survival, and increased risk of complications; on the other hand, there is an increased risk of cancer patients dying from COVID-19. A safe delay strategy is needed for this issue. Turage et al. analyzed 4 million cancer patients and found out that most cancer surgeries can safely be postponed for at least one month without having a drastic impact on tumor progression or survival rate [17].

American College of Surgeons (ACS) divided COVID-19 period into three phases: semi-urgent setting, a period where hospitals have enough intensive care units and COVID cases does not increase rapidly; an urgent setting where intensive care units and mechanical ventilators are limited, operating theater supplies are limited and there is a rapid incline of COVID patients; phase 3, where all intensive care units and mechanical ventilators are full [18].

In a semi-urgent setting, for breast malignancies and emergencies, ACS recommended operating on malignancy recurrence, triple-negative, and HER 2 positive patients. Breast abscess, hematoma drainage, ischemic mastectomy flap, and autologous tissue flap revision are suggested to be operated in an urgent setting in phase 3 [18].

For gastrointestinal tumors, early-stage rectal cancers for which adjuvant therapy is not recommended, rectal cancers after neoadjuvant chemoradiotherapy with no regression, nearly obstructing rectal cancer, cancers with the risk of local perforation are suggested to be operated in the semi-urgent setting. In an urgent setting, nearly obstructing colon cancer where the stent is not an option and cancers with local perforation, should be operated. In phase 3, only actively bleeding, perforated, and obstructed cancers are suggested for operation [18].

Emergency Surgery in the COVID-19 Period

Although elective surgeries are postponed in the COVID-19 pandemic, emergency surgeries such as the acute abdomen, trauma surgery, and emergency endoscopies cannot be delayed [19]. To deliver surgical care safely and effectively is the main goal. Nepogodiev et al. reviewed 13 articles and found out that reducing elective surgeries will reduce the risk of infection, provide more beds in general ward and intensive care units for COVID-19 patients and boost the number of doctors to take care of COVID-19 patients [20].

American College of Surgeons stated that mesenteric ischemia, perforated hollow organs, necrotizing fasciitis, incarcerated hernia, close loop obstruction and patients in septic or hemorrhagic shock should be operated without delay as emergency cases [18].

Uncomplicated appendicitis could be followed with oral antibiotherapy while appendicitis with abscess or perforation could undergo percutaneous drainage. However, if conservative management fails, surgery should be the only choice [18]. Necrotizing soft tissue infections or large soft tissue abscess and large perianal abscess should be treated in operating theater [18].

Surgical Education During the Pandemic

In this unprecedented time of the COVID-19 pandemic, residents had flexible working hours and shift based schedules to take care of patients in order to minimize the exposure risk. Other than their own department, they had to work directly with COVID-19 patients so, they were more exposed to getting infected. Moreover, since they were only able to get involved in emergency surgeries, they had a quantitative loss of operation experience, clinical judgment, teaching, leadership skills, and basic patient-physician relationship [21]. In many countries, residents were engaged in virtual education and online theoretical sessions to recover the loss of education and training. Continuing surgical education is difficult in this era. However, with new ways of training the lost time will be recovered in a way [22].

TELEMEDICINE

During the pandemic, telemedicine becomes popular since many healthcare givers were able to contact their followup patients through this route. It reduced the visit time, cost, and increase patient satisfaction [23, 24]. Through video calls or teleconferences, suitable patients could be followed.

In surgeries with low postoperative complication risks or in patients who are already diagnosed with a disease and just need a close followup, telemedicine is an ideal approach to seek healthcare guidance [9]. In the COVID-19 period, teleconferences reduce face-to-face contact and also contamination risk. It also decreases the burden on outpatient clinics. However, before the application of telemedicine services, technological infrastructure and patient privacy issues should be considered with care [25].

Although many physicians are doubtful about any superiority of telemedicine to traditional outpatient clinic visits, some publications are supporting the applicability and cost-effectiveness of telemedicine [26, 9].

We believe that the first patient visit should be done face-to-face during the pandemic period since physical evaluation, the stress level of a patient is crucial for clinical decision making. After the first visit, according to the disease status and patient's compliance, telemedicine could be used.

CONCLUDING REMARKS

In the COVID-19 pandemic, it is important to keep healthcare providers safe by using personal protective equipment with great care and thus reducing the risk of contamination. All surgeons from different subspecialties should be trained to recognize COVID-19 patients. First, when physicians from other specialties such as internal medicine, infectious diseases, ear-nose-throat get infected or exhausted, they will be replaced with physicians from other specialties such as surgery. Second, in patients undergoing emergency surgery due to perforated gallbladder, bowel or mesenteric ischemia, it should be kept in mind that there can be concurrent COVID-19 [20]. Third, after an emergency or elective surgery, the patient could get infected with COVID-19 when observed in the general ward. [20].

The surgeons should think of their safety first to keep on working during this unprecedented period. Guidelines and recommendations for each hospital or country should be prepared. Strict rules on how to transport a COVID-19 patient for operation and protection measures that need to be taken before, during, and after surgery should be established. Guidelines for elective and emergency surgeries during the COVID-19 period will help the physicians to decide when and how to operate.

REFERENCES

[1] Li, Q, Guan X., Wu P., Wang X., Zhou L., Tong Y et al., 2020. "Early Transmission Dynamics in Wuhan, China, of Novel Coronavirus–Infected Pneumonia," *New England Journal of Medicine.* 382(13): 1199–1207. https://doi.org/10.1056/NEJMoa20 01316.

[2] WHO, *"Country & Technical Guidance - Coronavirus Disease (COVID-19),"* April 24, 2020. https://www.who.int/emergencies/ diseases/novel-coronavirus-2019/technical-guidance.

[3] Borges do Nascimento I J, Cacic N, Abdulazeem H M, von Groote T C, Jayarajah U, Weerasekara I et al., "Novel Coronavirus Infection (COVID-19) in Humans: A Scoping Review and Meta-Analysis." *Journal of Clinical Medicine.* 9 (4): 941. https://doi.org/10.3390/ jcm9040941.

[4] Corman V., Landt O., Kaiser M., Molenkamp R., Meijer A., Chu D et al. "Detection of 2019 Novel Coronavirus (2019-NCoV) by Real-Time RT-PCR," *Eurosurveillance.* 25 (3). published online January 23, 2020. https://doi.org/ 10.2807/1560-7917.ES.2020.25.3. 2000045.

[5] Zhou F., Yu T., Du R., Fan G., Liu Y., Liu Z et al. "Clinical Course and Risk Factors for Mortality of Adult Inpatients with COVID-19 in Wuhan, China: A Retrospective Cohort Study." *Lancet.* 395(10229): 1054–62. https://doi.org/ 10.1016/S0140-6736(20)30566-3.

[6] Wong T., Lee C., Tam W., Lau J., Yu T., Lui S. et al. "Cluster of SARS among Medical Students Exposed to Single Patient, Hong Kong," *Emerging Infectious Diseases.* 10 (2):269–76. published online February 2004. https://doi.org/ 10.3201/eid1002.030452.

[7] Center for Disease Control, *"Interim Guidance for Healthcare Facilities: Preparing for Community Transmission of COVID-19 in the United States,"* Published online. February 29, 2020. https://www.cdc.gov/coronavirus/2019-ncov/hcp/guidance-hcf.html?CDC_AA_refVal=https%3A%2F%2F www.cdc.gov%2Fcoronavirus%2F2019-ncov%2Fhealthcare-facilities%2Fguidance-hcf.html.

[8] Karaca, A. S., Özmen M., Uçar A. D., Yastı A. Ç., Demirer S. "General Surgery Operating Room Practice in Patients with COVID-19," *Turk. J. Surg*. 2020; 36 (1): I-V.

[9] Kimberly H., Sherry M. W. "Telehealth Follow-up in Lieu of Postoperative Clinic Visit for Ambulatory Surgery: Results of a Pilot Program," *JAMA Surgery*. 148(9):823. published online. September 1, 2013. https://doi.org/10.1001/jamasurg.2013.2672.

[10] Brücher B., Nigri G., Tinelli A., Lapeña J. F., Basany E. E., Macri P et al. *COVID-19: Pandemic surgery guidance. 4open. 2020.* 3(1):19. https://doi.org/10.1051/fopen/2020002.

[11] Morris S. N., Fader A. N., Milad M. P., Dionisi H. J., Stephanie N. "Understanding the 'Scope' of the Problem: Why Laparoscopy Is Considered Safe during the COVID-19 Pandemic." *Journal of Minimally Invasive Gynecology*. 27(4):789–91. published online. May 2020. https://doi.org/10.1016/j.jmig.2020.04.002.

[12] Coccolini F., Perrone G., Chiarugi M., Di Marzo F., Ansaloni L., Scandroglio I et al. "Surgery in COVID-19 Patients: Operational Directives," *World Journal of Emergency Surgery*. 15(1): 25. published online. December 2020. https://doi.org/10.1186/s13017-020-00307-2.

[13] Wong J., Goh Q. Y., Tan Z., Lie S. A., Tay Y. C., Ng S. H., Soh C. R. "Preparing for a COVID-19 Pandemic: A Review of Operating Room Outbreak Response Measures in a Large Tertiary Hospital in Singapore." *Canadian Journal of Anesthesia/Journal Canadien d'anesthésie*. 67(6): 732–45. published online. June 2020. https:// doi.org/10.1007/s12630-020-01620-9.

[14] Moletta L., Pierobon E. S., Capovilla G., Costantini M., Salvador R., Merigliano S. "International Guidelines and Recommendations for Surgery during Covid-19 Pandemic: A Systematic Review." *International Journal of Surgery*. 79: 180–88. published online. (July 2020) https://doi.org/10.1016/j.ijsu.2020.05.061.

[15] Wang D., Hu B., Hu C., Zhu F., Liu X., Zhang J. Etal. "Clinical Characteristics of 138 Hospitalized Patients With 2019 Novel Coronavirus–Infected Pneumonia in Wuhan, China." *JAMA*. 323(11.9: 1061. published online. March 17, 2020. https://doi.org/10.1001/jama.2020.1585.

[16] Kampf G., Todt D., Pfaender S., Steinmann E. "Persistence of Coronaviruses on Inanimate Surfaces and Their Inactivation with Biocidal Agents." *The Journal of Hospital Infection*. 104 (3): 246–51, published online. March 2020. https://doi.org/10.1016/j.jhin.2020. 01.022.

[17] Turaga K. K., Girotra S. "Are We Harming Cancer Patients by Delaying Their Cancer Surgery During the COVID-19 Pandemic?," *Annals of Surgery*. Published Ahead of Print June 2, 2020. https://doi. org/10.1097/SLA.0000000000003967.

[18] American College of Surgeons, *"COVID 19: Elective Case Triage Guidelines for Surgical Care Updated,"* March 27, 2020.

[19] Gok A. F. K., Eryılmaz M., Ozmen M. M., Alimoglu O., Ertekin C., Kurtoglu M. H. "Recommendations for Trauma and Emergency General Surgery Practice During COVID-19 Pandemic." *Turkish Journal of Trauma and Emergency Surgery*. published online. 2020 https://doi.org/10.14744/tjtes.2020.79954.

[20] COVIDSurg Collaborative. "Global Guidance for Surgical Care during the COVID-19 Pandemic: Surgical Care during the COVID-19 Pandemic." *British Journal of Surgery*. 107 (9): 1097–1103. published online. August 2020. https://doi.org/10.1002/bjs.11646.

[21] Zheng J., Hundeyin M., He K., Sachs T., Hess D. T., Whang E. "General Surgery Chief Residents' Perspective on Surgical Education during the Coronavirus Disease 2019 (COVID-19) Pandemic." *Surgery*. 168 (2): 222–25. published online. August 2020. https://doi.org/10.1016/j.surg.2020.06.003.

[22] Dedeilia A., Sotiropoulos M. G., Hanrahan J. G., Janga D., Dedeilias P., Sideris M. "Medical and Surgical Education Challenges and Innovations in the COVID-19 Era: A Systematic Review." *In Vivo*. 34 (3): 1603–11. published online. June 2020. https://doi.org/10. 21873/ invivo.11950.

[23] Russo J. E., McCool R. R., Davies L. "VA Telemedicine: An Analysis of Cost and Time Savings." *Telemedicine and E-Health*. 22 (3): 209–15. published online. March 2016. https://doi.org/10.1089/ tmj.2015.0055.

[24] Cain S. M., Moore R., Sturm L., Mason T., Fuhrman C., Smith R. "Clinical Assessment and Management of General Surgery Patients via Synchronous Telehealth," *Journal of Telemedicine and Telecare*. 23(2): 371–75. published online. February 2017. https://doi.org/ 10.1177/1357633X16636245.

[25] Zheng F., Park K. W., Thi W. J., Ro C. C., Bass B. L., Yeh M. W. "Financial Implications of Telemedicine Visits in an Academic Endocrine Surgery Program." *Surgery*. 165(3) : 617–21. published online. March 2019. https://doi.org/10.1016/j. surg. 2018.08.017.

[26] Wade V. A., Karnon J., Elshaug A. G., Hiller J. E. "A Systematic Review of Economic Analyses of Telehealth Services Using Real-Time Video Communication." *BMC Health Services Research.* 10 (1): 233. published online. December 2010. https://doi.org/10. 1186/1472-6963-10-233.

In: Coronavirus Disease
Editor: Yildiz Dincer
ISBN: 978-1-53619-296-4

Chapter 17

CYTOKINE STORM AND OXIDATIVE STRESS IN SEVERE COVID-19

Yildiz Dincer*, PhD and Selin Yuksel, MSc
Istanbul University - Cerrahpasa, Cerrahpasa Medical Faculty, Department of Medical Biochemistry, Istanbul, Turkey

ABSTRACT

Some patients infected with the SARS-CoV-2 virus show rapid progress to acute respiratory distress syndrome, multi-organ failure, and death. Acute respiratory distress syndrome is a large concern of death in COVID-19. Current therapeutic strategies focus on the virus itself and antiviral drugs are used to manage the disease. Unfortunately, the benefits of antiviral drugs are not satisfactory in every patient. It seems that the excessive inflammatory response rather than the virus titer is more relevant to the death. A brisk immune response generally destroys the virus but can cause significant local and long-term damage in tissues. In severe COVID-19, acute respiratory distress syndrome and multi-organ failure are associated with cytokine storm. Cytokine storm triggers the production of reactive oxygen species storm in immune system cells to destroy the virus. Although a certain amount of reactive oxygen species is helpful in the regulation of immune response and killing viruses, an excessive amount of reactive oxygen species damages the cellular lipids, proteins, and DNA. Extensive damage by reactive oxygen species results in apoptosis. Apoptotic death of endothelial and epithelial cells in the lungs plays important role in the development of acute respiratory distress syndrome in COVID-19 patients. Here, we will summarize the current molecular understanding of the vicious circle between the cytokine storm and oxidative stress that is an executive factor for cells.

Keywords: COVID-19, cytokine storm, reactive oxygen species, oxidative stress

* Corresponding Author's Email: yldz.dincer@gmail.com.

INTRODUCTION

COVID-19 (coronavirus disease 2019) caused by the SARS-CoV-2 virus is spreading rapidly worldwide. No specific antiviral therapy and vaccine are available. Although many patients have mild or moderate symptoms, some patients show rapid progress to acute respiratory distress syndrome (ARDS), septic shock, multi-organ failure, and death [1]. In general, conditions such as advanced age, comorbidity, high body mass index are associated with severe disease. Besides, in COVID-19 survivors, life quality was observed to be low even 12 months after discharge from the hospital. Reduced lung function, reduced ability to exercise and mental health problems were seen in some survivors up to 6 months and beyond [2]. These long-term complications of COVID-19 in survivors indicate that not only acute executive conditions but also some long-term degenerative processes are triggered during the disease. Cytokine storm is a common feature in critically ill COVID-19 patients. Cytokine storm occurs due to uncontrolled activation of the immune system. It can lead to hyper inflammation, multi-organ failure, and can even die. Increased plasma levels of the cytokines including IL-2, IL-6, IL-7, IL-10, TNF-α, IFN-α, granulocyte-macrophage colony-stimulating factor (GM-CSF) were reported in severally ill COVID-19 patients [3].

CYTOKINE STORM IN COVID-19

Cytokine storm is a general term used to define abnormal cytokine release in response to infection and other stimuli. It occurs due to loss of regulatory control on proinflammatory cytokine production. The innate and adaptive immune responses activated by SARS-CoV-2 infection cause uncontrolled inflammatory responses leading to the cytokine storm [4]. Cytokines and chemokines are small peptides or glycoproteins that exert their actions by binding cell surface receptors. They act as signal molecule to activate immune system cells for chemotaxis and diapedesis and induce acute phase response. The overproduction of cytokines and chemokines increases the severity of the inflammation and a vicious cycle starts. The immune system is stimulated more than usual in patients with severe COVID-19. Especially if the patient had already got a chronic inflammation, the outcome gets worse. The cytokine storm can lead to excessive cellular damage that triggers apoptosis of epithelial and endothelial cells, vascular leakage, and finally results in acute respiratory distress syndrome (ARDS), multi-organ failure, and death [5]. The cytokine storm may be responsible for long-term complications of COVID-19 in survivors.

In viral infections, the body's first line of defense is the innate immune response. The SARS-CoV-2 virus induces a delayed elevation in the levels of proinflammatory cytokines and chemokines [6, 7]. In the early phase of SARS-CoV-2 infection, the release of cytokines and chemokines from respiratory epithelial cells, dendritic cells, and macrophages is delayed. Afterward, cells secrete low levels of antiviral factors, INF-α and INF-β, but high levels of proinflammatory cytokines such as interleukin (IL)-1 β, IL-6, and tumor necrosis factor (TNF) and chemokines such as C-C motif chemokine ligand (CCL)-2, CCL-3, and CCL-5 [8-10]. Publications indicate that interferon response is dysfunctional in critically ill patients during the pandemic COVID-19 [11]. IFN-1 α and IFN-1 β are the key molecules that trigger the innate immune response in the early stages of viral infections. IFN-1 α and IFN-1 β exert antiviral activity by the induction of numerous interferon-stimulated genes that antagonize viral replication by various mechanisms. However, along with the activation of immune cells, SARS-CoV-2 expresses proteins that inhibit the synthesis of IFN-1 α and IFN-1 β thus weakens the immune responses and provides an optimal environment for rapid replication of the virus [12]. The low IFN-1 level at the onset of the disease delays the body's antiviral response. Afterward, the rapid increase of cytokines and chemokines attracts a large number of neutrophils, monocytes, and pathogenic inflammatory mononuclear macrophages to the infection site. Neutrophils migrate through the blood vessels and are recruited to the site of infection. Monocytes move into tissues and differentiate into macrophages. Excessive infiltration of these phagocytic cells into the lungs causes tissue damage, likely oxidative damage.

Cytokine Storm-Induced Reactive Oxygen Species Production

When activated, all phagocytic cells bind and engulf pathogens to destroy. They can use oxygen-dependent and oxygen-independent mechanisms to kill pathogens. In oxygen-dependent systems, membrane-bound NADPH oxidase is activated, oxygen utilization increases (respiratory burst), and reactive oxygen species (ROS) are produced. ROS can cross the membranes of bacterial pathogens and destroy them by damaging their nucleic acids, proteins, and cell membranes. Superoxide anions produced by NADPH activity generate hydrogen peroxide (H_2O_2) via superoxide dismutase. The myeloperoxidase chlorinates H_2O_2 and produces hypochlorous acid (HClO) which is the strongest bactericidal agent. NADPH oxidase is a multi-protein complex that is made up of five components and a small GTPase protein, Rac2. Flavocytochrome b558 (cytb558) is found in the active site of the enzyme and transfers electrons from cytosolic NADPH to molecular oxygen. At resting state, cytb558 resides at the membranes of phagosomes, secretory vesicles, specific granules, and the plasma membrane. When neutrophils are activated, the regulatory cytosolic complex translocates to the membrane and interacts with cytb558 to activate NADPH oxidase. Activated GTP-bound Rac2 contributes to the assembly of the regulatory cytosolic complex [13]. Superoxide anions produced by the NADPH oxidase activity are the precursor in the generation of other ROS that all contribute to the destruction of the pathogens. In the presence of transition metal ions such as Fe^{2+} or Cu^{2+} superoxide anions can react with H_2O_2 to produce hydroxyl radical (OH^{-}.) that is the most active form of ROS.

Nitric oxide (NO) that is synthesized from arginine and NADPH by inducible nitric oxide synthase is the precursor of reactive nitrogen species (RNS). Superoxide anions can react with NO to produce peroxynitrite ($ONOO^{-}$), a strong oxidant. When the respiratory burst is triggered and superoxide anions are produced, if NO is present, peroxynitrite is generated as long as the respiratory burst lasts [14]. Superoxide anion is a short-lived ROS with limited diffusion within the cell, its cytotoxic effect occurs due to its derivatives including H_2O_2, hydroxyl radical, and peroxynitrite. Both peroxynitrite and NO are toxic to mitochondria [15] leading to mitochondrial dysfunction which in turn increases superoxide anion production. Mitochondrial dysfunction is a general mechanism of ROS production detected in most viral infections because several viruses induce oxidative stress to facilitate their replication in the host cell [16-18]. In viral infections, tissue damage occurs due to oxidative stress formed by cytokine storm and mitochondrial dysfunction. COVID-19 does share many similar symptoms with SARS and influenza. In an experimental study, viral replication increased rapidly and peaked on day 4, then reduced to baseline on day 8 in mice infected by the influenza virus. The lung damage index increased from day 2 and peaked from day 8 to day 10. Mice began to die from day 8 to day 14 [19]. ROS and NO in the infected mice started producing from day 5 and peaked on day 8 [20]. These results confirm the idea that cytokine storm triggers a ROS storm in COVID-19 and oxidative damage is responsible for worse outcomes in patients.

Pro-inflammatory cytokines including IL-6, TNF-α, IFN-α, IFNγ, and chemokines such as GM-CSF are up-regulated in COVID-19 patients [3]. IL-6, TNFα, GM-CSF, IFNγ can induce the production of ROS and RNS in neutrophils. IL-6 and IFNγ induce expression of NADPH oxidase. IFNγ triggers the production of superoxide anions by inducing NADPH oxidase 2 (NOX2) [21]. IL 6 induces expression of NOX2 in human aortic endothelial cells [22]. Nrf2 is a transcription factor that up-regulates the expressions of many antioxidant enzymes. It was reported that the overexpression of circulating IL-6 increases the ROS production and accumulation in the diaphragm muscle of adult NSE/IL-6 mice, by deregulating the nuclear factor erythroid 2-related factor 2-(Nrf2-) mediated antioxidant response [23]. Respiratory viral infections are associated with inhibition of NRF2-mediated pathways. These viruses have evolved to acquire the ability to suppress the Nrf2 pathway in their favor [24].

At the inflammation site, neutrophils express a large number of cell surface receptors including cytokine receptors such as tumor necrosis factor receptors (TNFRs), and toll-like receptors (TLRs). All receptors are G-protein-coupled. Ligand binding to these receptors can prime neutrophils for a more strong response if additional signals are available. Activation of these receptors induces tyrosine kinase and MAP Kinase activation. Both pathways stimulate the regulation of the NADPH oxidase components to cause activation of the enzyme. One group of the priming ligands are proinflammatory cytokines such as tumor necrosis factor TNF-α, GM-CSF, IL-1b, IL-8, and IL-18. IL-1b and IL-18 induce respiratory burst weakly but TNF-α and GM-CSF exert a strong priming effect [25]. TNF-α primes neutrophils for oxidative burst by inducing calcium flux and p38 MAPK-dependent mobilization of $cytb_{558}$ to the plasma membrane [26]. GM-CSF primes cells by inducing phosphorylation of certain residues on regulatory components which in turn promotes translocation and docking of the cytosolic complex to the membrane that is required for activation of NADPH oxidase [25, 27].

Oxidative Damage in COVID-19

ROS are highly active chemical compounds that easily react with other molecules and damage them. The harmful effects of ROS occur in a few ways: (1) ROS can act as signaling messengers to stimulate inflammatory pathways, (2) ROS can impair cellular integrity and intracellular metabolism by oxidizing lipids, proteins, and nucleic acids (3) ROS can trigger apoptosis and lead to cell death, and organ failure, (4) ROS can consume antioxidant reserve and make macromolecules more vulnerable. The interaction between cytokines and ROS constitutes a *vicious cycle* in which cytokines stimulate production ROS and then ROS form an oxidative signal that stimulates inflammatory signaling pathways. For instance, an increase in H_2O_2 level act as a signal to induce expression of the IL-2 and IL-4 and facilitate induction of the transcription factor NF-κB which mediates induction of pro-inflammatory cytokines.

The harmful effects of ROS are counteracted by antioxidant enzymes and non-enzyme antioxidant molecules. Antioxidants inactivate ROS and prevent oxidative stress. Oxidative stress is a state in which ROS production overwhelms cellular antioxidant capacity. Cytokine storm leads to oxidative stress in COVID-19 patients by stimulating ROS production. While high ROS causes the rapid depletion of antioxidants, they also suppress the antioxidant defense mechanism by modulating Nrf-2 and/or NF-kB pathways resulting in exacerbation of inflammation and oxidative stress [28]. According to preclinical studies, overproduction of ROS and disruption of the antioxidant system play a key role in the pathogenesis, progression, and severity of SARS-CoV infections [29-31].

ROS attack to membranes causes oxidation of membrane proteins and lipids which results in impaired membrane integrity and function. Oxidation of intra-cellular proteins leads to their denaturation and functional loss. Oxidized phospholipids were detected in human and animal lung cells infected with SARS viruses. Oxidized phospholipids can induce cytokine storm and lung injury in SARS-CoV infection [32]. On the other hand, the damaging effects of excessive ROS on the red blood cell membrane and heme group function play an important role in hypoxic respiratory failure observed in the most severe patients of COVID-19. Excess ROS can disrupt the lateral and transversal distribution and organization of red blood cell membrane lipids by oxidizing polyunsaturated fatty acids of phospholipids. This alteration affects the diffusion of oxygen and carbon dioxide and the deformability capacity of red blood cells in the capillary vessels which in turn favors thrombocytosis. Excess ROS can impair the function of hemoglobin to carry oxygen. Heme iron must be kept in the reduced state (Fe^{2+}) to bind oxygen. ROS excess can disrupt the Fe^{2+}/Fe^{3+} balance by oxidizing iron to a $Fe3^{+}$ state. $Fe3^{+}$ can not bind oxygen, resulting in less efficient oxygen transport despite a high oxygen supply [33].

Microvascular thrombosis is the most important aspect of severe COVID-19. COVID-19 infection appears to be hypercoagulability and vascular endothelial dysfunction [34, 35]. COVID-19 patients who present a hypercoagulability state characterized by longer prothrombin times, higher fibrinogen levels and inflammatory markers have statistically significantly worse outcomes [36]. Over-activation of neutrophils may be a potential explanation for the diffuse microvascular thrombosis and capillary leak syndrome observed in critical COVID-19 patients. Endothelial function plays a key role in the maintenance of vascular integrity and inhibition of excessive thrombosis. Oxidative stress that is induced by cytokine storm is one of the causes of endothelial dysfunction in COVID-19 [37, 38]. TNF-α can stimulate both mitochondrial and NADPH oxidase-mediated ROS and NO production in endothelial cells. TNF-α induced oxidative damage plays a critical role in endothelial dysfunction [39].

ROS interaction with nucleic acids causes oxidation of purine/pyrimidine bases and DNA strand breaks. All contribute the impaired cell metabolism and function. In the case of mild to moderate oxidative stress, DNA strand breaks, and oxidized bases are repaired by DNA repair systems. However massive oxidative DNA damage is fatal to the cells. When genomic damage exceeds the DNA repair capacity, apoptosis is triggered. Apoptosis is one form of programmed cell death. Apoptotic changes in endothelial cells were showed histologically in COVID-19 [40]. Apoptosis of endothelial and epithelial cells damages the pulmonary microvascular and alveolar epithelial cell barriers and disrupts oxygenation by triggering coagulopathy in the alveolar vascular bed and vascular fluid leaking to the lung tissue. Therefore, apoptosis appears to be the most important pathogenic mechanism underlying ARDS. In cell culture experiments, a viral protease (SARS-CoV $3CL^{pro}$) was found to trigger ROS production and apoptosis in the host cells [31, 41]. SARS-CoV $3CL^{pro}$ activates the NF-kB-dependent reporter gene in HL-CZ cells. ROS-activated NF-kB signaling induced by SARS-CoV $3CL^{pro}$ was suggested as a contributory factor in SARS-CoV pathophysiology [31]. All mitogen-activated protein kinases (MAPKs) are activated in the response of environmental stresses including oxidative stress and DNA damage derived from viral infections. A SARS-CoV's protease, the 3a protein, was found to be associated with the activation of apoptotic cell death through p38 MAPK activation [41]. In autopsy studies, hallmarks of apoptosis were observed in SARS-CoV-infected lung, spleen, and thyroid tissues [42].

In addition to ARDS, some patients develop various neurologic symptoms, ranging from hyposmia, headache, and dizziness to seizures and stroke. Severely affected patients are more prone to develop neurological damage than mild or moderate cases [43]. The neurological symptoms may be derived from the direct effects of the coronavirus on the nervous system and/or systemic effects of the disease. The local increased production of cytokines in the cerebral tissue can induce neuroinflammation, oxidative stress that are underlying pathogenic mechanisms of neurodegenerative diseases such as Alzheimer's disease and Parkinson's disease. Particularly in elderly individuals, neurological damage that occurs due to COVID-19 may lead to serious neurodegenerative diseases in the post-COVID-19 term.

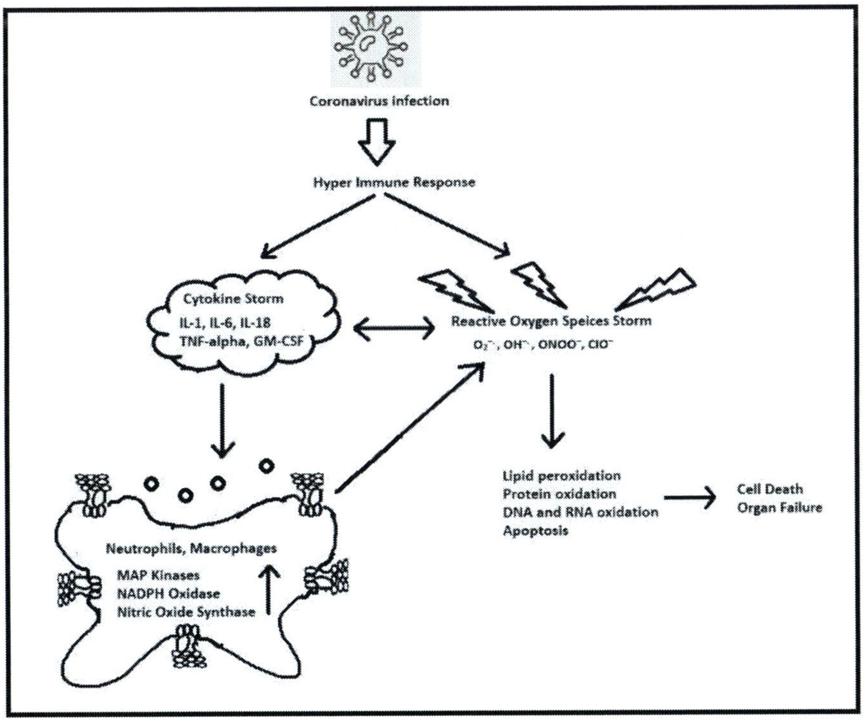

Figure 1. Cytokine storm-driven oxidative damage in severe COVID-19.

CONCLUSION

ARDS is a large concern of death in COVID-19. In severe COVID-19, the development of ARDS and multi-organ failure is associated with cytokine storm. When discussing the prevent ARDS and death in COVID-19, it is critical to understand that the closed-circuit between cytokine storm and oxidative stress is the executive factor for direct damage to cells and multiple organs. As a result of cytokine storm, the number of innate immune system cells increases in the inflammation zone and they produce an excessive amount of ROS and NRS to destroy the virus. In addition to killing viruses, ROS, and NRS damage cells by directly damaging or depleting cellular antioxidant reserves. The depletion of the antioxidant system exacerbates oxidative stress which in turn triggers apoptosis, causing cell death. Apoptotic death of endothelial and epithelial cells in the lungs is one of the most important causes of ARDS in critically ill COVID-19 patients. Elders and people suffering from diabetes, hypertension, and cardiovascular diseases have already a state of oxidative stress. SARS- CoV-2 infection will increase this stress. This may be the cause of the severity of COVID-19 in these categories of patients and elderly individuals. Astonishingly very few medical scientists mention the pivotal role of oxidative damage in patients with severe COVID-19. Current therapeutic approaches focus on the virus itself and try desperately to apply antiviral medicine. Unfortunately, the benefits of antiviral drugs are not satisfactory in every patient due to severe side effects. The suppression of the cytokine storm and oxidative stress may help to prevent tissue damage, save the patients' lives, and prevent complications after recovery. Drugs with antioxidant and anti-apoptotic properties may be helpful in the management of severe COVID-19 patients. In this context, anti-oxidative therapeutic strategy in COVID-19 was evaluated in the next chapter.

REFERENCES

[1] Kakodkar, P., Kaka, N., Baig, M. N. 2020. "A comprehensive literatüre review on the clinical presentation, and management of the pandemic coronavirus disease 2019 (COVID-19)." *Cureus*. 12(4):e7560.

[2] Ahmed, H., Patel, K., Greenwood, D. C., Halpin, S., Lewthwaite, P., Salawu, A., Eyre, L., Breen, A., O'Connor, R., Jones, A., Sivan, M. 2020. "Long-term clinical outcomes in survivors of severe acute respiratory syndrome (SARS) and middle east respiratory syndrome (MERS) coronavirus outbreaks after hospitalisation or ICU admission: a systematıc review and meta-analysis." *J. Rehabil. Med.* 52(5): jrm00063.

[3] Nasonov, E., Samsonov, M. 2020. "The role of interleukin 6 inhibitors in therapy of severe COVID-19." *Biomed. Pharmacother*. 131:110698.

[4] Cao, X. 2020. "COVID-19: immunopathology and its implications for therapy." *Nat. Rev. Immunol*. 20:269-70.

[5] Channappanavar, R., Perlman, S. 2017. "Pathogenic human coronavirus infections: causes and consequences of cytokine storm and immunopathology." *Semin. Immunopathol.* 39:529-39.

[6] Tynell, J., Westenius, V., Rönkkö, E., Munster, V. J., Melén, K., Österlund, P., Julkunen, I. 2016. "Middle East respiratory syndrome coronavirus shows poor replication but significant induction of antiviral responses in human monocyte-derivedmacrophagesand dendritic cells." *J. Gen. Virol.* 97(2):344-55.

[7] Zhou, J., Chu, H., Li, C., Wong, B. H. Y., Cheng, Z. S., Poon, V. K. M., Sun, T., Lau, C. C. Y., Wong, K. K. Y., Chan, J. Y. W., Chan, J. F. W., To, K. K. W., Chan, K. H., Zheng, B. J., Yuen, K. Y. 2014. "Active replication of Middle East respiratory syndrome coronavirus and aberrant induction of in-flammatory cytokines and chemokines in human macrophages: implications for pathogenesis. *J. Infect. Diseases*. 209(9):1331-42.

[8] Law, H. K. W., Cheung, C. Y., Ng, H. Y., Sia, S. F., Chan, Y. O., Luk, W., John, M., Nicholls, J. S., Peiris, M., Yu Lung Lau, Y. L. 2005. "Chemokineup-reg-ulation in SARS-coronavirus-infected, monocyte-derivedhuman dendritic cells." *Blood*. 106(7):2366-74.

[9] Cheung, C. Y., Poon, L. L. M., Ng, I. H. Y., Luk, W., Sia, S.F., Wu, M. H. S., Chan, K. H., Yuen, K. Y., Gordon, S., Guan, Y., Peiris, J. S. M. 2005. "Cytokine responses in severe acute respiratory syndrome coronavirus-in-fected macrophagesin vitro: possible relevance to pathogenesis." *J. Virol*. 79(12):7819-26.

[10] Lau, S. K. P., Lau, C. C. Y., Chan, K. H., Li, C. P. Y., Chen, H., Jin, D. Y., Chan, J. F. W., Woo, P. C. Y., Yuen, K. Y. 2013. "Delayed induc-tion of proinflammatory cytokines and suppression of innate antiviral response by the novel MiddleEast respiratory syndrome coronavirus: implications for pathogenesisand treatment." *J. Gen. Virol*. 94(Pt 12):2679-90.

[11] Blanco-Melo, D., Nilsson-Payant, B. E., Liu, W. C., Uhl, S., Hoagland, D., Møller, R., Jordan, T. X., Oishi, K., Panis, M., Sachs, D., Wang, T. T., Schwartz, R. E., Lim, J. K., Albrecht, R. A., tenOever, B. R. 2020. "Imbalanced host response to SARS-CoV-2 drives development of COVID-19." *Cell*. 181(5):1036-1045 e9.

[12] Hadjadj, J., Yatim, N., Barnabei, L., Corneau, A., Boussier, J., Smith, N., Péré, H., Charbit, B., Bondet, V., Chenevier-Gobeaux, C., Breillat, P., Carlier, N., Gauzit, R., Morbieu, C., Pène, F., Marin, N., Roche, N., Szwebel, T. A., Merkling, S. H., Jean-Marc Treluyer, J. M., Veyer, D., Mouthon, L., Blanc, C., Tharaux, P. L., Rozenberg, F., Fischer, A., Duffy, D. Rieux-Laucat, F., Kernéis, S., Terrier, B. 2020. "Impaired type I interferon activity and inflammatory responses in severe COVID-19 patients." *Science*. 369(6504):718-724.

[13] Nguyen, R. G. T., Erin R. Green, E. R., Mecsas, J. 2017. "Neutrophils to the ROScue: Mechanisms of NADPH oxidase activation and bacterial resistance." *Front. Cell Infect. Microbiol*. 7:373.

[14] Alvarez, M. N., Trujillo, M., Radi, R. 2002. "Peroxynitrite formation from biochemical and cellular fluxes of nitric oxide and superoxide." *Methods Enzymol.* 359:353-366.

[15] Ademowo, O. S., Dias, H. K. I., Burton, D. G. A., H. R. Griffiths, H. R. 2017. "Lipid (per) oxidation in mitochondria: an emerging target in the ageing process?" *Biogerontol.* 18:859-79.

[16] Okuda, M., Li, K., Beard, M. R., Scholle, F., Lemon, S. M., Weinman, S. A. 2002. "Mitochondrial injury, oxidative stress, and antioxidant gene expression are induced by hepatitis C virus core protein." *Gastroenterology.* 122(2):366-375.

[17] Wang, T., Campbell, R. V., Yi, M. K., Lemon, S. M., Weinman, S. A. 2010. "Role of hepatitis C virus core protein in viral-induced mitochondrial dysfunction." *J. Viral Hepat.* 17:784-793.

[18] Gjyshi, O, Bottero, V., Veettil, M. V., Dutta, S., Singh, V. V., Leela Chikoti, L., Chandran, B. 2014. "Kaposi's sarcoma-associated herpesvirus in-duces Nrf 2 during de novo infection of endothelial cells to create a micro-environment conducive to infection." *PLoS Pathog.* 10(10):e1004460.

[19] Akaike, T., Molla, A., Ando, M., Araki, S., Maeda, H. 1989. "Molecular mechanism of complex infection by bacteria and virüs analyzed by a model using serratial protease and influenza virus in mice." *J. Virol.* 63(5):2252-2259.

[20] Akaike, T., Ando, M., Oda, T., Doi, T., Ijiri, S., Araki, S., Maeda, H. 1990. "Dependence on O2-generation by xanthine oxidase of patho-genesis of influenza virus infection in mice." *J. Clin. Invest.* 85(3):739-745.

[21] Hodny, Z., Reinis, M., Hubackova, S., Pavla Vasicova, P., Bartek, J. 2015. "Interferon gamma/NADPH oxidase defense system in immunity and cancer." *Oncoimmunology.* 5(2):e1080416.

[22] Wang, Y., Nie, W., Yao, K., Wang, Z., He, H. 2016. "Interleukin 6 induces expression of NADPH oxidase 2 in human aortic endothelial cells via long noncoding RNA MALAT1." *Pharmazie.* 71(10):592-597.

[23] Forcina, L., Miano, C., Scicchitano, B. M., Rizzuto, E., Berardinelli, M. G., Benedetti, F. D., Pelosi, L., Musarò, A. 2019. "Increased Circulating Levels of Interleukin-6 Affect the Redox Balance in Skeletal Muscle." *Research Article.* 2019: Special Issue.

[24] Komaravelli, N., Ansar, M., Garofalo, R. P., Casola, A. 2017. "Respiratory syncytial virus induces NRF2 degradation through a promyelocytic leukemia protein-ring fi nger protein 4 dependent pathway." *Free Rad. Biol. Med.* 113:494-504.

[25] El-Benna, J., Hurtado-Nedelec, M., Marzaioli, V., Marie, J. C., Gougerot-Pocidalo, M. A., Dang, P. M. 2016. "Priming of the neutrophil respiratory burst: role in host defense and inflammation." *Immunol. Rev.* 273:180-193.

[26] Brown, G. E., Stewart, M. Q., Bissonnette, S. A., Elia, A. E., Wilker, E., Yaffe, M. B. 2004. "Distinct ligand-dependent roles for p38 MAPK in primingand activation of the neutrophil NADPH oxidase." *J. Biol. Chem.* 279:27059-27068.

[27] Dang, P., Stensballe, A., Boussetta, T., Raad, H., Dewas, C., Kroviarski, Y., Hayem, G., Jensen, O. N., Gougerot-Pocidalo, M. A., El-Benna, J. 2006. "A specific p47 phox-serine phosphorylated by convergent MAPKs mediates neutrophil NADPH oxidase priming at inflammatory sites." *J. Clin. Invest.* 116: 2033-2043.

[28] Komaravelli, N., Casola, A. 2014. "Respiratory Viral Infections and Subversion of Cellular Antioxidant Defenses." *J. Pharmacogenomics Pharmacoproteomics*. 5(4): 1000141.

[29] van den Brand, J. M. A., Haagmans, B. L., van Riel, D., Osterhaus, A. D. M. E., Kuiken, T. 2014. "The pathology and pathogenesis of experimental severe acute respiratory syndrome and influenza in animal models." *J. Comp. Pathol.* 151:83-112.

[30] Smith, J. T., Willey, N. J., Hancock, J. T. "Low dose ionizing radiation produces too few reactive oxygen species to directly affect antioxidant concentrations in cells." *Biol. Lett.* 8:594-597.

[31] Lin, C. W., Lin, K. H., Hsieh, T. H., Shiu, S. Y., Li, J. Y. 2006. "Severe acute respiratory syndrome coronavirus 3C-like protease-induced apoptosis." *FEMS Immunol. Med. Microbiol.* 46:375-380.

[32] Imai, Y., Kuba, K., Neely, G. G., Yaghubian-Malhami, R., Perkmann, T., Loo, G., Ermolaeva, M., Veldhuizen, R., Leung, Y. H. C., Wang, H., Liu, H., Sun, Y., Pasparakis, M., Kopf, M., Mech, C., Bavari, S., Peiris, J. S. M., Slutsky, A. S., Akira, S., Hultqvist, M., Holmdahl, R., Nicholls, J., Jiang, C., Binder, C. J., Penninger, J. M. 2008. "Identification of Oxidative Stress and Toll-like Receptor 4 Signaling as a Key Pathway of Acute Lung Injury." *Cell.* 133:235-249.

[33] Laforge, M., Elbim, C., Frère, C., Hémadi, M., Massaad, C., Nuss, P., Benoliel, J. J., Becker, C. 2020. "Tissue damage from neutrophil-induced oxidative stress in COVID-19." *Nat. Rev. Immunol.* 20:515-516.

[34] Evans, P. C., Rainger, G. E., Mason, J. C., Guzik, T. J., Osto, E., Stamataki, Z., Neil, D., Hoefer, I. E., Fragiadaki, M., Waltenberger, J., Weber, C., Bochaton-Piallat, M. L., Bäck, M. 2020. "Endothelial dysfunction in COVID-19: a position paper of the ESC Working Group for Atherosclerosis and Vascular Biology, and the ESC Council of Basic Cardiovascular Science." *Cardiovascular Research.* cvaa230.

[35] Benussi, A., Pilotto, A., Premi, E., Libri, I., Giunta, M., Agosti, C., Alberici, A., Baldelli, E., Benini, M., Bonacina, S., Brambilla, L., Caratozzolo, S., Cortinovis, M., Costa, A., Piccinelli, S. C., Cottini, E., Cristillo, V., Delrio, I., Filosto, M., Gamba, M., Stefano Gazzina, S., Gilberti, N., Gipponi, S., Imarisio, A., Invernizzi,

P., Leggio, U., Leonardi, M., Liberini, P., Locatelli, M., Masciocchi, S., Poli, L., Rao, R., Risi, B., Rozzini, L., Scalvini, A., di Cola, F. S., Spezi, R., Vergani, V., Volonghi, I., Zoppi, N., Borroni, B., Magoni, M., Pezzini, A., Padovani, A. 2020. "Clinical characteristics and outcomes of inpatients with neurologic disease and COVID-19 in Brescia, Lombardy, Italy." *Neurology*. 95(7):e910-e920.

[36] Tang, N. 2020. "Abnormal coagulation parameters are associated with poor prognosis in patients with novel coronavirus pneumonia." *J. Thromb. Haemost*. 18(4):844-847.

[37] D'Oria, R., Natalicchio, A., Perrini, S., Laviola, L., Giorgino, F. 2018. "Oxidative stress and reactive oxygen species in endothelial dysfunction associated with cardiovascular and metabolic diseases." *Vascular Pharmacology*. 100:1-19.

[38] Chen, X., Andresen, B. T., Hill, M., Zhang, J., Booth, F., Zhang, C. 2008. "Role of reactive oxygen species in tumor necrosis factor-alpha induced endothelial dysfunction." *Curr. Hypertens. Re*. 4(4): 245-255.

[39] Xia, Z., Liu, M., Wu, Y., Luo, T., Ouyang, J., McNeill, J. H. 2006. "N-acetylcysteine attenuates TNF-alpha-induced human vascular endothelial cell apoptosis and restores eNOS expression." *Eur. J. Pharmacol*. 550:134-142.

[40] Varga, Z., Flammer, A. J., Steiger, P., Haberecker, M., Andermatt, R., Zinkernagel, A. S., Mehra, M. R., Schuepbach, R. A., Ruschitzka, F., Moch, H. 2020. "Endothelial cell infection and endotheliitis in COVID-19." *Lancet*. 395(10234): 1417-1418.

[41] Padhan, K., Minakshi, R., Towheed, M. A. B., Jameel, S. 2008. "Severe acute respiratory syndrome coronavirus 3a protein activates the mitochondrial death pathway through p38 MAP kinase activation." *J. Gen. Virol*. 89:1960-1969.

[42] Krahling, V., Stein, D. A., Spiegel, M., Weber, F., Mühlberger, E. 2009. "Severe Acute respiratory syndrome coronavirus triggers apoptosis via protein kinase R but is resistant to its antiviral activity." *J. Virol*. 83:2298-2309.

[43] Mao, L., Wang, M., Chen, S., He, Q., Chang, J., Hong, C., Zhou, Y., Wang, D., Li, Y., Jin, H., Hu, B. 2020. "Neurological manifestations of hospitalized patients with COVID-19 in Wuhan, China: a retrospective case series study." *JAMA Neurol*. 77(6):683-690.

In: Coronavirus Disease
Editor: Yildiz Dincer
ISBN: 978-1-53619-296-4

Chapter 18

ANTIOXIDANT AGENTS IN THE TREATMENT OF COVID-19

Mujgan Cengiz*, PhD
Department of Medical Biology, Cerrahpasa Medical Faculty,
Istanbul University Cerrahpasa, Istanbul, Turkey

ABSTRACT

SARS-CoV-2 (Severe Acute Respiratory Syndrome Coronavirus-2) belongs to the beta coronavirus family and shows an important global spread that is forcing the worldwide health care capacity, economic and social public life. It was referred that this deadly infection (COVID-19) has resulted in more than 1 million deaths and a lot of multiorgan failure around the world. The virus seriously affected people of old age, chronic cardiac problems, chronic respiratory syndromes, and hypertension. But in some cases, the disease may have a moderate or asymptomatic indication. Oxidative stress occurs because of an imbalance in the organism between the formation of the oxidizing system and antioxidant mechanisms. After the production of free radicals, antioxidant enzymes such as glutathione, melatonin, quercetin, curcumin, and vitamins, play an important role in neutralizing the effects of free radicals. The imbalance of oxidative stress and accumulating free radicals may get involved in the formation of cancers, degenerative diseases, hypertension, diabetes mellitus, heart and vessel diseases, and virus infections, especially RNA viruses like HIV 1, SARS, MERS, and coronaviruses.

A common approach in COVID-19 infection is the disruption of the antioxidant balance so free radicals can be exposed and accumulate in the organism. The depletion of the glutathione content, which is the most common antioxidant molecule of the tissues, causes the organism to increase the inflammation.

* Corrresponding Author's Email: mcengiz@istanbul.edu.tr.

In this article, we will discuss the role of free radical mechanisms in the formation of infection by COVID-19 and the treatment of the disease by different antioxidants such as GSH, melatonin, vitamins (C, D, E, A), and food additives.

Keywords: COVID-19, antioxidants, glutathione, vitamin, flavinoid

INTRODUCTION

Free radicals are chemical products that carry an unshared electron in its outer orbit. They are formed by the release of an electron from a non-radical atom or molecule, or by the addition of an electron to an atom or molecule. Free radicals are produced in animals and plants during aerobic metabolism and reduce the effects of the antioxidant activity or amount of compounds, as to behave as antioxidants (albumin, melatonin, urea, glutathione, vitamin D), exogenic antioxidants (vitamin E, vitamin C, vitamin A, polyphenols, curcumin), and enzymes (superoxide dismutase (SOD), glutathione peroxidase (GPx), glutathione S transferase (GST), catalase (CAT). Dietary antioxidants are beneficial in protecting against free radicals. Decreasing amounts of them cause the death of cells by lipid peroxidation, protein and DNA damage. They play an important role in preventing many diseases in humans, e.g., infection diseases, cardiovascular diseases, and cancer. Antioxidant enzymes and other non-enzyme antioxidants exhibit synergistic effects in scavenging free radicals.

Large different kinds of chemical carcinogens, viruses cause the formation of DNA and protein hazards and require activation by enzyme systems like cytochrome P450 [1]. In opposite to this situation, phase 2 xenobiotic-metabolizing enzymes and compounds such as Glutathione related enzymes (Glutathione peroxidase, glutathione s transferase, glutathione reductase), NAT (N-Acetyl Transferase), epoxides hydroxylase, sulfotransferase, GSH and NO takes place in the detoxification of chemicals, viruses, and consequently, known to be protective [2].

For a long time, the association of the environmental risk factors such as viruses was interesting for researchers. They increase oxidative stress that is triggered by various viral infections such as reactive oxygen species (ROS) production that disrupts the cell membrane integrity, and mitochondrial dysfunction [3]. Most of these viruses are RNA viruses which are, herpes viruses, respiratory viruses, HIV 1, viral hepatitis, and coronaviruses. Coronaviruses are single-stranded and encapsulated viruses which shown in 3 types: the classic coronaviruses, responsible for mild respiratory infections in general, the SARS-CoV and second one MERS-CoV (Middle Eastern respiratory syndrome) seen in epidemics of severe respiratory infections, and the third one; new coronavirus (caused by SARS-CoV-2) spread in December 2019 responsible for an infectious disease called COVID-19 which is currently accomplishing a worldwide pandemic [4].

Generally, viral infections produce an augmentation in the production of free radicals and a reduction of antioxidant capacity in the organisms in which they live [5]. This was previously shown in a study of HIV infection [6]. Oxidative stress caused by RNA virus infections can take part in the formation of several aspects of viral disease pathogenesis which are apoptosis, disruption of the immune system, viral replication, increased inflammatory response. SARS-CoV-2, MERS-CoV, and COVID-19 infections increase oxidative stress and ROS increases in the cell and disrupt the mitochondria after the cells get infected with these viruses. The release of acute-response cytokines (TNF and IL-1β), chemotactic cytokines (Il 1, Il 6, IL-8, and MCP-1) increases (Figure 1).

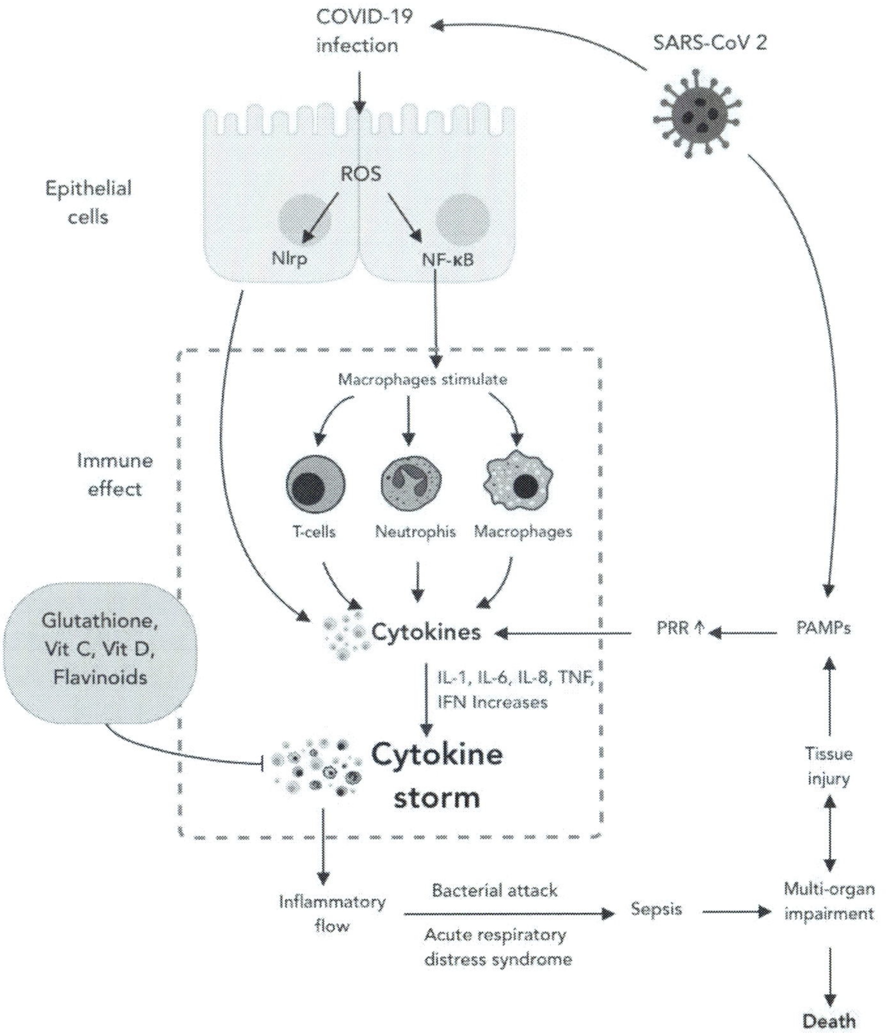

Figure 1. Mechanism of SARS-CoV-2 after entering to the organism. Pattern recognition receptors (PRR), pathogen-associated molecular patterns (PAMPs). Interleukin (IL). TNF(tumor necrosis factor).

Increasing these cytokines causes a shock by hyper inflammation and generates a lot of ferritin by the reaction of Fe^{2+} by hydrogen peroxide and increases OH- radicals, ROS and Fe^{3+}. Because of this dysfunction, interleukins increase in the organism, and the cytokine storm begins [7]. In studies, the oxidative storm also investigates that lipid peroxidation and protein oxidation may disrupt the alveolar membranes and cause serious respiratory problems [8]. Elderly people and patients with hypertension, diabetes, obesity, and cardiovascular diseases are affected by the virus more than healthy and young people do because of the existing accumulation of oxidative stress [9].

In the people infected by COVID-19, the antioxidant therapy aims to reduce the number of oxygen radicals by reducing oxidative stress with substances such as Glutathione and its precursors like N acetylcysteine, melatonin, vitamin C, vitamin D, some substances like curcumin and quercetin.

Examples of Medicaly Used Antioxidants

Glutathione

GSH (glutathione) consists of a tripeptide (cysteine, glycine, and glutamate) and is the most abundant antioxidant in the whole body and has a master role in most of the organisms to reduce the oxidative stress caused by an increase of ROS (reactive oxygen species) [10]. As a substrate of the GSH redox cycle, it is useful in scavenging singlet oxygen with hydroxyl radicals. In addition to directly scavenging free radicals; it also acts enzymatically with GPx. GSH plays a vital role in keeping enzymes and other cellular components in the cells in a reduced state. GSH is mostly synthesized in the liver and about 40% of it is excreted in bile. It is spread % 85 in the cytosol, the lesser amount at the subcellular parts of the cell which are; mitochondria, endoplasmic reticulum, and nucleus [11]. Its amount is measured 0.1-10 mM in living cells [12]. It reduces the amounts of ROS by using the reduced GSH to form oxidized GSSG (glutathione disulfide). Another important GSH function is to support the maintenance of the intracellular redox balance and thiol levels in the cell [13, 14] In the case of inflammation diseases, intrinsic oxidative stress has been found as depletion of total free thiol levels (free sulfhydryl, free thiols, and glutathione) [14]. It is found in most cells especially in upper and lower respiratory tract epithelial cells fluids and it protects the nose throat and lungs from pro-inflammatory processes. Glutathione has increased the immune response at herpes and influenza by blocking their replication [14].

The glutathione synthesis may increase by the GCS (gamma-glutamyl synthetase), this is a rate-limiting step for the synthesis and causes a rapid increase at the amount of the GSH. The other synthesis way is the induction of GCS by Nrf2 (The nuclear factor erythroid 2-related factor 2). Nrf2 is a transcription factor that increases the expression of a group of antioxidant, anti-inflammatory, neuroprotective protein [15].

In a study, N acetylcysteine, a GSH precursor, was given to two COVID-19 infected patients and it is found that this treatment inhibited the cytokine storm by blocking NF Kappa B (Figure 1) [16]. They applied glutathione to the patients infected by COVID-19, they showed the relieving of the respiratory symptoms. The increasing amount of GSH induce the Nrf2 and this inhibits the excess cytokine production that causes cytokine storm. In this study, the authors also used potent Nrf2 activators such as curcumin and sulforaphane.

In another study from Russia, it is postulated that increased age may reduce the synthesis of glutathione and the antioxidant protection may disrupt because of this reason [17].

According to various studies, this hypothesis recommends that the SARS-CoV-2 virus shows a major risk for people with endogenous glutathione deficiency, anyhow which of the factors old age, chronic disease, comorbidity, smoking, cardiovascular diseases, and obesity were responsible for this defect [18, 19, 20]. The hypothesis shows a new explanation into the etiology and mechanisms responsible for the serious appearance of COVID-19 infection and proves the right promising statutory for powerful treatment and controlling of the illness through glutathione rescuing with N-acetylcysteine and reduced glutathione.

Onward the antiviral influence of glutathione is non-standard, there is cause to count on that glutathione is also effective against COVID-19. Therefore, increasing glutathione levels in COVID-19 patients would be an encouraging perspective for saving the health of the new coronavirus for SARS-CoV-2 infection also.

Melatonin

Melatonin (*N*-acetyl-5-Methoxytryptamine) is a natural antioxidant molecule synthesized from tryptophan in the pineal gland and all organs of the body because its synthesis occurs in the mitochondria [21]. It neutralizes antioxidant molecules ten times more than vitamins C and E that binds only one. The antioxidant effects of melatonin are connected to the increased activity of superoxide dismutase, glutathione S transferase, reductase, peroxidase, and catalase [22, 23].

COVID-19 caused long-term stress in people resulting in anxiety and sleep defects.

Sleep defects may have negative effects on the immune system [24]. Prolonged anxiety causes a decrease in the amount of the immune cell and increases immunosuppressive mechanisms (increases T Cells). Inflammation and oxidative stress are implicated together in COVID-19 pathogenesis [25]. Oxidative stress-sensitive genes were stimulated in the peripheral blood mononuclear cells of SARS-CoV-2 infected patients [26]. Melatonin is found as a free radical scavenger and antioxidant at researches [27]. The metabolites of melatonin are cyclic-3-hydroxymelatonin (c3OHM), N1-acetyl-N2-formyl-5-methoxykynuramine (AFMK), and N1-acetyl-5-methoxykynuraminem (AMK) are produced by true scavenging free radicals. These metabolites have also been indicated to have protective properties of the melatonin [28]. Besides this, melatonin and its metabolites act as anti-excitatory agents that reduce prooxidant enzyme activity, inducing glutathione synthesis, and it elevates antioxidant enzyme synthesis. Furthermore, melatonin plays a significant action in ameliorating mitochondrial function with mention to the promotion of mitochondrial complex I and complex IV activities and inhibits of electron loss [29].

According to the studies, melatonin can not destroy the virus directly but it has an indirect antioxidant and immune system enhancer [28, 30]. In a study performed by respiratory virus models, melatonin caused a serious decrease in acute lung oxidative injury, depressed pro-inflammatory cytokine release, and inflammation in the cell [31].

Nevertheless for using this supplement the safety and side effects should be investigated. Metionin's characteristics scavenging free radicals show antioxidant property and increase in the immune system and may cause its potential decrease of COVID-19 infection.

A significant number of the long and short term of clinical studies suggest the safe use of melatonin up to 100 fold higher its physiologic concentration [32, 33]. Further, the brain is the organ where the number of drugs at the lowest level after melatonin administration, which could excuse the use of high doses for the potential treatment of SARS-CoV-2 [32].

Vitamin C

Ascorbic acid (vitamin C) is a very vital vitamin for the overall health and development of humans and other animals because it protects these organisms from serious diseases. It exists especially in vegetables and fruits [34]. It's synthesized from glucose in the liver of different mammalian species, permitting the preservation of physiological levels at the organisms. However in some species, including humans, it does not have the functional enzyme for the last step of the synthesis that's why they have to use exogenous sources of ascorbic acid [35]. It has very different effects on the rearranging the immune system of the organisms. The most important function and need for using of vitamin C is its antioxidant property to decrease the reactive oxygen radicals, which responsible for free radical hazards, biomolecular, cellular, and tissue damage related diseases, as well as cancer, atherosclerosis, and virus infections [36, 37]. Vitamin C also has been shown to increase the migration of neutrophils to the infection region, stimulating phagocytosis, and ROS generation [38]. Because of the required high need, it's recommended that the human daily intake of vitamin C (60 mg) is the highest of all vitamins [39].

The antiviral properties of ascorbic acid were known and it was searched around for a long time before [40, 41]. It has been applied to patients who were infected by influenza and herpes and found healing for these patients [42]. COVID-19 pneumonia is a serious disease with the risk of death with chronic organ disorders. This helps to provoke severe lung injury which causes Acute Respiratory Distress Syndrome (ARD S), causes a deadly injury in the lungs. This process inhibits adequate oxygen to enter into the lungs and at last cause death. Coronaviruses increase oxidative stress that promotes cellular damage and the results in organ failure. It is thought that pulmonary failure (ARDS) is the main reason for COVID-19's action on humans. This causes to increase in oxidative stress markedly because of the productıon of free radicals and cytokines. This action causes important cellular injury, organ damage, and death. The application of anti-oxidizing agents forward with known antioxidant property counts on to have a serious role in stopping these medical symptoms. Although evidence for the consumption of vitamin C for healing COVID-19 infections is not strong enough, there were studies from investigations of vitamin C in other respiratory diseases to begin conducting [43]. In a meta-analysis published by Ran, it is concluded that daily supplementation in vitamin C with more than daily doses decreases the time of period having a catching cold [44]. In acute lung injury and ARDS as seen in COVID-19 infections, overage neutrophil aggregation in the inflammatory region causes lung tissue damage via the release of necrotic cell ingredient [44], and vitamin C is declared to prohibit this action [45]. The antiviral characteristics of vitamin C may support depress symptoms and death seen in COVID-19 cytokine storm and could be a promising candidate for the treatment [46].

Vitamin D

Vitamin D is a steroid hormone that classically regulates bone calcium and phosphate metabolism, modulates the immune system, and its insufficiency is related to increased autoimmunity as well as enhances sensitivity to infection [47]. Its decreased amount is an important health problem seen all age range worldwide. In the last years, the relationships between low levels of vitamin D and various diseases has been shown by several studies, it increases innate and adaptive immunity, secretes antiviral peptides and augments mucosal resistance, improves membrane permeability [48, 49]. The studies have shown that the vitamin D3 synthesized in the skin by the UVB radiation is converted to the 25(OH)D in the liver and it has changed to its active form 1,25-dihydroxy vitamin D in the kidney and other organs [49]. In human normal serum 25(OH)D levels in between 40-60 ng/mL (100-150 nmol/L) [50].

These vitamin D amounts are stable with the published studies for decreasing the risk of various types of immune system diseases, cancers, cardiovascular diseases [51, 52, 53]. Several reviewers consider that the relationship between low level of serum 25(OH)D and the effectiveness and severity of respiratory tract infection in children and adults [54, 55, 56]. At a prospective study in healthy individuals, it is found that the acute respiratory tract infection reduced at the patients which have high levels of vitamin 25 (OH) D (38 ng/mL) in their serum [56]. In another study carried out in New Zeland children aged less than 2 years, showed the severity and hospitalization of acute respiratory infection percentage higher at the vitamin D deficiency [55]. This may explain the preventive effects of sufficient vitamin D status against respiratory viral infection. 1,25(OH)2D shows anti-viral activities by increasing innate immunity by enhancing the antimicrobial peptides and regulates inflammatory reply to viral infection by adjusting of toll-like receptor generation and NK cells production, inhibiting excess expression of proinflammatory cytokines [54]. Besides the immune modulatory and anti-viral influences, 1,25(OH)2D may act as to the disposition of the renin-angiotensin pathway and decreases the angiotensin-converting enzyme-2 expression, which may act as the subjects cell receptor which regulates infection of SARS-CoV-2 [56]. In a study done at African American and obese individuals, it is observed high morbidity, mortality and increased hospitalization at these subjects may be depends on their vitamin D deficiency [58].

Flavinoids

Flavonoids have a lot of secondary metabolites, that are found in vegetables, seeds, fruit, and beverages, like red wine and green tea [59]. There are very different kinds of structurally identified flavonoid molecules such as hesperidin and quercetin.

These chemicals are synthesized in plants to protect them from stressful mediums and play an important role in defending the plant cells from pathogens and insects [59].

The prophylactic characteristics of flavonoids implicate antibacterial, antioxidant, anti-inflammatory, and antiviral functions. Flavonoids work to defend the organisms from a group of DNA and RNA viruses [60].

After spreading the COVID-19 pandemic worldwide, the interest of researchers to the potential therapeutics other than antiviral drugs, the utilization of flavonoids against coronavirus infection concentrated on the SARS-CoV-2 virus [60, 61].

Hesperidin is a common flavon glucoside which used as an herbal medicine continually. It is mainly found in citrus fruit such as lemon, orange, and grapefruit [62]. It has various activities against the viruses. It's the antiviral and anti-inflammatory activity has been attributed to it an antioxidant property and reduce the pro-inflammatory cytokine production. In a study after SARS-CoV 2 pandemic, it has been shown that

COVID-19 uses the ACE-2 receptor for entering the organism the serine protease TMPRSS2 for priming of S-protein. Recently in a work Camostat mesylate used which a serine protease inhibitor drug blocked virus entry and was used as a COVID-19 treatment has been shown in research [63].

Another flavonoid compound quercetin was studied for their chemical activity in searching capillary wall resistance [64]. The *in vitro* and *in vivo* investigation shows that Quercetin affects the organism as a free radical scavenger, which gives two electrons by o-quinone/quinine methide [65], studies also in agreement that quercetin as a potent antioxidant [65, 66].

An important flavonoid naringenin has the chemical name of 4' 5 7-trihydroxyflavone, is accepted as a very important flavonoid, mostly a flavanone, because of its potential biological activities such as antioxidant, anti-inflammatory, and antiviral food additive. In a recent meta-analysis, it was indicated that naringenin may show curative effects against COVID-19 via inhibition of COVID-19 main protease, 3-chymotrypsin-like protease (3CLpro), and decreasing of angiotensin-converting enzyme receptors activity [67].

CONCLUSION

In a conclusion During the COVID-19 pandemics, as in all other health conditions, or saving health, it is recommended sustainable nutrition which affluence in antioxidant food. Glutathione, melatonin, Vitamin C, and D play an important role in regulating the immune system. But it can not evaluate these supplemental amounts of the vitamins that might give an efficacy. Some reports show the benefit of intra-venous utilization of vitamin C at the high dose in hospitalized COVID-19 patients [43, 68]. Vitamin D insufficiency has been associated with an increased probability of respiratory tract infection, therefore it is sensible, even in enough of specific data, to give vitamin D to healthy individuals and COVID-19 patients [48, 55, 57]. Flavinoids also found increased cell defense mechanisms against the COVID-19 virus [61, 62]. The diet is also important nutritional supplements, researches recommend advice for preventing and healing COVID-19, but the important size of clinical research data is required to support that suggestion.

REFERENCES

[1] Correia, M. A. 2001. "Drug Biotransformation." In: Katzung B. G., editor. *Basic and Clinical Pharmacology*. Lange Medical Books, Int ed 52-56.

[2] Becket, G. J., Haydes, J. D. 1993. "Glutathione S. Transferases: biomedical applications." *Adv Clin Chem.* 30:281-380.

[3] Reshi, M. L., Che, S. Y., Ruey, H. J. 2014. "RNA Viruses: ROS-Mediated Cell Death." *Int J Cell Biol.*; 2014: 467452. Published online 2014 May 8. doi: https://10.1155/2014/467452. PMC4034720.

[4] Zhou, P., Yang, X. L., Wang, X. G., Hu, B., Zhang, L., Zhang, W., et al., 2020. "A pneumonia outbreak associated with a new coronavirus of probable bat origin." *Nature* 579, 270-273. doi: https://10.1038/s41586-020-2012-7.

[5] Peterhans, E., Grob, M., Bürge T, Zanoni R. 1987. "Virus-induced formation of reactive oxygen intermediates in phagocytic cells." *Free Radical Research Communications*. 3(1-5):39-46.

[6] Ivanov, A. V., Valuev-Elliston, V. T, Ivanova, O. N., Kotchetkov, S. N., Starodubova, E. S., Bartoschsch, B. et al., 2016. "Oxidative Stress during HIV Infection: Mechanisms and Consequences." *Oxid Med Cell Longev*. 2016:8910396.

[7] Channappanavar, R., Perlman, S., 2017. "Pathogenic human coronavirus infections: causes and consequences of cytokine storm and immunopathology," Semin. *Immunopathol.* 39 (2017) 529-539.

[8] Xu, Z., Shi, L., Wang, Y., Zhang, J., Huang, L., Zhang, C. et al., 2020. "Pathological findings of COVID-19 associated with acute respiratory distress syndrome." *The Lancet Respiratory Medicine*. 8(4):420-422.

[9] Kregel, K. C. and Zhang, H. J. 2007. "An integrated view of oxidative stress in aging: basic mechanisms, functional effects, and pathological considerations." *Am J Physiol Regul Integr Comp Physiol* 292: R18-R36, First published August 17, 2006; doi: https://10.1152/ajpregu.00327.2006.

[10] Meister, A., Anderson, M. E. 1983." Glutathione." *Annu Rev Biochem*. 52:711-60.

[11] Lv, H., Zhen, C., Liu, J., Yang, P., Hu, L., Shang, P. 2019. "Unraveling the potential role of glutathione in multiple forms of cell death in cancer therapy." *Oxid Med Cell Longev*. p: 3150145.

[12] Gérard-Monnier, D., Chaudiere, J. 1996. "Metabolism and antioxidant function of glutathione." *J Pathol Biol (Paris).* Jan; 44(1):77-85.

[13] Zinellu, A., Zinellu, E., Sotgiu, E., Fois, A. G., Paliogiannis, P., Scano, V., Piras, B., et al., 2020. "Systemic transsulfuration pathway thiol concentrations in chronic obstructive pulmonary disease patients." *Eur. J. Clin. Investig*., e13267.

[14] Fraternale, A., Paoletti, M. F., Casabianca, A., Nencioni, L., Garaci, E., Palamara, A. T. et al., 2009. "GSH and analogs in antiviral therapy." *MolecularAspects of Medicine*. 2009; 30(1-2):99-110.

[15] Cengiz, M., Kurt, E., Bayoğlu, B. 2019. "Effects of valproic acid treatment on Nrf2 gene expression and oxidative stress levels in lithium- pilocarpine rat model of epilepsy." *International Molecular medicine symposium by bosphorus*, Istanbul, Turkiye, 16-18 May 2019, 105-105.

[16] Horowitz, R. I., Freeman, P. R., Bruzzese, J. 2020. "Efficacy of glutathione therapy in relieving dyspnea associated with COVID-19 pneumonia: A report of 2 cases." *Respir Med Case Rep*. 2020; 30: 101063. Published online 2020 Apr 21.

[17] Polonikov, A. 2020. "Endogenous Deficiency of Glutathione as the Most Likely Cause of Serious Manifestations and Death in COVID-19 Patients." *ACS Infect Dis*. 2020 May 28: acsinfecdis.0c00288. Published online 2020 May 28. doi: https://10.1021/acsinfecdis.0c00288 PMCID: PMC7263077.

[18] Li, B., Yang, J., Zhao, F., Zhi, L., Wang, X., Liu, L., Bi, Z. et al. 2020. "Prevalence and impact of cardiovascular metabolic diseases on COVID-19 in China." *Clinical research in cardiology: official journal of the German Cardiac Society*, 109(5), 531-538. https://doi.org/10.1007/s00392-020-01626-9.

[19] Sardu, C., Gambardella, J., Morelli, M. B., Wang, X., Marfella, R., & Santulli, G. 2020. "Hypertension, Thrombosis, Kidney Failure, and Diabetes: Is COVID-19 an Endothelial Disease? A Comprehensive Evaluation of Clinical and Basic Evidence." *Journal of clinical medicine*, 9(5), 1417. https://doi.org/10.3390/jcm9051417.

[20] Shahid, Z., Kalayanamitra, R., McClafferty, B., Kepko, D., Ramgobin, D., Patel, R., Aggarwal, C. S., et al.2020. "COVID-19 and Older Adults: What We Know." *Journal of the American Geriatrics Society*, 68(5), 926-929. https://doi.org/10.1111/jgs.16472.

[21] Zhang, R., Wang, X., Ni, L., Di, X., Ma, B., Niu, S., Liu, C., et al. 2020. "COVID-19: Melatonin as a potential adjuvant treatment." *Life sciences*, 250, 117583. https://doi.org/10.1016/j.lfs.2020.117583.

[22] Cengiz, M., Alansal, N. O., Tuncdemir, M., Tanriverdi, G., & Bayoglu, B. 2016. "Evaluation of effects of melatonin and caffeic acid phenethyl ester on acute potassium dichromate toxicity and genotoxicity in rats." *Indian journal of pharmacology*, 48(4), 407-411. https://doi.org/10.4103/0253-7613.186213.

[23] Reiter, R., Tang, L., Garcia, J. J., & Muñoz-Hoyos, A. 1997. "Pharmacological actions of melatonin in oxygen radical pathophysiology." *Life sciences*, 60(25), 2255-2271. https://doi.org/10.1016/s0024-3205(97)00030-1.

[24] Kang, L., Li, Y., Hu, S., Chen, M., Yang, C., Yang, B. X., Wang, Y., et al. 2020. "The mental health of medical workers in Wuhan, China dealing with the 2019 novel coronavirus." *The lancet. Psychiatry*, 7(3), e14. https://doi.org/10.1016/S2215-0366(20)30047-X.

[25] Merad, M., Martin, J. C. 2020. "Pathological inflammation in patients with COVID-19: a key role for monocytes and macrophages." *Nat Rev Immunol*. 2020 May 6: 1-8. doi: https://10.1038/s41577-020-0331-4.

[26] Shao, H., Lan, D., Duan, Z., Liu, Z., Min, J., Zhang, L., Huang, J., 2006. "Upregulation of mitochondrial gene expression in PBMC from convalescent

SARS patients." *Journal of clinical immunology*, 26(6), 546-554. https://doi.org/10.1007/s10875-006-9046-y.

[27] Galano, A., Castañeda-Arriaga, R., Pérez-González, A., Tan, D. X., & Reiter, R. J. 2016. "Phenolic Melatonin-Related Compounds: Their Role as Chemical Protectors against Oxidative Stress." *Molecules* (Basel, Switzerland), 21(11), 1442. https://doi.org/10.3390/molecules21111442.

[28] Reiter, R. J., Mayo, J. C., Tan, D. X., Sainz, R. M., Alatorre-Jimenez, M., Qin, L., 2016. "Melatonin as an antioxidant: under promises but over delivers." *J. Pineal Res*. 61 (3), 253-278.

[29] Juybari, K. B., Hosseinzadeh, A., Ghaznavi, H., Kamali, M., Sedaghat, A., Mehrzadi, S., Naseripour, M. 2019. "Melatonin as a modulator of degenerative and regenerative signaling pathways in injured Retinal Ganglion Cells." *Curr. Pharm. Des*. 25 (28), 3057-3073.

[30] Reiter, R. J., Ma, Q. and Sharma, R. 2020. "Treatment of ebola and other infectious diseases: melatonin 'goes viral'." *Melatonin Research*. 3, 1 (Mar. 2020), 43-57. doi: https://doi.org/10.32794/mr11250047.

[31] Ben-Nathan, D., Maestroni, G. J., Lustig, S., Conti, A. 1995. "Protective effects of melatonin in mice infected with encephalitis viruses." *Arch Virol.* 1995; 140(2):223-30. doi: https://10.1007/BF01309858.PMID:771035.

[32] Andersen, L. P., Werner, M. U., Rosenkilde, M. M., Fenger, A. Q., Petersen, M. C., Rosenberg, J., Gogenur, I. 2016 "Pharmacokinetics of high-dose intravenous melatonin in humans." *J Clin Pharmacol* 56:324-329. https://doi.org/10.1002/jcph.592.

[33] Seabra, M. L., Bignotto, M., Pinto, L. R. Jr., Tufik, S. 2000 "Randomized, double-blind clinical trial, controlled with placebo, of the toxicology of chronic melatonin treatment." *J Pineal Res* 29:193-200. https://doi.org/10.1034/j.1600-0633.2002.290401.x.

[34] Pisoschi, A. M., Pop, A., Negulescu, G. P., & Pisoschi, A. 2011. "Determination of ascorbic acid content of some fruit juices and wine by voltammetry performed at pt and carbon paste electrodes." *Molecules (Basel, Switzerland)*, 16(2), 1349-1365. https://doi.org/10.3390/molecules16021349.

[35] Nishikimi, M., Kawai, T., Yagi, K. 1992. "Guinea pigs possess a highly mutated gene for L-gulono-γ-lactone oxidase, the key enzyme for L-ascorbic acid biosynthesis missing in this species." *J. Biol. Chem*. 1992, 267, 21967-21972.

[36] El Halabi, I., Bejjany, R., Nasr, R., Mukherji, D., Temraz, S., Nassar, F. J., et al. 2018. "Ascorbic Acid in Colon Cancer: From the Basic to the Clinical Applications." *International journal of molecular sciences*, 19(9), 2752. https://doi.org/10.3390/ijms19092752.

[37] Al-Khudairy, L., Flowers, N., Wheelhouse, R., Ghannam, O., Hartley, L., Stranges, S., & Rees, K. 2017. "Vitamin C supplementation for the primary prevention of

cardiovascular disease." *The Cochrane database of systematic reviews*, 3(3), CD011114. https://doi.org/10.1002/14651858.CD011114.pub2.

[38] Carr, A. C., & Maggini, S. 2017. "Vitamin C and Immune Function." *Nutrients*, 9(11), 1211. https://doi.org/10.3390/nu9111211.

[39] Levine, M. 1986 "New concepts in the biology and biochemistry of ascorbic acid." *N. Eng. J. Med.*, 314, 892-902.

[40] Klenner, F. R. 1948. "Virus pneumonia and its treatment with vitamin C." *Southern medicine and surgery*, 110(2), 36-38.

[41] Naidu, K. A. 2003. "Vitamin C in human health and disease is still a mystery? An overview." *Nutrition journal*, 2, 7. https://doi.org/10.1186/1475-2891-2-7.

[42] Colunga Biancatelli, R. M. L., Berrill, M., Marik, P. E., 2020. "The antiviral properties of vitamin C." *Expert Rev Anti Infect Ther* 18, 99-101.

[43] Cheng, R. Z. 2020 "Can early and high intravenous dose of vitamin C prevent and treat coronavirus disease 2019. (COVID-19)?" *Med. Drug Discov* 2020, 5, 100028.

[44] Ran, L., Zhao, W., Wang, J., Wang, H., Zhao, Y., Tseng, Y., Bu, H. 2018. "Extra Dose of Vitamin C Based on a Daily Supplementation Shortens the Common Cold: A Meta-Analysis of 9 Randomized Controlled Trials." *Biomed. Res. Int.*, 1837634.

[45] Fan, E. K. Y., Fan, J. 2018. "Regulation of alveolar macrophage death in acute lung Inflammation." *Respiratory Research* volume 19, Article number: 50 (2018)

[46] Boretti, A., & Banik, B. K. 2020. "Intravenous vitamin C for reduction of cytokines storm in acute respiratory distress syndrome." *PharmaNutrition*, 12, 100190. https://doi.org/10.1016/j.phanu.2020.100190.

[47] Dankers, W., Colin, E. M., van Hamburg, J. P., & Lubberts, E. 2017. "Vitamin D in Autoimmunity: Molecular Mechanisms and Therapeutic Potential." *Frontiers in immunology*, 7, 697. https://doi.org/10.3389/fimmu.2016.00697.

[48] Ali, N. 2020. "Role of vitamin D in preventing of COVID-19 infection, progression and severity." *Journal of infection and public health*, S1876-0341(20)30531-1. Advance online publication. https://doi.org/10.1016/j.jiph.2020.06.021/.

[49] Gruber-Bzura, B. M. 2018. "Vitamin D and Influenza-Prevention or Therapy?" *International journal of molecular sciences*, 19(8), 2419. https://doi.org/10.3390/ijms19082419.

[50] Wacker, M., and Holick, M. F. 2013. "Sunlight and Vitamin D: A global perspective for health." *Dermato-endocrinology*, 5(1), 51-108. https://doi.org/10.4161/derm.24494.

[51] Li, J., Chen, N., Wang, D., Zhang, J., & Gong, X. 2018. "Efficacy of vitamin D in treatment of inflammatory bowel disease: A meta-analysis." *Medicine*, 97(46), e12662. https://doi.org/10.1097/MD.0000000000012662.

[52] Holick, M. F. 2018. "The Death D-fying Vitamin." *Mayo Clinic proceedings*, 93(6), 679-681. https://doi.org/10.1016/j.mayocp.2018.04.014.

[53] Dudenkov, D. V., Mara, K. C., Petterson, T. M., Maxson, J. A., & Thacher, T. D. 2018. "Serum 25-Hydroxyvitamin D Values and Risk of All-Cause and Cause-Specific Mortality: A Population-Based Cohort Study." *Mayo Clinic proceedings*, 93(6), 721-730. https://doi.org/10.1016/j.mayocp.2018.03.006.

[54] Gunville, C. F., Mourani, P. M., & Ginde, A. A. 2013. "The role of vitamin D in prevention and treatment of infection." *Inflammation & allergy drug targets*, 12(4), 239-245. https://doi.org/10.2174/18715281113129990046.

[55] Ingham, T. R., Jones, B., Camargo, C. A., Kirman, J., Dowell, A. C., Crane, J., Stanley, et al. 2014. "Association of vitamin D deficiency with severity of acute respiratory infection: A case-control study in New Zealand children." *Eur. Respir. J.* 2014; 44:439.

[56] Sabetta, J. R., DePetrillo, P., Cipriani, R. J., Smardin, J., Burns, L. A., & Landry, M. L. 2010. "Serum 25-hydroxyvitamin d and the incidence of acute viral respiratory tract infections in healthy adults." *PloS one*, 5(6), e11088. https://doi.org/10.1371/journal.pone.0011088.

[57] Cui, C., Xu, P., Li, G., Qiao, Y., Han, W., Geng, C. et al. 2019. "Vitamin D receptor activation regulates microglia polarization and oxidative stress in spontaneously hypertensive rats and angiotensin II-exposed microglial cells: Role of renin-angiotensin system." *Redox Biol.* 2019; 26:101295. doi: https://10.1016/j.redox.2019.101295.

[58] Mendy, A., Apewokin, S., Wells, A. A., and Morrow, A. L. 2020. "Factors Associated with Hospitalization and Disease Severity in a Racially and Ethnically Diverse Population of COVID-19 Patients." *medRxiv: the preprint server for health sciences*, 2020.06.25.20137323. https://doi.org/10.1101/2020.06.25.20137323.

[59] Russo, M., Spagnuolo, C., Tedesco, I., & Russo, G. L. 2010. "Phytochemicals in cancer prevention and therapy: truth or dare?" *Toxins*, 2(4), 517-551. https://doi.org/10.3390/toxins2040517.

[60] Jo, S., Kim, S., Shin, D. H., & Kim, M. S. 2020. "Inhibition of SARS-CoV 3CL protease by flavonoids." *Journal of enzyme inhibition and medicinal chemistry*, 35(1), 145-151. https://doi.org/10.1080/14756366.2019.1690480.

[61] Mani, J. S., Johnson, J. B., Steel, J. C., Broszczak, D. A., Neilsen, P. M., Walsh, K. B., & Naiker, M. 2020. "Natural product-derived phytochemicals as potential agents against coronaviruses: A review." *Virus research*, 284, 197989. https://doi.org/10.1016/j.virusres.2020.197989.

[62] Haggag, Y. A., El-Ashmawy, N. E., & Okasha, K. M. 2020. "Is hesperidin essential for prophylaxis and treatment of COVID-19 Infection?" *Medical hypotheses*, 144, 109957. Advance online publication. https://doi.org/10.1016/j.mehy.2020.109957.

[63] Hoffmann, M., Kleine-Weber, H., Schroeder, S., Krüger, N., Herrler, T., Erichsen, S., Schiergens., et al.. 2020. "SARS-CoV-2 Cell Entry Depends on ACE2 and

TMPRSS2 and Is Blocked by a Clinically Proven Protease Inhibitor." *Cell*, 181(2), 271-280.e8. https://doi.org/10.1016/j.cell.2020.02.052.

[64] Gábor, M. 1988. "Szent-Györgyi and the bioflavonoids: new results and perspectives of pharmacological research into benzo-pyrone derivatives. Commemoration on the 50th anniversary of the award of the Nobel Prize." *Progress in clinical and biological research*, 280, 1-15.

[65] Awad, H. M., Boersma, M. G., Vervoort, J., & Rietjens, I. M. 2000. "Peroxidase-catalyzed formation of quercetin quinone methide-glutathione adducts." *Archives of biochemistry and biophysics*, 378(2), 224-233. https://doi.org/10.1006/abbi.2000.1832.

[66] Terao, J. 1999. "Dietary flavonoids as antioxidants *in vivo*: conjugated metabolites of (-)-epicatechin and quercetin participate in antioxidative defense in blood plasma." *The journal of medical investigation*: JMI, 46(3-4), 159-168.

[67] Tutunchi, H., Naeini, F., Ostadrahimi, A., and Hosseinzadeh-Attar, M. J. 2020. "Naringenin, a flavanone with antiviral and anti-inflammatory effects: A promising treatment strategy against COVID-19." *Phytotherapy research*: PTR, 10.1002/ptr.6781. Advance online publication. https://doi.org/10.1002/ptr.6781.

[68] Erol, A. 2020. "High-dose Intravenous Vitamin C Treatment for COVID-19." *OSF Preprints*. February 26. doi: https://10.31219/osf.io/p7ex8.

In: Coronavirus Disease
Editor: Yildiz Dincer

ISBN: 978-1-53619-296-4

Chapter 19

VACCINE DEVELOPMENT STUDIES FOR COVID-19

Yesim Tok[1], MD and Gökhan Aygün[1,*], MD
[1]Istanbul University- Cerrahpasa, Cerrahpasa Medical Faculty, Department of Medical Microbiology, Istanbul, Turkey

ABSTRACT

The ongoing coronavirus disease (COVID)-19 pandemic caused by severe acute respiratory syndrome coronavirus 2 (SARS-CoV-2) has affected people worldwide both sociologically and economically. This crisis might be controlled by a safe, tolerable, and immunogenic vaccine. Multiple vaccines are in development, and some of them are even in phase III trials but, no approved efficacious vaccine is currently available. Vaccines protect from infection, reduce symptom development, lower mortality rates, and reduce the extent of virus circulation. Therefore, hopefully in the near future, when the vaccine is roll-out, we can overcome this pandemic by informing the people correctly on vaccine safety and importance for public health and by vaccinating susceptible people in the most effective policies.

Keywords: COVID-19, SARS-CoV-2, vaccine, pandemic

INTRODUCTION

The first SARS-CoV-2 case identified in December 2019 within a month, the genetic sequence of the virus became available (MN908947.3). On 11 March 2020, the World Health Organization (WHO) declared the SARS-CoV-2 outbreak as a pandemic. Since

[*] Corresponding Author's Email: gokhanaygun67@yahoo.com.

then, the virus has infected millions of people globally [1]. Current public health interventions aimed at blocking the spread of SARS-CoV-2 have been limited to nonpharmaceutical interventions (NPIs), including travel-associated quarantines, contact tracing, mask usage, and implementation of social distancing regulations. These measures have had various degrees of success worldwide. While critical to slowing viral spread, some of these NPIs have resulted in widespread job loss and economic hardship. Considering the substantial political and economic costs associated with NPIs, long-term and effective solutions are needed [2, 3].

In this context, the vaccine remains the most promising solution. Thanks to devoted research efforts worldwide, vaccine development is well underway, with more than 100 vaccine candidates in clinical trials, including candidates in phase III trials. Clinical trials for SARS-CoV-2 vaccines evaluate both the safety and efficacy of vaccine candidates. Ethically, a vaccine cannot be licensed if it does not provide a direct protective benefit to the vaccine. Direct protective benefits of vaccines include protection from infection, reduced symptom development, and lower mortality rates [4].

For vaccine-preventable diseases, not all susceptible individuals can be immunized for various reasons, such as they are too young or too old to be vaccinated, they have co-morbidities and weakened immune systems or they reject the vaccination for cultural, traditional, or religious reasons. The question then is what is the minimum proportion of those we can vaccinate that we need to vaccinate so that those that we cannot vaccinate can be protected from developing severe disease or dying of the disease. The notion of herd immunity in the transmission dynamics is associated with the indirect protection against acquisition of a communicable disease, members of the community receive when a large percentage of the population has become immune to the infectious disease due to natural recovery from prior infection or vaccination. The consequence of herd immunity is that individuals who are not immune (e.g., those who cannot be vaccinated or those who have not been infected yet) receive some protection against the acquisition of the disease. The safest and fastest way to achieve herd immunity is obviously vaccination [5]. This indirect effect decreases the infection risk of both vaccinated and unvaccinated susceptible individuals by reducing the extent of virus circulation in a community. Virus circulation can decrease because vaccinated individuals are less susceptible to infection, or because vaccinated individuals have shorter durations of infection or lower viral loads that reduce their infectiousness. Vaccination campaigns can significantly reduce the number of infections and deaths in subpopulations that remain unvaccinated, even when the vaccination percentage is quite low [6]. The vast majority of the global population remains susceptible to the virus and we are likely well below the herd immunity threshold, despite the staggering rates of infection that some regions have already experienced. Therefore the indirect effects of vaccine candidates are critically important to consider when evaluating SARS-CoV-2 vaccine candidates and formulating strategies for their roll-out. Clinical trials to test vaccine effectiveness do not evaluate population-level effects. Quantifying both the direct and indirect effects of vaccines on population-level outcomes, such as disease incidence and mortality, requires evaluating data after a vaccine has been in use for some time. Therefore, mathematical models are needed to assess the potential indirect effects in advance.

With the hope of producing a vaccine in the near future comes the difficult task of deciding who to vaccinate first as vaccine shortages are inevitable. According to our knowledge on COVID-19 so far, children are less susceptible to infection than middle-aged adults (20 to 65 years old), while older adults (older than 65) were relatively more susceptible. Studies showed that a vaccine with an effectiveness ≥50% would be enough to substantially mitigate the ongoing pandemic provided that a high percentage of the population is optimally vaccinated [7]. When minimizing deaths, for low vaccine effectiveness (VE), it is optimal to allocate vaccine to high-risk (older) age-groups first. In contrast, for higher vaccine effectiveness, there is a switch to allocate vaccine to high-transmission (younger) age-groups first for high vaccination coverage [8]. Any vaccine with medium to high effectiveness (VE ≥ 50%) would be able to considerably slow the epidemic while keeping the burden on healthcare systems manageable, as long as a high proportion of the population is optimally vaccinated. Moreover, once VE = 70%, the attack rate drop and full containment of the epidemic would be possible [9].

Vaccine Development and Clinical Trials

Despite many organizations have announced plans to start efficacy testing for their candidate vaccines, an approved vaccine is not expected until 2021, even with substantially compressed development timelines, smooth proceeding of clinical trials, and not accounting for possible failures [10]. Unlike typical therapeutics that are administered to sick patients, vaccines are intended for the healthy. Therefore, confirming the safety and effectiveness of a vaccine is of critical importance [11]. The two primary methods for demonstrating vaccine safety and efficacy are through either a vaccine efficacy randomized clinical trial (RTC) or a vaccine immunogenicity RTC. In the former, large numbers of recruited healthy volunteers are randomly selected to receive either the vaccine or a placebo and then monitored for some time. At the end of the surveillance period, the difference in the proportion of infections between the treatment and control arms is computed to demonstrate the ability of vaccine prevention. In a vaccine immunogenicity RCT, the primary endpoint is an immunity measurement or marker which is known to correlate with protection against infection or disease. This type of trial involves a smaller number of volunteers and requires a shorter follow-up period, and as a result, is quicker and less costly. Given that SARS-CoV-2 is a novel pathogen for which we do not yet know how to determine whether a subject is protected, vaccine efficacy must be confirmed using the longer and more costly vaccine efficacy RCT. Follow-up continues for all participants and includes a collection of serious adverse events for 6 months, and COVID-19 infection and multiple additional immunogenicity measurements through up to two years. Later phases of the study prioritize enrollment of more diverse populations, including those with chronic underlying health conditions and from racial/ethnic groups adversely affected by COVID-19 [12].

A human challenge trial (HCT), in which volunteers are randomized into either the vaccine or placebo arm and then infected deliberately with a live virus in a controlled setting, has been proposed as an alternative to accelerate the vaccine development process. Upon challenge, HCTs can quickly demonstrate the safety and efficacy of candidate vaccines in preventing infection or disease.

Depending on sample size, HCTs could also help to establish functional immune correlates of protection to inform the design of future vaccines. Since an HCT allows comparison of immune responses in vaccinated and unvaccinated individuals, precise measurements of post-vaccination viral loads, characterization of immune responses (innate, adaptive, cell-mediated) and antibody titers, and close monitoring and care of patients, it can help establish the correlates of protection and prove vaccine efficacy concurrently.

Moreover, a properly designed HCT can determine the transmission risk of the infected in a controlled setting with minimal exposure to investigators and the public.

While concerns have been raised regarding the ethics and morality of HCTs, it is generally accepted that HCTs are ethically permissible when the benefits to society outweigh acknowledged risks [13], and they have been deemed acceptable for developing vaccines for multiple infectious diseases such as influenza [14], malaria [15], typhoid [16], cholera [17], and dengue fever [18]. To the best of our knowledge, there have been no published studies of a quantitative analysis of the potential societal value of a COVID-19 HCT.

Vaccine Technologies and Targets

RNA vaccine technology which has been preferred for vaccine candidates so far has enabled rapid vaccine development in response to this pandemic. RNA vaccines provide flexibility in the design and expression of vaccine antigens that can mimic antigen structure and expression during natural infection. RNA is required for protein synthesis, does not integrate into the genome, is transiently expressed, and is metabolized and eliminated by the body's natural mechanisms and, therefore, is considered safe. RNA vaccines for the prevention of infectious diseases and treatment of cancer have been shown in clinical trials to be safe and well-tolerated. In general, vaccination with RNA elicits a robust innate immune response. RNA directs expression of the vaccine antigen in host cells and has intrinsic adjuvant effects. A strength of the RNA vaccine manufacturing platform, irrespective of the encoded pathogen antigen, is the ability to rapidly produce large quantities of vaccine doses against a new pathogen. Most RNA vaccine candidates encode the receptor-binding domain (RBD) of the SARS-CoV-2 spike protein, a key target of virus-neutralizing antibodies [19]. Another well-known vaccine design strategy is incompetent virus vectors, which stabilized SARS-CoV-2 Spike (S) protein. These candidates are selected based on their immunogenicity and manufacturability profile. Vector vaccines are also used for Ebola, RSV, HIV, and Zika viruses [20].

COVID-19 Vaccine Effects and Adverse-Effects

Phase III findings from ongoing vaccine trials being published, recently. Up to these results, after administration of prime and boost doses for RTCs, IgG concentrations, and SARS-CoV-2 neutralizing titers (in neutralization assays) in sera increased, TH1 skewed T cell immune responses with specific CD8+ and CD4+ T cell expansion. Interferon (IFN)γ was produced by a high fraction of specific CD8+ and CD4+ T cells. No serious adverse events were reported. Local injection site reactions and systemic events (mostly flu-like symptoms) were dose-dependent, generally mild to moderate, and transient. Symptoms such as fever, fatigue, chills, headache, muscle pain, joint pain, injection site pain, and tenderness occurred within 7 days after each dose. Reactogenicity resolved spontaneously or could be managed with simple measures (e.g., paracetamol). Whereas no relevant change in routine clinical laboratory values occurred after vaccination, temporary reduction of blood lymphocyte counts -related redistribution of lymphocytes into lymphoid tissues- and a transient increase in C-reactive protein (CRP) were observed in a dose-dependent manner in vaccinated participants. CRP is a well-known inflammatory serum protein previously described as a biomarker for various infectious disease vaccines and an indicator of vaccine adjuvant activity [21].

Concluding Remarks

Immunization programs are only successful when there are high rates of acceptance and coverage. To accomplish this, it is critical to understand risk perceptions about COVID-19, acceptance of a COVID-19 vaccine, and confidence in media sources, specifically those used to obtain information about the COVID-19 pandemic. We must clearly understand the hesitancy and acceptance of a COVID-19 vaccine to develop evidence-based interventions. This will allow healthcare professionals and health officials to develop messaging to best address concerns and educate all people, especially vulnerable groups [22]. Since the beginning of the COVID-19 pandemic, our government has taken precautions, plans have been made, taken into account the risk that immunization services may be interrupted and there may be an increase in other vaccine-preventable diseases. Immunization is an indispensable part of the healthcare system and is carried out in our healthcare institutions without interruption following the COVID-19 pandemic period measures. Parents should follow the vaccination programs of their children, and when the vaccination time comes, they should contact family physicians and get information about vaccination practices. Children must be vaccinated during the COVID-19 pandemic, too. It has been reported by the World Health Organization that there are currently no known medical contraindications to vaccination of people with COVID-19, either. Also, studies show that the effect of mass influenza vaccination on the spread of COVID-19 and other influenza-like pathogens co-circulating during an influenza season [23]. Therefore, increasing influenza vaccine uptake, or enhancing the public health interventions, would facilitate the management of outbreaks of SARS-CoV-2 and other respiratory pathogens circulating during the peak flu season.

REFERENCES

[1] WHO. "*Coronavirus disease (COVID-19) Situation Report-161*". Accessed June 30th (2020).

[2] Flaxman, S., Mishra, S., Gandy, A., Unwin, H., Coupland, H., Mellan, T., Zhu, H., Berah, T., Eaton, J., Perez Guzman, P., Schmit, N., Cilloni, L., Ainslie, K., Baguelin, I., Blake, M., Boonyasiri, A., Boyd, O., Cattarino, L., Ciavarella, C., Cooper, L., Cucunuba Perez, Z., Cuomo-Dannenburg, G., Dighe, A., Djaafara, A., Dorigatti, I., Van Elsland, S., Fitzjohn, R., Fu, H., Gaythorpe, K., Geidelberg, L., Grassly, N., Green, W., Hallett, T., Hamlet, A., Hinsley, W., Je_rey, B., Jorgensen, D., Knock, E., Laydon, D., Nedjati Gilani, G., Nouvellet, P., Parag, K., Siveroni, I., Thompson, H., Verity, R., Volz, E., Walters, C., Wang, H., Wang, Y., Watson, O., Winskill, P., Whittaker, X. Xi., C., Walker, P., Ghani, A., Donnelly, C., Riley, S., Okell, L., Vollmer, M., Ferguson, N. and Bhatt, S. "*Report 13: Estimating the number of infections and the impact of non-pharmaceutical interventions on COVID-19 in 11 European countries*". 2020.

[3] An Pan, Li Liu, Chaolong Wang, Huan Guo, Xingjie Hao, Qi Wang, Jiao Huang, Na He, Hongjie Yu, Xihong Lin, Sheng Wei and Tangchun Wu. "Association of public health interventions with the epidemiology of the COVID-19 outbreak in Wuhan, China". *JAMA,* 323(19):1915, May 2020.

[4] *FDA drug development process*. https://www.fda.gov/patients/ drug-development-process/step-3-clinical-research#phases. Accessed 17 July 2020.

[5] Anderson, Roy M. and May, Robert M. "Vaccination and herd immunity to infectious diseases". *Nature,* 318(6044):323{329, 1985.

[6] Eichner, Martin, Schwehm, Markus, Eichner, Linda and Gerlier, Laetitia. "Direct and indirect effects of inuenza vaccination". *BMC Infectious Diseases,* 17(1), April 2017.

[7] Matrajt, Laura, Eaton, Julie, Leung, Tiffany, Brown, Elizabeth R. "*Vaccine optimization for COVID-19, who to vaccinate first?*" https://doi.org/10.1101/2020.08.14.20175257.

[8] Bubar, Kate M., Kissler, Stephen M., Lipsitch, Marc, Cobey, Sarah, Grad, Yonatan H., Larremore, Daniel B. "*Model-informed COVID-19 vaccine prioritization strategies by age and serostatus*". https:// doi.org/10.1101/2020.09.08.20190629.

[9] Bartsch, Sarah M., O'Shea, Kelly J., Ferguson, Marie C., Bottazzi, Maria Elena, Cox, Sarah N., Strych, Ulrich, McKinnell, James A., Wedlock, Patrick T., Siegmund, Sheryl S., Hotez, Peter J., Lee, Bruce Y. "*How Efficacious Must a COVID-19 Coronavirus Vaccine be to Prevent or Stop an Epidemic by Itself*". https://doi.org/10.1101/2020.05.29.20117184.

[10] Abutaleb, Y., Dawsey, J., McGinley, L. and Johnson, C. Y. "Trump pushing officials to speed up already-ambitious coronavirus vaccine timeline". *Washington Post,* Jun. 2020, accessed: 2020-06-15. [Online]. Available: https://www.washingtonpost.com/health/2020/ 06/ 17/trump-coronavirus-vaccine.

[11] Burton, T. M. "Fda to require proof virus vaccine is effective before approving its Use". *The Wall Street Journal,* Jun. 2020. [Online]. Available: https://www.wsj.com/articles/fda-to-issue-guidance-on-covid-19-vaccine-approval-11593516090.

[12] International Federation of Pharmaceutical Manufacturers and Associations. "The complex journey of a vaccine". International Federation of Pharmaceutical Manufacturers and Associations, *Tech. Rep.,* Jul. 2019. [Online]. Available: https://www.ifpma.org/wp-content/uploads/2019/07/IFPMA-ComplexJourney-2019 FINAL.pdf.

[13] Shah, S. K., Miller, F. G., Darton, T. C., Duenas, D., Emerson, C., Lynch, H. F., Jamrozik, E., Jecker, N. S., Kamuya, D., Kapulu, M. et al. "Ethics of controlled human infection to address covid-19". *Science,* vol. 368, no. 6493, pp. 832{834, 2020.

[14] Sherman, A. C., Mehta, A., Dickert, N. W., Anderson, E. J. and Rouphael, N. "The future of u: A review of the human challenge model and systems biology for advancement of influenza vaccinology". *Frontiers in Cellular and Infection Microbiology*, vol. 9, p. 107, 2019.

[15] Stanisic, D. I., McCarthy, J. S. and Good, M. F. "Controlled human malaria infection: applications, advances, and challenges". *Infection and Immunity,* vol. 86, no. 1, 2018.

[16] Raymond, M., Gibani, M. M., Day, N. P. and Cheah, P. Y. "Typhoidal salmonella human challenge studies: Ethical and practical challenges and considerations for low-resource settings". *Trials,* vol. 20, no. 2, pp. 1{7, 2019.

[17] Shirley, D.-A. T. and McArthur, M. A. "The utility of human challenge studies in vaccine development: Lessons learned from cholera". *Vaccine: Development and Therapy*, vol. 2011, no. 1, p. 3, 2011.

[18] Yan, W. "*Challenge accepted: Human challenge trials for dengue*". 2015.

[19] Mulligan, Mark J. et al. "*Phase 1/2 Study to Describe the Safety and Immunogenicity of a COVID-19 RNA Vaccine Candidate* (*BNT162b1*) *in Adults 18 to 55 Years of Age: Interim Report*". https://doi.org/10.1101/2020.06.30.20142570.

[20] Sadoff, Jerald et al. "*Safety and immunogenicity of the Ad26.COV2.S COVID-19 vaccine candidate: Interim results 1 of a phase 1/2a, double-blind, randomized, placebo-controlled trial*". https://doi.org/10.1101/2020.09.23.20199604.

[21] Sahin, Ugur et al. "*Concurrent human antibody and TH1 type T-cell responses elicited by a COVID-19 RNA vaccine*". https://doi.org/10.1101/2020.07.17.20140533.

[22] Malik, Amyn A., McFadden, Sarah Ann M., Elharake, Jad and Omer, Saad B. "*Determinants of COVID-19 Vaccine Acceptance in the U.S.*". https://doi.org/10.1101/2020.05.22.20110700.

[23] Iboi, Enahoro, Ngonghala, Calistus N. and Gumel, Abba B. "*Will an imperfect vaccine curtail the COVID-19 pandemic in the U.S.?*" https://doi.org/10.1101/2020.05.10.20097428.

In: Coronavirus Disease
Editor: Yildiz Dincer

ISBN: 978-1-53619-296-4

Chapter 20

MOLECULAR APPROACHES IN COVID-19 TREATMENT

Mehmet Güven[1], PhD and Bahadır Batar[2,*], PhD
[1]Department of Medical Biology, Cerrahpasa Faculty of Medicine, Istanbul University-Cerrahpasa, Istanbul, Turkey
[2]Department of Medical Biology, Tekirdag Namik Kemal University Faculty of Medicine, Tekirdag, Turkey

ABSTRACT

Coronaviruses are a family of enveloped RNA viruses that cause diseases in various mammals and birds. Severe acute respiratory syndrome coronavirus 2 (SARS-CoV-2) is a novel coronavirus identified as the cause of a global infectious disease called coronavirus disease 2019 (COVID-19). To date, there are currently no specific antiviral drugs that have been shown to effectively treat COVID-19. Moreover, vaccines based on viral-encoded peptides may not be effective against COVID-19, as virus mutations could make them futile. Many therapeutic strategies can be predicted in controlling and preventing the SARS-CoV-2 infections, such as oligonucleotide-based therapy, neutralizing monoclonal antibody therapy, autophagy pathway as therapeutic targets, chimeric antigen receptor T-cell (CAR-T) therapy, and mesenchymal-derived exosome therapy. Synthetic oligonucleotide-based therapeutic options containing small interfering RNA (siRNA) and antisense oligonucleotide (ASO) target the virus itself and mediate the silencing of its genome. Neutralizing monoclonal antibodies that target the receptor-binding motif (RBM) can prevent the virus from binding to angiotensin-converting enzyme 2 (ACE2), and are therefore promising antiviral drugs. On the other hand, vaccines and drugs can be developed to target the spike (S) glycoprotein of the coronavirus.

---

* Corresponding Author's Email: bbatar@nku.edu.tr.

Autophagy plays an important role in viral infection. Autophagosomes can induce apoptotic cell death of virally infected cells and disrupt the virus replication cycle. CAR-T treatment is a successful therapeutic option for patients with relapsed and/or refractory hematologic malignancies. Increased interleukin-6 (IL-6) is related to cytokine storm syndrome (CSS) in COVID-19 patients. CAR-T therapy is used successfully in the blocking of IL-6. Therefore, IL-6 can be a specific target for CAR-T therapy in SARS-CoV-2 infected patients. Mesenchymal-derived exosomes demonstrate anti-inflammatory and immunomodulatory effects. MSC-derived exosomes can modulate the activity of T cells. MSC-derived exosomes may inhibit pro-inflammatory cytokines and increase the levels of anti-inflammatory cytokines such as IL-10 in SARS-CoV-2 infection. MSC-derived exosomes have been considered a specific therapeutic option for COVID-19 patients. Future preclinical and clinical investigations are needed to understand the critical roles of these therapy approaches in COVID-19.

Keywords: angiotensin-converting enzyme 2, autophagosomes, CAR-T, exosomes, monoclonal antibody, antisense oligonucleotide, SARS-CoV-2

INTRODUCTION

Therapeutic drugs affect molecular compounds, cellular pathways, and cellular processes for the treatment of diseases. Small molecule targets and peptides are the basic types of medical use.

RNA molecules containing antisense oligonucleotides (ASO) and small interfering RNAs (siRNA) are promising approaches for clinical trials [1]. These options can be used to inhibit and disrupt the virus RNA genome. Moreover, several mRNAs and microRNAs (miRNAs) are assessed for vaccination [2]. Besides, ribosomal RNA (rRNA)-targeted antibiotics are designed for the control of infections [3]. If these oligonucleotides are effectively delivered into the lungs, they can stop the infection.

Another promising option is neutralizing monoclonal antibodies that can be used as therapeutics. The major target of these agents is the viral spike (S) that mediates the binding of the virus to the angiotensin-converting enzyme 2 (ACE2) membrane receptor on the host cell. S1 subunit and S2 subunit are the two subunits of the viral S protein. The S1 subunit has two primary structural domains, receptor-binding domain (RBD) and N-terminal domain (NTD). The S2 subunit acts on virus-cell membrane interaction and fusion. Neutralizing monoclonal antibodies to the S protein provide immune protection against SARS-CoV and MERS-CoV [4, 5]. It is possible to produce efficacy humanized monoclonal antibodies. The SARS-CoV-2 infection could be prevented and treated by human monoclonal antibodies [6]. ACE2 receptor would be also created as an antibody-like molecule. For this strategy, a soluble form of the ACE2 receptor would bind to the S molecule of SARS-CoV-2 and neutralize the virus [7].

Coronaviruses can target the autophagy pathway and promote viral replication [8]. Stressful conditions upregulate autophagy. Autophagy provides cellular homeostasis and involves the organization of numerous molecules. These molecules are generally called autophagy-related (ATG) proteins. Autophagosome formation is a major process for the canonical autophagy pathway. Autophagosome fuses with the lysosome and performs enzymatic degradation.

Autophagy plays a role in regulating pathogen degradation mechanisms. Thus, autophagy is a major part of the immunity against pathogens, such as viruses.

Severe COVID-19 patients have elevated serum levels of IL-6. Increased IL-6 plays a key role in cytokine storms. Chimeric antigen receptor T-cell (CAR-T) immunotherapy appears to control and prevent cytokine storms in SARS-CoV-2 infected patients [9].

Exosomes contain several molecules such as mRNAs, tRNAs, proteins, and microRNAs (miRNAs). Mesenchymal-derived exosomes exhibit immunomodulatory and anti-inflammatory responses. Molecular components of exosomes can regulate immune reactions [10]. Thus, in COVID-19, mesenchymal-derived exosomes can be used as a therapeutic option.

Many drugs are known for clinical evaluation of COVID-19. However, more attention has been paid to these treatment strategies.

Oligonucleotides as Therapeutic Drugs

In recent years, it has been made promising progress in the understanding of viral genomics and target-based drugs have been designed for silencing viral gene expression as new therapeutic approaches. Oligonucleotide-based therapeutics have significant anti-viral properties [11]. Oligonucleotide-based therapies, such as ASOs and siRNAs neutralize the viral mRNA molecules.

ASOs are single-stranded DNA or RNA molecules. These oligonucleotides are approximately 15-20 nucleotides in length. ASOs bind to target mRNA and block its function or gene transcription. ASOs have been commonly used in the studies of gene functions and the development of new therapeutics [12]. ASO was first used to block HIV replication [13]. Treatment on ASO strategy requires knowledge of the DNA sequence. Therefore ASOs would be improved against the SARS-CoV-2 DNA sequence and block viral infection.

siRNA also called short interfering RNA or silencing RNA is a double-stranded non-coding RNA molecule. siRNA is approximately 20-25 base pairs in length. Gene expression can be regulated by siRNAs. siRNA-based therapeutic molecules have been designed and applied for antiviral diseases [14]. siRNA-mediated treatment can be an effective option for combating with COVID-19.

The SARS-CoV-2 viral genome is approximately 30 kb long. This genome consists of fourteen open reading frames (ORFs) and codes twenty-seven structural and nonstructural proteins [15]. Ribosome translates ORF1a and ORF1b into a single large poly-protein. The ORF1a contains two viral cysteine proteases, papain-like protease (nsp3) and 3-chymotrypsin-like protease (3CL). The sequence in which codes the nsp3 has been less conserved, however sequence which codes the protease 3CL (nsp5) has been highly conserved. In recent, the protease has been a major drug target for multiple antiviral pathogens. Thus, the nsp5 coding sequence can be treated as a potential target for siRNA-based therapeutics.

Viral RNA dependent RNA polymerase (Rd-Rp) is the other possible target. Rd-Rp is located in the ORF1b and encompasses 13-16 kbp on the viral genome. Rd-Rp site is a highly conserved genome of SARS-CoV-2. Therefore, this region can be evaluated as a potential target for siRNA.

Currently, nanoparticles based carriers and viral vectors have been used as delivery systems for siRNA. In 2003, a siRNA drug was developed targeting SARS-CoV and H5N1 influenza genome by Sirnaomics, Inc. (Maryland, USA). Furthermore, in 2017, Alnylam Pharmaceuticals (USA) and Vir Biotechnology have developed six siRNA against infectious diseases [16]. Nevertheless, more effective carriers should be identified for the targeted specific delivery of the drug.

Mechanisms Related to Cell Entry of SARS-CoV-2 as Therapeutic Targets

The scientific community has little knowledge of the molecular pathogenesis of SARS-CoV-2. Viruses must enter host cells before they can initiate their life cycle. Therefore, one of the critical steps for the development of effective therapeutics for COVID-19 is to clearly understand the exact mechanism of how the virus enters the human body. The majority of viruses have developed strategies to invade the cell by a process called receptor-dependent endocytosis [17]. Knowledge about the receptor recognition mechanisms of coronaviruses is critical for the development of targeted antiviral treatments focused on blocking that pathway. The cell entry mechanism of SARS-CoV -2 has been extensively studied.

The crown-like appearance of coronaviruses is caused by spike proteins, which are necessary for the viruses to enter the target cell by endocytosis. Three spike proteins assemble into trimers on the virus surface to form a crown-like appearance. The SARS-CoV-2 coronavirus uses a spike protein to bind to the ACE2 receptor on the cell surfaces. Therefore, the distribution and expression of ACE2 may be critical for the target organ of the SARS-CoV-2 [18].

The spike protein is composed of two subunits; S1 and S2. The S1 subunit contains two distinctive domains, the N-terminal domain, and the C-terminal domain. These domains of the S1 subunit can function as receptor-binding domains (RBD). The S2 subunit is the most conserved region of the protein and responsible for mediating membrane fusion between the virus and the host cell membrane. After the spike protein of SARS-CoV-2 binds to ACE2 through its RBD, the S protein priming, allowing the fusion of viral and cellular membranes and viral entry into the cell is done by a protease enzyme [19]. Recent studies revealed that the transmembrane serine proteinase 2 (TMPRSS2), furin, trypsin, and elastase prime the S proteins and provided evidence that successive S protein cleavage at two sites is required for S protein priming. After cleavage, the spike protein S1 segment remains attached to ACE2, while the spike protein S2 segment anchors the viral and cellular membranes, inducing fusion, and viral entry [20].

The ACE2/SARS-CoV-2 complex undergoes endocytosis, which is typically mediated by the acidic endosomal pH, resulting in the fusion of the viral and endosomal membranes and release of the viral genome into the cytosol for productive infection. The results revealed that the cellular entry of SARS-CoV-2 is through clathrin-mediated endocytosis [17].

This discovery is important in the search for several inhibitors targeting the endocytic pathway including endosome and lysosome in the treatment of COVID-19. Several inhibitors targeting the endocytic pathway appear to have therapeutic potential including lysosomotropic agents, clathrin-mediated endocytosis inhibitors, and endosomal/ lysosomal protease inhibitors [21].

Chloroquine and hydroxychloroquine, often in combination with a second-generation macrolide, are probably the most well-studied lysosomotropic agent that accumulates in the acidic organelles such as endosomes and lysosomes and neutralizes their pH. They have widely used malaria drugs that have yielded mixed results for the treatment of COVID-19.

Chlorpromazine (CPZ) inhibits membrane fusion processes on clathrin-dependent endocytosis and thereby prevents the entry of the virus into host cells [21]. Therefore, it can be used for the treatment of COVID-19. The inhibition of SARS-CoV-2 by CPZ was suggested in an in vitro study using cell lines. The first clinical study on the treatment of COVID-19 of CPZ has started in Paris. The results in this study suggest that CPZ is unlikely to have the therapeutic potential in the treatment of COVID-19 [22].

Cathepsins are endosomal and lysosomal proteases that play important roles in various cellular processes including both the endocytic pathway and autophagy. Several studies suggested that the inhibitors of cathepsin proteases such as teicoplanin acts to inhibit entry of the virus [23].

The endocytosis route of SARS-CoV-2 involves key proteins involved in endosome formation. The phosphatidylinositol 3-phosphate 5-kinase (PIKfyve) synthesizes a class of phosphoinositides that are required in the maturation process of endosomes. The activity of PIKfyve has been discovered to be essential in the SARS-CoV-2. Apilimod and Vacuolin-1, small molecule inhibitors of PIKfyve were found to significantly reduce SARS-CoV-2 entry. These results suggest the potential for targeting PIKfyve in developing new antiviral molecules against SARS-CoV-2 [24].

The other target is proton pumps that drive protons into endosomes and lysosomes, lowering the pH. Thus, the acidic environment that is required for pH-dependent protease activity is provided. Zohreh et al. hypothesized that metformin may be an effective treatment of COVID-19-related pulmonary fibrosis because it a potential regulator of Vacuolar ATPase and endosomal Na+/H+ exchangers, and additionally a regenerative agent for lung fibrosis [25].

Two pore segment channel 2 (TPC2) is a calcium release channel expressed in lysosomal membranes. An article by Ou et al. demonstrated that the activity of human TPC2 is a key player for SARS-CoV-2 cell entry [24]. They suggested that the blocking TPC2 activity by tetrandrine, an inhibitor for TPC2, decreased entry of SARS-CoV-2 S pseudovirions.

SARS-CoV-2 cell entry depends on ACE2 and TMPRSS2. TMPRSS2 is a member of transmembrane protease serines, which are a family of proteins with conserved serine protease domains located on the cell membrane. TMPRSS2 is expressed by human lung cells. Therefore, it is thought that TMPRSS2 plays an important part in virus entry into respiratory system cells. Also, TMPRSS2 happens to be present near the spike-ACE2 binding interface. This cleavage must occur after spike S1 Subunit -ACE2 binding. If it occurs before, the virus is less able to infect the cell. TMPRSS2 inhibitors (Nafamostat, Bromhexine, Aprotinin, Camostat) play a key role in the treatment of COVID-19 disease. The protease inhibitor camostat mesylate is already in clinical use for the treatment of pancreatitis. It was known to inhibit TMPRSS2 and effectively protected the mice against death caused by SARS-CoV infection [26].

SARS-CoV-2 has a high binding capacity for ACE2 – between 10-20 times more than the original coronavirus. This means it is much easier for SARS-CoV-2 to get into human cells compared to the original coronavirus. The structures of SARS-CoV-2 RBD that are essential for ACE2 binding showed that it contains a core and an RBM. The RBD is the most immunogenic region of COVID-19 spike protein and contains major neutralization epitopes, which induce most of the host immune responses [24]. Therefore, these epitopes may serve as subunit vaccines against coronavirus infections. Therefore, it presents a major challenge to both vaccination and antibody-drug. A structure-based strategy for SARS-CoV-2 RBD may help design subunit vaccines. The hot spot residues at the SARS-CoV-2 RBM are important for SARS-CoV-2 binding to ACE2 receptors.

Monteil et al. suggested that human recombinant soluble ACE2 can significantly block the early stages of SARS-CoV-2 infections in artificial human tissues [27]. Thus, an antibody-drug with a significantly higher RBD binding affinity than ACE2 can block viral attachment. On the other hand, vaccines and drugs can be developed to target the S2 subunits of the spike glycoprotein of the coronavirus. However, the success of this approach may be limited because the spike S2 subunit is less immunogenic than the SARS-CoV-2 Spike S1 protein RBD.

Another potential drug target might be the cellular enzymes that attach fatty acids to a cluster of cysteines in the cytoplasmic tail of spike protein. However, enzymes that attach acyl chains to S have not been identified.

Autophagy Pathway as Therapeutic Targets

Autophagy is conserved in all eukaryotic cells. Autophagy is a constitutive pathway, also it is activated by endoplasmic reticulum stress, starvation, and pathogen infections. Autophagy involves the formation of autophagosomes. Autophagosomes enclose cytoplasmic components, such as protein aggregates and organelles. Furthermore, autophagosomes deliver these components to lysosomes for degradation. Therefore, autophagy is one of the major degradation pathways.

The autophagy pathway is regulated by several proteins encoded by autophagy-related genes (ATGs). The autophagy process is performed through many stages. First, class III phosphatidylinositol 3-kinase (PtdIns3K) protein complex forms autophagy-specific phagophore. Second, the ULK complex expands the phagophore. Also, the Atg8 protein family maturates the phagophore. Then, cytoplasmic components are recruited through autophagic receptors followed by the fusion of vesicles with endosomes. The vesicle-endosome complex is called as amphisome. Last, amphisome fuses with a lysosome and subsequently, degradation occurs.

Coronaviruses like other RNA viruses stimulate the development of double-membrane vesicles (DMVs), a hallmark of autophagy [28]. These vesicles mimic autophagosomes. The fusion of viral DMVs with lysosomes (also with late endosomes) results in viral acidification which induces viral replication or virion maturation [29]. Some coronaviruses release their genome into the cytoplasm of the host cell during the entry of the virus [30]. SARS-CoV replicates and transcribes its genome through the autophagic pathway.

The fusion of DMV-lysosome is a crucial stage in the autophagy pathway. The fusion between the autophagy pathway and DMVs may occur during the life cycles of coronaviruses [31]. Coronavirus DMVs play a role as the RNA synthesis site for coronaviruses [32].

Chloroquine, an anti-malarial drug, is a lysosomotropic agent. It neutralizes endosomes and lysosomes. Chloroquine mainly blocks the autophagic pathway by impairing autophagosome fusion with the lysosome and inhibits the lysosomal degradation activity [33]. The acidic subcellular compartments, lysosomes, and endosomes, are neutralized by chloroquine. Besides, chloroquine can stimulate autophagy-independent dysfunctions of endosomal-lysosomal systems. Thus, chloroquine may affect on the fusion between autophagosome and lysosome [33].

It is well known that chloroquine has anti-viral effects, such as anti-CoVs, anti-HIV, and anti-influenza [34]. It has been suggested that chloroquine treatment suppressed the viral infection in SARS-CoV-infected Vero E6 cells [35]. Also, a recent study revealed that chloroquine inhibits the SARS-CoV-2 infection in Vero E6 cells [36]. In another study, chloroquine has been tested for COVID-19 treatment. The first evidence on in vitro assay showed that they could act on anti-SARS-CoV-2 [37].

The mechanisms of the chloroquine effect are not known clearly during SARS-CoV2 infection. Also, the clinical efficacy of chloroquine is unclear and needs further studies.

Autophagy regulates innate and adaptive immunity. Activation of autophagy can induce the immune system [38]. Targeting the immune system, such as autophagy that regulates immunity could be a therapeutic approach against SARS-CoV-2 infection.

A viral-infected body encounters infection through the innate immune system also the adaptive immune responses are carried out by recruiting virus-specific T lymphocytes and B lymphocytes, respectively. Cell-mediated and humoral immune responses are stimulated. These immune responses both potentiate inflammatory effects and neutralize against viral invasion.

Macrophages and dendritic cells, antigen-presenting cells (APC), present the viral antigen to T cells through human leukocyte antigen (HLA). Activated T cells are transformed into CD8 + T cells and CD4 + T cells. These cells activate both cell-mediated and humoral immune responses. CD8 + T cells disrupt virus-infected cells. CD4 + T cells play a pivotal role in priming CD8 + T cells and B cells. Th1 cells, one of the subsets of CD4+, both stimulate natural killer (NK) cells and CD8 + T cells or remain as memory T cells. However, CD4 + Th2 cells activate B cells to be converted into plasma B cells. Then, B cells produce SARS-CoV-2-specific IgM and IgG antibodies [39]. These antibodies bind and neutralize SARS-CoV-2. Many B cells form immune memory.

Some of the viruses block autophagy by inhibiting autophagy-inducing pathways, AKT1/BECN1, to stimulate viral replication [40]. A recent study has confirmed that SARS-CoV-2 infection also inhibited autophagy [41]. Also, this study suggested that autophagy stimulation revealed the potentiality against this infection [41].

Fasting activates autophagy [42], which induces immunity [43]. Therefore, fasting may control and prevent to COVID-19 [44]. However, to date, there is no experimental evidence that determined the effects of fasting against SARS-CoV-2 infection.

Chimeric Antigen Receptor T-Cell Therapeutic Strategy for COVID-19

T cells play a key role in the initiation of antiviral immune responses. Investigations in lymphocytes of COVID-19 patients are beginning to emerge [45]. Lymphopenia is one of the major hallmarks of severe COVID-19. T cells, B cells, and natural killer (NK) cells are affected by lymphopenia [46]. It has been demonstrated that SARS-CoV-2 has an impact on T cell function [47]. Patients with severe COVID-19 are most likely to have a reduced number of lymphocytes, monocytes, eosinophils, and basophils. COVID-19 patients have decreased Th cell counts and suppressor T cell counts. These findings show the importance of the T cell-based immunotherapies for COVID-19.

Immunotherapy has promising success in cancer, autoimmune diseases, and other immune system-related diseases [48, 49]. Immunotherapy can be accepted to improve immune responses in COVID-19. It has been well known for the success of interferons in viral infections, so several studies investigate the efficacy of interferon-alpha-1b and alpha-2b for the treatment of COVID-19 [47].

Chimeric antigen receptor T-cell (CAR-T) immunotherapy, adoptive cell therapy, is extensively used for the treatment of patients with hematologic malignancies due to their immune dysregulation and long-term immune reconstitution. Current, CAR-T cell therapy has made promising progress in the treatment of refractory and/or relapsed (R/R) hematological malignancies. Targeting the CD19 CAR-T cell therapy has shown efficient remission in non-Hodgkin lymphoma (NHL) and acute lymphocytic leukemia (ALL) [50].

Importantly, antigen-specific T cells were developed against chronic viral infections. HBV-specific T cells were renewed by CAR-T cells [51]. Bohne et al. first produced CAR-T cells targeting the hepatitis B surface antigen (HBsAg). CAR-T cells were developed to recognize a determinant of HBsAg and to direct aa37-43 in the preS1 peptide. Thus, HBsAg-positive primary human hepatocytes were able to target, and specifically, HBV-infected target cells were eliminated [52]. HIV-targeted CAR-T cells have been generated for the treatment of HIV/AIDS. In recent years, anti-HIV neutralizing antibodies (bNAbs), and bNAb-based CAR-T therapy has been developed as a potential treatment strategy to control HIV infection [53].

To date, numerous immune cell-based immunotherapeutic options against SARS-CoV-2 are being significantly improved. A study demonstrated that CAR-NK cells may have the potential to treat patients with severe COVID-19 [54]. NK cells are extracted from peripheral blood and can be modified to express CAR.

NK cell therapy has a significant anti-tumor effect, which is the direct activity of NK cells on the immune system [55]. Thus, COVID-19, a viral infection associated with immune dysregulation, can be treated with regenerative medicine and its immunoregulatory actions [56].

COVID-19 patients exhibit increased serum inflammatory cytokines. Interleukin-6 (IL-6) seems to play an important role in COVID-19 associated cytokine storm syndrome (CSS). Based on the successful use of IL-6 receptor blockade for CAR-T cell therapy-related cytokine release syndrome (CAR T-cell CRS), similar strategies using tocilizumab, an anti–IL-6 receptor antibody, are being investigated in COVID-19 [9].

CAR-T immunotherapy might be considered for severe COVID-19 patients at increased risk of complications. If patients are affected by hematological diseases and are suffering from relapsed and/or refractory diseases, CAR-T might be useful to control SARS-CoV-2 infection [57].

Mesenchymal Stem Cells-Derived Exosomes in COVID-19 Treatment

Cell-based therapies aim to control or prevent the damage and disease by repairing and/or replacing the injured cells and tissues. Also, many cell-based therapies contribute to stopping degenerative and pathophysiologic progress [58].

Mesenchymal stem cell (MSC) treatment is one of the major therapy among stem cell-based therapies. MSCs are widely used in regenerative medicine. These cells can repair damaged tissues and organs. Also, MSCs have anti-apoptotic, anti-inflammatory, pro-inflammatory immune reactions. MSCs regulate the immune responses through the transforming growth factor b1 (TGFβ1), which can stimulate the Treg proliferation, activate IL-6, which inhibits the neutrophil proliferation, and induce the prostaglandin E2 (PGE2), which prevents the antigen presentation by dendritic cells and T-effector cell proliferation [59, 60]. MSCs play an important role in immunomodulatory activity [61]. These features have revealed that MSCs are clinically significant.

MSC treatment has been effectively applied to treat many disorders such as degenerative, inflammatory, and metabolic diseases. Furthermore, MSCs are used for cancer therapy. Moreover, Recently, it has been suggested that the transplantation of MSCs enhanced the pulmonary function of COVID-19 patients [62]. Many reports revealed that MSC treatment is associated with low mortality and morbidity rates in COVID-19 patients [63]. The MSCs could use in immunomodulatory effects and differentiation potency for the COVID-19 treatment [64]. MSC treatment of COVID-19 patients is limited.

The exosomes are released from all types of cells, including stem cells [65]. The exosomes are membrane-enclosed extracellular vesicles (EVs). The exosomes include several molecules, such as miRNAs, tRNAs, long noncoding RNAs (lncRNAs), growth factors, proteins, and lipids. Molecular structures of exosomes can affect the immune regulations and epigenetic alterations [10]. Exosomes can be used as promising therapeutic approaches.

MSC-derived exosomes can be useful for repairing damaged tissues and organs. MSC-derived exosomes provide several advantages in comparison to traditional cell-based therapies. MSC-derived exosomes are safer and more stable than cells [66]. In addition to these advantages, MSC-derived exosomes increase their therapeutic potential, exosomes could be modulated with several types of cargos, such as mRNA, miRNA, and proteins [67].

MSC-derived exosomes can modulate the function of T cells. It has been found that MSC-derived exosomes treatment both enhanced the interleukin-10 (IL-10) and TGF-β1 expression levels, therefore the function of immunosuppressive regulatory T cells increased [68]. Moreover, MSC-derived exosomes reduced the levels of inflammatory cytokines, eosinophils, infiltrated mast cells, IgE, and CD86+ and CD206+ cells [69].

Many infected COVID-19 patients have a multiorgan injury. MSC-derived exosomes are known to reduce lung injury in asthmatic models and acute respiratory distress syndrome (ARDS) [68, 70]. Thus, Organ and tissue damage related to COVID-19 can be treated by MSC-derived exosomes.

Preclinical and clinical findings support the investigational MSC-derived exosomes application due to their anti-inflammatory and immunomodulatory abilities. MSC-derived exosomes can be a useful treatment strategy to reduce the effect of SARS-CoV-2 infection.

Conclusion

Currently, no therapeutic approach is approved for COVID-19. The development of diverse therapeutic strategies directing SARS-CoV-2 is needed for the treatment of patients with COVID-19. Oligonucleotide-based therapy, neutralizing monoclonal antibody therapy, autophagy pathway as therapeutic targets, chimeric antigen receptor T-cell (CAR-T) therapy, and mesenchymal-derived exosome therapy are novel therapeutic options against SARS-CoV-2 infection. The use of biomolecules associated with these novel therapeutics can provide significant results for the treatment of COVID-19 patients.

References

[1] Crooke, S. T., Witztum, J. L., Bennett, C. F. and Baker, B. F. (2018). RNA-targeted therapeutics. *Cell Metab* 27:714–739.

[2] Lieberman, J. (2018). Tapping the RNA world for therapeutics. *Nat Struct Mol Biol* 25:357–364.

[3] Lin, J., Zhou, D., Steitz, T. A., Polikanov, Y. S. and Gagnon, M. G. (2018). Ribosome-targeting antibiotics: modes of action, mechanisms of resistance, and implications for drug design. *Annu Rev Biochem* 87:451–478.

[4] Zhu, Z. et al. (2007). Potent cross-reactive neutralization of SARS coronavirus isolates by human monoclonal antibodies. *Proc Natl Acad Sci USA* 104:12123–12128.

[5] Tang, X. C. et al. (2014). Identification of human neutralizing antibodies against MERS-CoV and their role in virus adaptive evolution. *Proc Natl Acad Sci USA* 111:E2018–E2026.

[6] Jiang, S., Hillyer, C. and Du, L. (2020). Neutralizing antibodies against SARS-CoV-2 and other human coronaviruses. *Trends Immunol* 41:355–359.

[7] Kruse, R. L. (2020). Therapeutic strategies in an outbreak scenario to treat the novel coronavirus originating in Wuhan, China. *F1000Res* 9:72.

[8] Jackson, W. T. (2015). Viruses and the autophagy pathway. *Virology* 479-480:450–456.

[9] Hoiland, R. Y. et al. (2020). Amelioration of COVID-19 related cytokine storm syndrome: Parallels to chimeric antigen receptor-T cell cytokine release syndrome. *Br J Haetemol* 190(3):e150-e154.

[10] Id, L. M. and Sadovsky, Y. (2019). The biology of extracellular vesicles: The known unknowns. *PLoS Biol* 17:e3000363.

[11] Sridharan. K., Gogtay, N. J. (2016). Therapeutic nucleic acids: current clinical status. *Br J Clin Pharmacol* 82(3):659–672.

[12] Bennett, C. F. (2019). Therapeutic antisense oligonucleotides are coming of age. *Annu Rev Med* 70:307–321.

[13] Matsukura, M. (1987). Phosphorothioate analogs of oligodeoxynucleotides: inhibitors of replication and cytopathic effects of human immunodeficiency virus. *Proc Natl Acad Sci USA* 84(21):7706–7710.

[14] Liu, C. et al. (2020). Research and development on therapeutic agents and vaccines for COVID-19 and related human coronavirus diseases. *ACS Cent Sci* 6:315-331.

[15] Wu, F. et al. (2020). A new coronavirus associated with human respiratory disease in China. *Nature* 579:265-282.

[16] Ghosh, S., Firdous, S. M. and Nath, A. (2020). siRNA could be a potential therapy for COVID-19. *EXCLI J* 19:528-531.

[17] Wang, H., Yang, P., Liu, K., Guo, F., Zhang, Y., Zhang, G. and Jiang, C., (2008). SARS coronavirus entry into host cells through a novel clathrin- and caveolae-independent endocytic pathway. *Cell Res* 18:290-301.

[18] Shang, J., Wan, Y., Luo, C., Ye, G., Geng, Q., Auerbach, A. and Li, F. (2020). "Cell entry mechanisms of SARS-CoV-2." *Proc Natl Acad Sci USA* 117:11727-11734.
[19] Shang, J., Ye, G., Shi,, K., Wan Y., Luo, C., Aihara, H., Geng, Q., Auerbach, A. and Li, F. (2020). Structural basis of receptor recognition by SARS-CoV-2. *Nature* 581:221-224.
[20] Sun, J., He, WT., Wang, L., Lai, A., Ji, X., Zhai, X., Li, G., Suchard, MA., Tian, J., Zhou, J., Veit, M. and Su, S. (2020). COVID-19: Epidemiology, Evolution, and Cross-Disciplinary Perspectives. *Trends Mol Med* 26:483-495.
[21] Yang, N. and Shen, H. M. (2020). Targeting the Endocytic Pathway and Autophagy Process as a Novel Therapeutic Strategy in COVID-19. *Int J Biol Sci* 16:1724-1731.
[22] Plaze, M. et al. (2020). Repurposing chlorpromazine to treat COVID-19: The reCoVery study. *Encephale* 46:169-172.
[23] Baron, S. A, Devaux, C., Colson, P., Raoult, D. and Rolain, J. M. (2020). Teicoplanin: an alternative drug for the treatment of coronavirus COVID-19? *Int J Antimicrob Agents* 55:105944.
[24] Ou, X. et al. (2020). Characterization of spike glycoprotein of SARS-CoV-2 on virus entry and its immune cross-reactivity with SARS-CoV. *Nat Commun* 11:1620.
[25] Esam, Z. 2020. A proposed mechanism for the possible therapeutic potential of Metformin in COVID-19. *Diabetes Res Clin Pract* 25:108282.
[26] Amini Pouya, M., Afshani, S. M., Maghsoudi, A. S., Hassani, S. and Mirnia, K. (2020). Classification of the present pharmaceutical agents based on the possible effective mechanism on the COVID-19 infection. *Daru* 30:1-20.
[27] Monteil, V. al. (2020). Inhibition of SARS-CoV-2 infections in engineered human tissues using clinical-grade soluble human ACE2. *Cell* 181:905–913.
[28] Jackson, W. T. et al. (2005). Subversion of cellular autophagosomal machinery by RNA viruses. *PLoS Biol* 3:e156.
[29] Richards, A. L., Jackson, W. T. and Jung, J. U. (2012). Intracellular vesicle acidification promotes maturation of infectious poliovirus particles. *PLoS Pathog* 8:e1003046.
[30] Milewska, A. et al. (2018). Entry of human coronavirus NL63 into the cell. *J Virol* [Internet] 92.
[31] Prentice, E. et al. (2004). Coronavirus replication complex formation utilizes components of cellular autophagy. *J Biol Chem* 279:10136–10141.
[32] Snijder, E. J. et al. (2020). A unifying structural and functional model of the coronavirus replication organelle: tracking down RNA synthesis. *PLoS Biol* 18:e3000715.

[33] Mauthe, M., Orhon, I., Rocchi, C. (2018). Chloroquine inhibits autophagic flux by decreasing autophagosome-lysosome fusion. *Autophagy* 14:1435–1455.

[34] Savarino, A., Di Trani, L., Donatelli, I., Cauda, R. and Cassone, A. (2006). New insights into the antiviral effects of chloroquine. *Lancet Infect Dis* 6:67-69.

[35] Vincent, M. J. et al. (2005). Chloroquine is a potent inhibitor of SARS coronavirus infection and spread. *Virol J* 2:69.

[36] Wang, M. et al. (2020). Remdesivir and chloroquine effectively inhibit the recently emerged novel coronavirus (2019-nCoV) in vitro. *Cell Res* 30(3):269-271.

[37] Liu, J. et al. (2020). Hydroxychloroquine, a Less Toxic Derivative of Chloroquine, Is Effective in Inhibiting SARS-CoV-2 Infection in Vitro. *Cell Discovery* 16:1-4.

[38] Cui, B., Lin, H., Yu, J., Yu, J. and Hu Z. (2019) Autophagy and the immune response. *Adv Exp Med Biol* 1206:595–634.

[39] Nikolich-Zugich, J., Knox, K. S., Rios, C. T., Natt, B., Bhattacharya, D. and Fain, M. J. (2020). SARS-CoV-2 and COVID-19 in older adults: what we may expect regarding pathogenesis, immune responses, and outcomes. *GeroScience* 42(2):505-514.

[40] Orvedahl, A. et al. (2007). HSV-1 ICP34.5 confers neurovirulence by targeting the Beclin 1 autophagy protein. *Cell Host Microbe* 1(1):23–35.

[41] Gassen, N. C. et al. (2020). Analysis of SARS-CoV-2-controlled autophagy reveals spermidine, MK-2206, and niclosamide as putative antiviral therapeutics. *bioRxiv* doi: https://doi.org/10.1101/ 2020.04.15.997254.

[42] Alirezaei, M. et al. (2010). Short-term fasting induces profound neuronal autophagy. *Autophagy* 6(6):702–710.

[43] Brandhorst, S. et al. (2015). A periodic diet that mimics fasting promotes multi-system regeneration, enhanced cognitive performance, and healthspan. *Cell Metab* 22(1):86–99.

[44] Hannan, A. et al. (2020). Intermittent fasting, a possible priming tool for host defense against SARS-CoV-2 infection: Crosstalk among calorie restriction, autophagy and immune response. *Immunol Lett* 226:38-45.

[45] Vardhana, S. A. and Wolchok, J. D. (2020). The many faces of the anti-COVID immune response. *J Exp Med* 217(6):e20200678.

[46] Mazzoni, A. et al. (2020). Impaired immune 591 cell cytotoxicity in severe COVID-19 is IL-6 dependent. *J Clin Invest* 130(9):4694-4703.

[47] Qin, C. et al. (2020). Dysregulation of immune response in patients with COVID-19 in Wuhan, China. *Clin Infec Dis* 71(15):762-768.

[48] Fong, K. Y. (2002). Immunotherapy in autoimmune diseases. *Ann Acad of Med Singap* 31(6):702–706.

[49] Naran, K., Nundalall, T., Chetty, S. and Barth, S. (2018). Principles of immunotherapy: Implications for treatment strategies in Cancer and infectious diseases. *Front Microbiol* 9:3158 –3158.

[50] Ali, N. (2019). Haematology F. Chimeric antigen T cell receptor treatment in hematological malignancies. *Blood Res* 54(2):81–83.

[51] Bertoletti, A., Tan, A. T. and Koh, S. (2017). T-cell therapy for chronic viral hepatitis. *Cytotherapy* 19:1317–1324.

[52] Bohne, F. et al. (2008). T cells redirected against hepatitis B virus surface proteins eliminate infected hepatocytes. *Gastroenterology* 134:239–247.

[53] Qi, J., Ding, C., Jiang, X. and Gao, Y. (2020). Advances in Developing CAR T-Cell Therapy for HIV Cure. *Front Immunol* 11:361.

[54] Ma, M., Badeti, S., Geng, K. and Liu, D. (2020). Efficacy of Targeting SARS-CoV-2 by CAR-NK Cells. *bioRxiv* 2020.08.11. 247320.

[55] Yoon, S. R., Kim, T. D. and Choi, I. (2015). Understanding of molecular mechanisms in natural killer cell therapy. *Exp Mol Med* 47(2):e141.

[56] Saghazadeh, A. and Rezaei, N. (2020). Immune-epidemiological parameters of the novel coronavirus–a perspective. *Expert Rev Clin Immunol* 16(5):1–6.

[57] Hu, Y. et al. (2020). CAR T-cell treatment during the COVID-19 pandemic: Management strategies and challenges. *Curr Res Transl Med* 68(3):111-118.

[58] Sleem, A. and Saleh, F. (2020). Mesenchymal stem cells in the fight against viruses: face to face with the invisible enemy. *Curr Res Transl Med* 68(3):105-110.

[59] Patel, S. A., Meyer, J. R., Greco, S. J., Corcoran, K. E., Bryan, M. and Rameshwar, P. (2010). Mesenchymal stem cells protect breast cancer cells through regulatory T cells: role of mesenchymal stem cell-derived TGF-beta. *J Immunol* 184:5885-5894.

[60] Raffaghello, L. et al. (2008). Human mesenchymal stem cells inhibit neutrophil apoptosis: a model for neutrophil preservation in the bone marrow niche. *Stem Cells* 26:151-162.

[61] Zheng, G. et al. (2018). Mesenchymal stromalcellderived extracellular vesicles: regenerative andimmunomodulatory effects and potential applications in sepsis. *Cell Tissue Res* 374(1):1–15.

[62] Leng, Z. et al. (2020). Transplantation of ACE2-mesenchymal stem cells improves the outcome of patients with COVID-19 pneumonia. *Aging Dis* 11:216.

[63] Tobaiqy, M. et al. (2020). Therapeutic management of patients with COVID-19: a systematic review. *Infect Prevent Practice* 2(3): 100061.

[64] Holchun, A. (2020). Cell-Based Therapy for Severe COVID-19 Patients: Clinical Trials and Cost-Utility. *Stem Cell Rev Rep* (in print).

[65] Cheng, L., Zhang, K., Wu, S., Cui, M. and Xu, T. (2017). Focus on mesenchymal stem cell-derived exosomes: opportunities and challenges in cell-free therapy. *Stem Cell Int* 2017:6305295.

[66] Qin, Y., Sun, R., Wu, C., Wang, L. and Zhang, C. (2016). Exosome: A Novel Approach to Stimulate Bone Regeneration through Regulation of Osteogenesis and Angiogenesis. *Int J Mol Sci* 17:712.

[67] Sun, D. Z., Abelson, B., Babbar, P. and Damaser, M. S. (2019). Harnessing the mesenchymal stem cell secretome for regenerative urology. *Nat Rev Urol* 16:363–375.

[68] Du, Y. M., Zhuansun, Y. X., Chen, R., Lin, L., Lin, Y. and Li, J. G. (2018). Mesenchymal stem cell exosomes promote immunosuppression of regulatory T cells in asthma. *Exp Cell Res* 363(1):114–120.

[69] Cho, B. S., Kim, J. O., Ha, D. H. and Yi, Y. W. (2018). Exosomes derived from human adipose tissue-derived mesenchymal stem cells alleviate atopic dermatitis. *Stem Cell Res Ther* 9(1):187.

[70] Fujita, Y., Kosaka, N., Araya, J., Kuwano, K. and Ochiya, T. (2015) Extracellular vesicles in lung microenvironment and pathogenesis. *Trends Mol Med* 21:533-542.

About the Editor

Yildiz Dincer
Member of Academic Board
Istanbul University-Cerrahpasa, Cerrahpasa Medical Faculty,
Department of Medical Biochemistry

Prof. Yildiz Dincer (Ph.D.) got her M.Sc. and Ph.D. degrees at Istanbul University Cerrahpasa Medical Faculty, Department of Medical Biochemistry, Istanbul, Turkey. She studied as a scholarship researcher in Imperial Research Fund-Clare Hall Laboratories, the UK in 1999, and gained experience in the field of DNA repair by working in the team of Dr. Tomas Lindahl who shared the 2015 Nobel Prize in Chemistry for work on DNA repair. Dr. Dincer maintains an active research program studying oxidative DNA damage, DNA repair, antioxidants, and epigenetic mechanismsin cancer, diabetes, and Alzheimer's disease. Dr. Dincer published many articles and book chapters. She served as the editor of various edited collections on topics including iron deficiency, chemical carcinogens, chemotherapeutics, tumor markers, epigenetics, and Alzheimer's Disease.

INDEX

#

A

B

C

D

E

F

G

H

I

J

K

L

M

N

O

P

Q

R

S

X